Synthetic and Biosynthetic Approaches to Marine Natural Products

Synthetic and Biosynthetic Approaches to Marine Natural Products

Special Issue Editor
Asunción Barbero

MDPI • Basel • Beijing • Wuhan • Barcelona • Belgrade • Manchester • Tokyo • Cluj • Tianjin

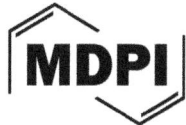

Special Issue Editor
Asunción Barbero
Universidad de Valladolid
Spain

Editorial Office
MDPI
St. Alban-Anlage 66
4052 Basel, Switzerland

This is a reprint of articles from the Special Issue published online in the open access journal *Marine Drugs* (ISSN 1660-3397) (available at: https://www.mdpi.com/journal/marinedrugs/special_issues/synthetic-biosynthetic).

For citation purposes, cite each article independently as indicated on the article page online and as indicated below:

LastName, A.A.; LastName, B.B.; LastName, C.C. Article Title. *Journal Name* **Year**, *Article Number*, Page Range.

ISBN 978-3-03928-466-5 (Pbk)
ISBN 978-3-03928-467-2 (PDF)

© 2020 by the authors. Articles in this book are Open Access and distributed under the Creative Commons Attribution (CC BY) license, which allows users to download, copy and build upon published articles, as long as the author and publisher are properly credited, which ensures maximum dissemination and a wider impact of our publications.
The book as a whole is distributed by MDPI under the terms and conditions of the Creative Commons license CC BY-NC-ND.

Contents

About the Special Issue Editor vii

Preface to "Synthetic and Biosynthetic Approaches to Marine Natural Products" ix

Stefano Serra
A General Strategy for the Stereoselective Synthesis of the Furanosesquiterpenes Structurally Related to Pallescensins 1–2
Reprinted from: *Materials* 2019, 17, 245, doi:10.3390/md17040245 1

Qinghao Jin, Zhiyang Fu, Liping Guan and Haiying Jiang
Syntheses of Benzo[d]Thiazol-2(3H)-One Derivatives and Their Antidepressant and Anticonvulsant Effects
Reprinted from: *Materials* 2019, 17, 430, doi:10.3390/md17070430 15

Danqiong Huang, Wenfu Liu, Anguo Li, Chaogang Wang and Zhangli Hu
Discovery of Geranylgeranyl Pyrophosphate Synthase (GGPPS) Paralogs from *Haematococcus pluvialis* Based on Iso-Seq Analysis and Their Function on Astaxanthin Biosynthesis
Reprinted from: *Materials* 2019, 17, 696, doi:10.3390/md17120696 25

Carlos Díez-Poza, Patricia Val, Francisco J. Pulido and Asunción Barbero
Synthesis of Polysubstituted Tetrahydropyrans by Stereoselective Hydroalkoxylation of Silyl Alkenols: En Route to Tetrahydropyranyl Marine Analogues
Reprinted from: *Materials* 2018, 16, 421, doi:10.3390/md16110421 39

Hao-yun Shi, Yang Xie, Pei Hu, Zi-qiong Guo, Yi-hong Lu, Yu Gao and Cheng-gang Huang
Asymmetric Synthesis of the C15–C32 Fragment of Alotamide and Determination of the Relative Stereochemistry
Reprinted from: *Materials* 2018, 16, 414, doi:10.3390/md16110414 51

Alessia Caso, Ilaria Laurenzana, Daniela Lamorte, Stefania Trino, Germana Esposito, Vincenzo Piccialli and Valeria Costantino
Smenamide A Analogues. Synthesis and Biological Activity on Multiple Myeloma Cells
Reprinted from: *Materials* 2018, 16, 206, doi:10.3390/md16060206 71

Iván Cheng-Sánchez, José A. Torres-Vargas, Beatriz Martínez-Poveda, Guillermo A. Guerrero-Vásquez, Miguel Ángel Medina, Francisco Sarabia and Ana R. Quesada
Synthesis and Antitumor Activity Evaluation of Compounds Based on Toluquinol
Reprinted from: *Materials* 2019, 17, 492, doi:10.3390/md17090492 85

Seoung Rak Lee, Dahae Lee, Hee Jeong Eom, Maja Rischer, Yoon-Joo Ko, Ki Sung Kang, Chung Sub Kim, Christine Beemelmanns and Ki Hyun Kim
Hybrid Polyketides from a *Hydractinia*-Associated *Cladosporium sphaerospermum* SW67 and Their Putative Biosynthetic Origin
Reprinted from: *Materials* 2019, 17, 606, doi:10.3390/md17110606 101

Yi Gong and Xiaoling Miao
Short Chain Fatty Acid Biosynthesis in Microalgae *Synechococcus* sp. PCC 7942
Reprinted from: *Materials* 2019, 17, 255, doi:10.3390/md17050255 117

Chamilani Nikapitiya, S.H.S. Dananjaya, H.P.S.U. Chandrarathna, Mahanama De Zoysa and Ilson Whang
Octominin: A Novel Synthetic Anticandidal Peptide Derived from Defense Protein of *Octopus minor*
Reprinted from: *Materials* **2020**, *18*, 56, doi:10.3390/md18010056 133

Qinxue Jing, Xu Hu, Yanzi Ma, Jiahui Mu, Weiwei Liu, Fanxing Xu, Zhanlin Li, Jiao Bai, Huiming Hua and Dahong Li
Marine-Derived Natural Lead Compound Disulfide-Linked Dimer Psammaplin A: Biological Activity and Structural Modification
Reprinted from: *Materials* **2019**, *17*, 384, doi:10.3390/md17070384 149

About the Special Issue Editor

Asunción Barbero was born in Burgos, Spain. She studied Chemistry at the University of Valladolid and received her Ph.D. degree at the same university, working with Prof. Pulido. She joined Prof. Ian Fleming's group at the University of Cambridge as a Marie Curie fellow for two years working in the study of stereocontrol in organic synthesis using silicon chemistry. She returned to Valladolid as Assistant Professor, was promoted to Associate Professor in 2001, and to full Professor in 2019. Since 2013, she has been the Coordinator of the Grade of Chemistry at the University of Valladolid. She has co-authored around 60 international scientific publications and has delivered several invited and plenary lectures. Her current interests include the use of organosilicon compounds in the synthesis of heterocycles.

Preface to "Synthetic and Biosynthetic Approaches to Marine Natural Products"

The ocean is the natural habitat for abundant multicellular plants or animals and unicellular bacteria. These organisms are excellent producers of secondary metabolites that have important biological properties. A group of marine natural products of special interest is the heterocycles. The chemical structures and biological properties of this compound type have attracted the attention of the scientific community, which has attempted to synthesize and biosynthesize this class of molecules.

This Special Issue of *Marine Drugs* collects a series of papers describing synthetic or biosynthetic approaches to marine natural products or analogs that contain a heterocyclic moiety in their structure.

Asunción Barbero
Special Issue Editor

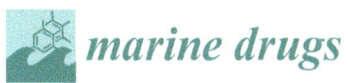

Article

A General Strategy for the Stereoselective Synthesis of the Furanosesquiterpenes Structurally Related to Pallescensins 1–2

Stefano Serra

Consiglio Nazionale delle Ricerche (C.N.R.) Istituto di Chimica del Riconoscimento Molecolare, Via Mancinelli 7, 20131 Milano, Italy; stefano.serra@cnr.it; Tel.: +39-02-2399 3076

Received: 22 March 2019; Accepted: 23 April 2019; Published: 25 April 2019

Abstract: Here, we describe a general stereoselective synthesis of the marine furanosesquiterpenes structurally related to pallescensins 1–2. The stereoisomeric forms of the pallescensin 1, pallescensin 2, and dihydropallescensin 2 were obtained in high chemical and isomeric purity, whereas isomicrocionin-3 was synthesized for the first time. The sesquiterpene framework was built up by means of the coupling of the C_{10} cyclogeranyl moiety with the C_5 3-(methylene)furan moiety. The key steps of our synthetic procedure are the stereoselective synthesis of four cyclogeraniol isomers, their conversion into the corresponding cyclogeranylsulfonylbenzene derivatives, their alkylation with 3-(chloromethyl)furan, and the final reductive cleavage of the phenylsulfonyl functional group to afford the whole sesquiterpene framework. The enantioselective synthesis of the α-, 3,4-dehydro-γ- and γ-cyclogeraniol isomers was performed using both a lipase-mediated resolution procedure and different regioselective chemical transformations.

Keywords: pallescensin 1; pallescensin 2; dihydropallescensin 2; isomicrocionin-3; pallescensone; furanosesquiterpenes; stereoselective synthesis; lipase-mediated resolution; cyclogeranylsulfonylbenzene isomers

1. Introduction

The furanosesquiterpenes are a large family of terpenoids that have been isolated from different natural sources. Among these compounds, those possessing a chemical framework consisting of a mono-cyclofarnesyl moiety linked to the 3-furyl moiety (compounds of type **1**, Figure 1) constitute a small subclass whose components occurs only in marine environments.

The first studies of these natural products date back to 1970s when pallescensin-1 (**2**) and pallescensin-2 (**4**) were isolated from the sponge *Dysidea pallescens* [1], together with other structurally related sesquiterpenes. Afterward, these compounds were also detected in other sponges [2,3] and in some nudibranchs that feed on sponges [4]. Moreover, the pallescensin-1 isomers isomicrocionin-3 (**3**) [3] and dihydropallescensin-2 (**5**) [2,4–7] were isolated contextually to the above-mentioned studies as well as during the course of researches finalized to the characterization of metabolites derived from marine organisms. In addition, the ketone derivative pallescensone (**6**) was obtained from the dichloromethane extract of the New Zealand sponge *Dictiodendrilla cavernosa* [8], and later, from different nudibranch species [9,10].

Almost immediately after their identification, both the chemical structure and the absolute configuration of the pallescensin-1 (**2**) and of the pallescensin-2 (**4**) were confirmed by chemical synthesis [11]. Thereafter, several new synthetic approaches [12–19] provided compounds **2**, **5**, and **6** both in racemic and in enantioenriched forms. Curiously, isomicrocionin-3 (**3**) has not been prepared yet, whereas pallescensis-2 (**4**) has been synthesized only in racemic form.

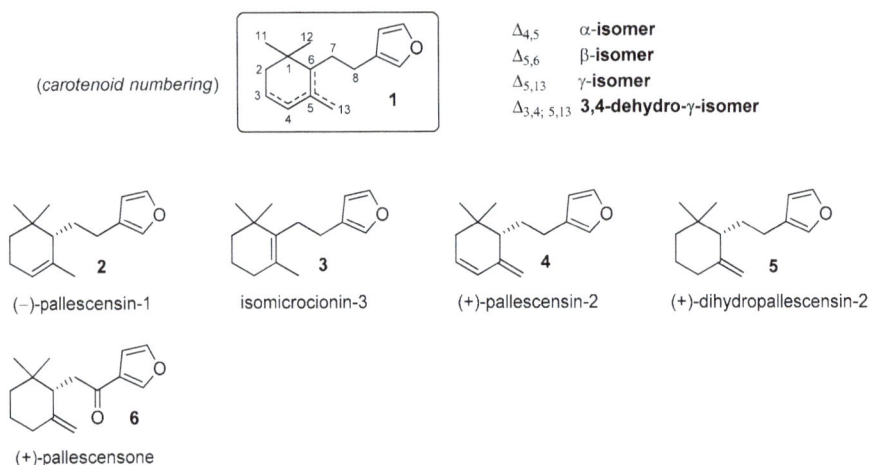

Figure 1. Representative examples of natural furanosesquiterpenes showing molecular framework of type **1**.

The reported syntheses were studied in order to confirm a proposed chemical structure or to assign the absolute configuration to a given metabolite. Overall, the preparation of the sesquiterpenes **2–6** was studied on a case-by-case basis. Therefore, a reliable and general synthetic approach to this class of compounds is still lacking. In addition, some of these sesquiterpenes have shown biological activity, but the limited amount of the available natural material precluded their comprehensive evaluation. For example, compounds **5** and **6** were isolated from nudibranch mollusks and are thought to possess antifeedant activity against their predators [4–10]. This ability was experimentally confirmed only on the whole dichloromethane extract of the mollusks [10], thus the determination of the real antifeedant contribute of each furanosesquiterpene could not be determined. Similarly, the antibacterial activity [3] of the pallescensin-1 (**2**) and the inhibitory activity against human tyrosine protein phosphatase 1B (hPTP1B) [7] of the dihydropallescensin-2 (**5**) were evaluated only for the natural occurring (S) enantiomers. Since the enantiomeric composition of a given compound could affect its biological properties, it is clear that the reported data are not enough to give a proper characterization of the biological activity of these metabolites. Overall, the aforementioned considerations point to the need of a general and stereoselective synthetic method for the preparation of all the isomeric forms of these furanosesquiterpenes.

By taking advantage of our previously acquired expertise in the enantioselective synthesis of monocyclofarnesyl terpenoids [20–23] and cyclogeraniol isomers [24], we decided to devise a synthetic procedure that could comply with the above-described requirements.

Our synthetic plan is exemplified by the retrosynthetic analysis described in Figure 2. Accordingly, we envisioned to prepare the target molecules of type **1** through the reductive cleavage of the phenylsulfonyl derivatives of type **7**, which can be in turn obtained by alkylation of the cyclogeranylsulfonylbenzene derivatives **8** with 3-(chloromethyl)furan **9**. The latter lithium salt can be prepared by reaction of a commercially available alkyllithium reagent (e.g., BuLi) with the cyclogeranylsulfonylbenzene derivatives, in turn synthesizable from the corresponding enantiopure cyclogeraniol isomers **10**. Of course, none of the above-described chemical transformations should involve side reactions, such as the double bond isomerization or the racemization, which could end up with decreasing the isomeric purity of the chemical intermediates, and thus, of the target compounds **1**.

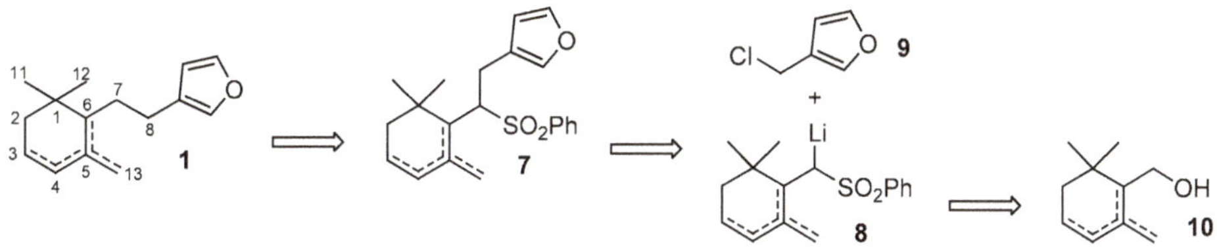

Figure 2. The proposed retrosynthetic analysis for the stereoselective synthesis of the furanosesquiterpenes possessing molecular framework of type **1**.

Herein, we describe the accomplishment of this synthetic plan, whose effectiveness was confirmed by the stereoselective preparation of some selected furanosesquiterpenes, namely (S)-pallescensin-1 (−)-**2**, isomicrocionin-3 (**3**), (R)-pallescensin-2 (−)-(**4**), and (R)-dihydropallescensis-2 (−)-(**5**). The limits of the presented approach were also discussed as highlighted with the stereoselective synthesis of (R)-pallescensone (−)-(**6**), which again required a building block of type **10** as starting material but with the use of a different synthetic path.

2. Results and Discussion

According to our retrosynthetic analysis, we started with the stereoselective preparation of the cyclogeraniol isomers **10**. The α-cyclogeraniol enantiomers were already prepared using both asymmetric synthesis [25] and resolution procedure [26]. Since racemic α-cyclogeraniol is easily synthesizable from ethyl geraniate [24], the lipase-mediated resolution procedure is the most suitable approach for the preparation of both the enantiomeric forms (Figure 3) of the alcohol **10a**.

In order to find out a proper enzyme to be employed in this process, we investigated the reactivity of (±)-**10a** toward irreversible acetylation using vinyl acetate as acyl donor in the presence of lipase catalyst. We checked three different commercial enzymes, namely porcine pancreatic lipase (PPL), *Candida rugosa* lipase (CRL), and lipase from *Pseudomonas* sp., (lipase PS). These preliminary experiments indicated that only lipase PS catalyzed the esterification reaction with an enantioselectivity acceptable to perform a proper enantiomers separation (enantiomeric ratio E = 9.2). Our findings agree with previous reported studies on the same enzymatic transformation [26], which assessed an enantiomeric ratio of 12.9 for lipase PS.

Accordingly, our resolution procedure furnished the enantioenriched alcohols (S)-(+)-**10a** and (R)-(−)-**10a** that were converted in the corresponding sulfones (S)-(+)-**11a** and (R)-(−)-**11a**, respectively. This chemical transformation was accomplished by means of a high yielding, three steps procedure [27], consisting of the reaction of alcohol **10a** with tosyl chloride, nucleophile substitution of the obtained tosylate with potassium thiophenate in dry DMF, followed by sodium molybdate catalysed oxidation of the resulting sulfide using an excess of hydrogen peroxide in methanol. Other synthetic methods, usually employed for the transformation of a hydroxyl functional group into a phenylsulfonyl group, afford sulfones **11** in inferior yields. For example, the reaction of the diphenyldisulfide/tributylphosphine reagent [28] with 3,4-dehydro-γ-cyclogeraniol or with γ-cyclogeraniol give the expected sulfide derivatives close to a significant amount of elimination side products. For this reason, we decided to employ exclusively the above-described thiophenate displacement procedure for the synthesis of the four sulfones **11a–d**.

Concerning β-cyclogeraniol, we selected β-cyclocitral **12** as starting compound. The latter aldehyde is commercially available since it is employed both as building block for carotenoids synthesis and as flavor ingredient [29,30]. The reduction of **12** with NaBH$_4$ in methanol afforded quantitatively β-cyclogeraniol **10b** that was converted into sulfone **11b** according to the general procedure described above.

For the stereoselective synthesis of γ-isomers **11c** and **11d**, we used diol **13** as a common starting compound. According to our previous studies [24], the latter racemic diol is preparable in high diastereoisomeric purity starting from α-cyclogeraniol. The following lipase PS mediated resolution procedure afforded diols (4R,6S)-(−)-13 and (4S,6R)-(+)-13 in high enantiomeric purity. Each one of these two enantiomers was transformed into the corresponding enantiomeric forms of the acetates 14 and 15. Accordingly, the chemical acetylation of the diol 13 enantiomers afforded the corresponding diacetates that were submitted to two different chemical reactions, aimed to the cleavage of the secondary allylic acetate group. The regioselective elimination of the latter group was accomplished refluxing the diacetates in dioxane, in presence of calcium carbonate and palladium acetate catalyst [31]. This process allow the conversion of the diols (−)-13 and (+)-13 into diene derivatives (+)-14 and (−)-14, respectively. Similarly, the diacetate derivatives of the diols (−)-13 and (+)-13 were reduced using triethylammonium formate, in refluxing tetrahydrofuran (THF) and in presence of the palladium catalyst to afford γ-cyclogeraniol acetate enantiomers (+)-15 and (−)-15, respectively [24]. It is worth noting that both reactions proceeded without appreciable formation of other isomers deriving from double bonds isomerization.

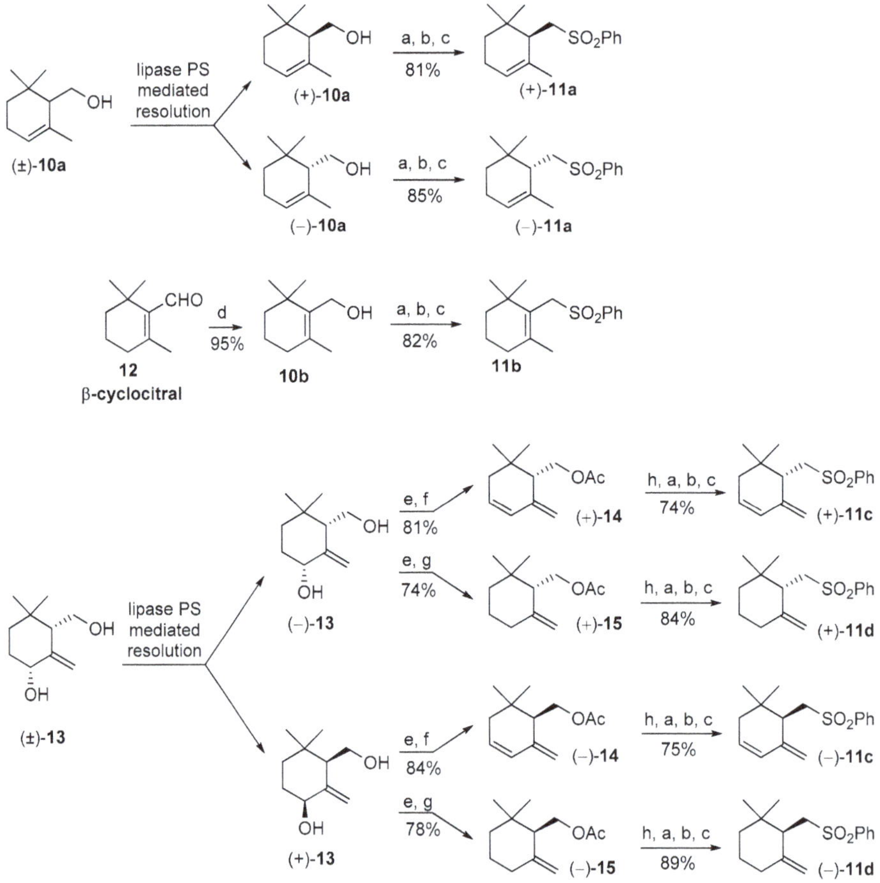

Figure 3. Synthesis of the stereoisomeric forms of the cyclogeranylsulfonylbenzene derivatives **11a-d** starting from the racemic cyclogeraniol derivatives **10a** and **13** and from β-cyclocitral **12**. Reagents and conditions: (**a**) TsCl, Py, CH$_2$Cl$_2$, DMAP catalyst, rt (room temperature), 4 h; (**b**) K$_2$CO$_3$, DMSO, PhSH, rt, 12 h; (**c**) H$_2$O$_2$, MeOH, (NH$_4$)$_2$MoO$_4$ catalyst, 0 °C then rt, 8 h; (**d**) NaBH$_4$, MeOH, 0 °C; (**e**) Ac$_2$O, Py, DMAP catalyst, rt, 8 h; (**f**) CaCO$_3$, PPh$_3$, Pd(OAc)$_2$ catalyst, dioxane, reflux, 5 h; (**g**) HCOOH, Et$_3$N, (PPh$_3$)$_2$PdCl$_2$ catalyst, PPh$_3$, THF, reflux, 6 h; (**h**) NaOH, MeOH, reflux.

This aspect is of pivotal relevance in natural product synthesis, where the biological activity of a given product is often dependent on its isomeric composition. Finally, the obtained acetates enantiomers (+)- and (−)-**14**, (+)- and (−)-**15** were hydrolyzed using sodium hydroxide in methanol, and the obtained alcohols were transformed into sulfones (+)- and (−)-**11c**, (+)- and (−)-**11d**, respectively, according to the general procedure used for the synthesis of compounds **11a** and **11b**.

The obtained sulfones were then used as chiral building blocks for the stereoselective synthesis of the marine furanosesquiterpenes structurally related to pallescensins. Although we prepared both enantiomers of the compounds **11a**, **11c**, and **11d**, the isomers (−)-**11a**, (−)-**11c**, and (−)-**11d** were those available in higher enantiomeric purity, according to the resolution procedures of alcohol **10a** and diol **13**. Therefore, we decided to use the latter sulfone enantiomers for the furanosesquiterpenes synthesis.

As described in the retrosynthetic analysis, compounds (−)-**11a**, **11b**, (−)-**11c**, and (−)-**11d** were treated with n-butyllithium (nBuLi) and the resulting lithium salts were alkylated using 3-(chloromethyl)furan **9**. The obtained derivatives **7a-d** were not isolated and were treated with lithium naphthalenide at low temperature (−70 °C) in order to remove the phenylsulfonyl group through its regioselective reduction. Both alkylation step and phenylsulfonyl group cleavage proceeded with high chemical yields and compounds (−)-**11a**, **11b**, (−)-**11c**, and (−)-**11d** were efficiently and stereoselectively converted into (−)-pallescensin-1 (**2**), isomicrocionin-3 (**3**), (−)-pallescensin-2 (**4**), and (−)-dihydropallescensin-2 (**5**), respectively (Figure 4).

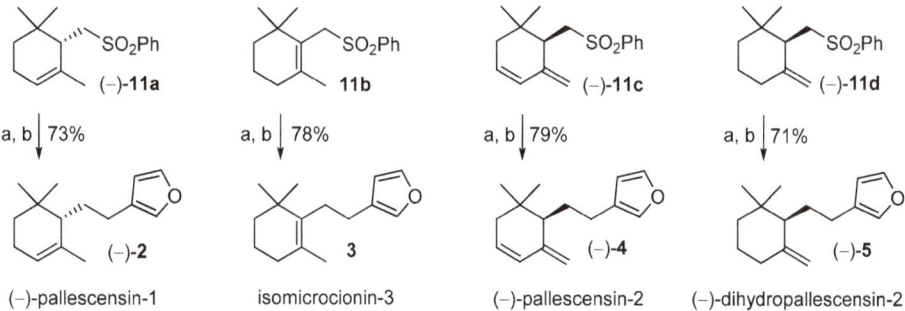

Figure 4. Use of the cyclogeranylsulfonylbenzene derivatives **11a–d** in the stereoselective synthesis of the furanosesquiterpenes (−)-pallescensin-1 (**2**), isomicrocionin-3 (**3**), (−)-pallescensin-2 (**4**), and (−)-dihydropallescensis-2 (**5**). Reagents and conditions: (**a**) nBuLi, THF dry, −60 °C, then **9** in DMPU, rt, 2 h; (**b**) lithium naphthalenide, THF dry, Et$_2$NH, −75 °C, 1 h.

The proposed synthesis of compounds **2**, **4**, and **5** compare favorably over the previously reported stereoselective methods [11,15,18,19] since the overall yields are higher, the approach is operationally simple, and it afforded the target compounds in high stereoisomeric purity.

Isomicrocionin-3 was not synthesized before. Therefore, the comparison of the analytical data of synthetic **3** with those recorded for the natural sesquiterpene isolated from *Fasciospongia* sp. [3] allows us confirming the chemical structure previously assigned to isomicrocionin-3.

Furthermore, as mentioned in the introduction, pallescensis-2 (**4**) was synthesized only in racemic form [11] and the (S) absolute configuration was tentatively assigned to the dextrorotatory isomer. This assumption is based on the observation that both (+)-pallescensin-2 and (−)-pallescensin-1 were isolated from the same sponge (*Dysidea pallescens*) and the absolute configuration of (−)-pallescensin-1 was already assigned by chemical correlation with (S)-(−)-α-cyclocitral. (S)-(−)-**2** and (+)-**4** most likely possess the same absolute configuration because they were formed through a common biosynthetic pathway. According to our synthetic procedure, we established a chemical correlation between (4S,6R)-4-hydroxy-γ-cyclogeraniol (+)-**13** and (−)-pallescensin-2 (**4**), thus confirming unambiguously that (−)-pallescensin-2 (**4**) possesses (R) absolute configuration.

The very good results described above prompted us to investigate a possible exploitation of the sulfone alkylation approach for the synthesis of pallescensone (**6**), a sesquiterpene ketone structurally related to dihydropallescensin-2 (**5**). As described previously [27,32], the lithium salt of a given phenylsulfonyl derivative can be acylated using anhydrous magnesium bromide and the alkyl ester of the corresponding acyl moiety. The following cleavage of the phenylsulfonyl group by means of lithium naphthalenide at low temperature provides the acylated derivative. Unfortunately, we found that the reaction of phenylsulfone **11d** with 3-furoic acid methyl ester afforded the acylated sulfone in very low yield.

This disappointing result is most likely due to the steric hindrance around the new formed bond, which does not allow phenylsulfonyl and ketone functional groups to adopt vicinal conformation with formation of the magnesium complex, whose chemical stability secure the product formation.

For that reason, we decided to study a different approach for the stereoselective synthesis of ketone **6**. Taking advantage of the above-described process for the preparation of the enantioenriched γ-cyclogeraniol derivatives (Figure 3), we selected the enantiomeric forms of compound **15** as chiral building blocks for pallescensone synthesis. More enantiopure isomer (−)-**15** was used as starting compound (Figure 5) and the devised synthetic procedure provided pallescensone (**6**) after six steps, in good overall yield (43%).

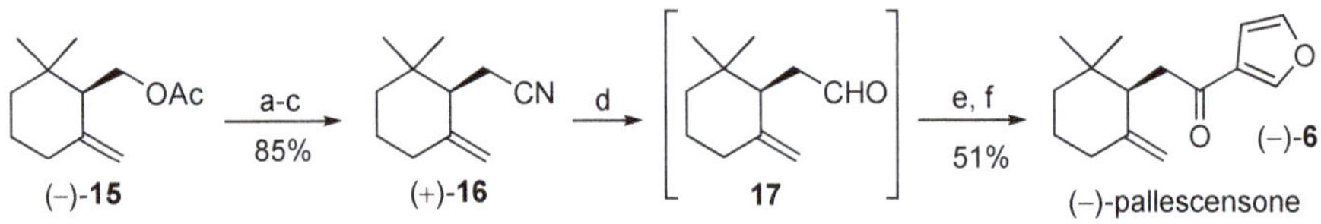

Figure 5. Stereoselective synthesis of (−)-pallescensone (**6**) starting from γ-cyclogeraniol acetate (−)-**15**. Reagents and conditions: (**a**) NaOH, MeOH, reflux; (**b**) TsCl, Py, CH$_2$Cl$_2$, DMAP catalyst, rt, 4 h; (**c**) NaCN, DMSO dry, 80–90 °C, 5 h; (**d**) DIBAL, toluene, −70 °C, 30 min; (**e**) 3-furyllithium, −70 °C, THF dry, 20 min; (**f**) IBX, DMSO dry, 40 °C, 4 h.

Accordingly, acetate (−)-**15** was hydrolyzed using sodium hydroxide in methanol and the obtained γ-cyclogeraniol was treated with tosyl chloride and pyridine, in presence of the DMAP catalyst. The nucleophilic substitution of the tosyl functional group with the cyanide group was performed by reaction with sodium cyanide in dimethylsulfoxide (DMSO), heating at 80–90 °C to afford cyanide (+)-**16** in 85% overall yield. The latter compound was then reduced at low temperature (−70 °C) using DIBAL in toluene. The resulting aldehyde **17** was not purified and was treated with freshly prepared 3-furyllithium in THF. The obtained crude carbinol was dissolved in dry DMSO and was treated with an excess of IBX [33] to afford (−)-(R)-pallescensone (**6**) in 51% overall yield from **16**.

The ^{1}H- and ^{13}C-NMR spectroscopic data of the synthesized compound **6** were superimposable with those reported for the synthetic [18,19] and the natural [8] sesquiterpene, whereas the measured optical rotation value, $[α]^{20}_D = -34.4$ (c 1.1, CH$_2$Cl$_2$), show comparable value and opposite sign of the naturally occurring (S)-pallescensone, $[α]^{20}_D = +36$ (c 1.0, CHCl$_3$).

Finally, it should be considered that the enantiomeric forms of γ-homocyclogeranial **17** were used as a chiral building blocks not only for the synthesis of pallescensone, but also for the preparation of other sesquiterpenes [18,34] or sesquiterpene analogues [35], thus expanding the prospective utility of this synthon in natural products synthesis.

3. Materials and Methods

3.1. Materials and General Methods

All moisture- and air-sensitive reactions were carried out using dry solvents under a static atmosphere of nitrogen.

All solvents and reagents were of commercial quality and were purchased from Sigma-Aldrich (St. Louis, MO, USA) with the exception of β-cyclogeraniol, 3-(chloromethyl)furan and IBX. β-Cyclogeraniol was prepared by reduction of β-cyclogeranial using $NaBH_4$ in methanol. 3-(Chloromethyl)furan was obtained starting from furan-3-carboxylic acid by means of reduction with $LiAlH_4$ and reaction of the obtained carbinol with mesyl chloride in presence of s-collidine and LiCl [36,37]. IBX was prepared starting from o-iodobenzoic acid, according to the literature [33].

Lipase from *Pseudomonas cepacia* (PS), 30 units/mg, was purchased from Amano Pharmaceuticals Co., Tokyo, Japan. Enantioenriched α-cyclogeraniol 10a and cis-4-hydroxy-γ-cyclogeraniol 13 were prepared by means of the lipase PS-mediated resolution of the corresponding racemic compounds, as previously described by Vidari [26] and Serra [24], respectively.

3.2. Analytical Methods and Characterization of the Chemical Compounds

^1H and ^{13}C-NMR spectra and DEPT (Distortionless enhancement by polarization transfer) experiments: $CDCl_3$ solutions at room temperature using a Bruker-AC-400 spectrometer (Billerica, MA, USA) at 400, 100, and 100 MHz, respectively; ^{13}C spectra are proton-decoupled; chemical shifts in ppm relative to internal $SiMe_4$ (0 ppm).

Thin-layer chromatography (TLC) involved the use of Merck silica gel 60 F_{254} plates (Merck Millipore, Milan, Italy), while column chromatography involved the use of silica gel.

Melting points were measured on a Reichert apparatus equipped with a Reichert microscope and are uncorrected.

Optical rotations were measured on a Jasco-DIP-181 digital polarimeter (Jasco, Tokyo, Japan).

Mass spectra were recorded on a Bruker ESQUIRE 3000 PLUS spectrometer (ESI detector, Billerica, MA, USA) or by GC-MS analyses.

GC-MS analyses involved the use of an HP-6890 gas chromatograph equipped with a 5973 mass detector, using an HP-5MS column (30 m × 0.25 mm, 0.25-μm film thickness; Hewlett Packard, Palo Alto, CA, USA) with the following temperature program: 60° (1 min), then 6°/min to 150° (held at 1 min), then 12°/min to 280° (held 5 min); carrier gas: He; constant flow 1 mL/min; split ratio: 1/30; t_R given in minutes.

The values of t_R for each compound are as follows: t_R(2) 18.70, t_R(3) 19.14, t_R(4) 18.47, t_R(5) 18.48, t_R(6) 21.81, t_R(9) 3.90, t_R(10a) 10.59, t_R(10b) 11.32, t_R(11a) 25.85, t_R(11b) 26.03, t_R(11c) 25.71, t_R(11d) 25.86, t_R(14) 14.02, t_R(15) 13.86, t_R(16) 14.71.

3.3. Stereoselective Preparation of (R) and (S) Enantiomers of 3,4-Dehydro-γ-cyclogeraniol Acetate 14 and γ-Cyclogeraniol Acetate 15

3.3.1. (R)-3,4-Dehydro-γ-cyclogeraniol Acetate (−)-14

A sample of diol (+)-13, (0.5 g, 2.9 mmol; $[α]^{20}_D$ = +29.5 (c 2.8, $CHCl_3$); 98% ee by chiral GC) was converted to the corresponding diacetate by treatment with pyridine (10 mL), DMAP (50 mg, 0.4 mmol) and Ac_2O (10 mL) at rt for 8 h. After removal of the solvents, the crude diacetate was dissolved in dioxane (20 mL) and treated under N_2 with $Pd(OAc)_2$ (50 mg, 0.2 mmol), $CaCO_3$ (1 g, 10 mmol), and PPh_3 (270 mg, 1 mmol). The resulting heterogeneous mixture was stirred under reflux for 5 h (TLC monitoring). The mixture was then cooled to room temperature, diluted with diethyl ether (100 mL), and filtered. The filtrate was washed successively with saturated aqueous $NaHCO_3$ solution (50 mL) and brine, dried (Na_2SO_4), and evaporated. The residue was purified by chromatography (n-hexane/Et_2O 95:5–8:2) and bulb-to-bulb distillation to give pure 3,4-dehydro-γ-cyclogeraniol acetate (−)-14 = (R)-(6,6-dimethyl-2-methylenecyclohex-3-enyl)methyl acetate (480 mg, 84% yield) as a colourless oil; $[α]^{20}_D$ = −69.9 (c 3.3, $CHCl_3$); 99% of chemical purity by GC. ^1H NMR (400 MHz, $CDCl_3$) δ 6.08 (d, J = 9.8 Hz, 1H), 5.70-5.63 (m, 1H), 4.95 (s, 1H), 4.86 (s, 1H), 4.23 (dd, J = 10.7, 4.6 Hz, 1H), 3.93 (dd, J = 10.7, 9.1 Hz, 1H), 2.21 (dd, J = 9.1, 4.6 Hz, 1H), 2.05 (d, J = 18.6 Hz, 1H), 2.02 (s, 3H), 1.83 (dd, J = 18.6, 5.2 Hz, 1H), 1.02 (s, 3H), 0.92 (s, 3H). ^{13}C NMR (100 MHz, $CDCl_3$) δ 171.0 (C), 143.3 (C), 127.5 (CH), 127.3 (CH),

114.2 (CH$_2$), 64.2 (CH$_2$), 50.0 (CH), 37.0 (CH$_2$), 31.8 (C), 28.4 (Me), 27.3 (Me), 21.0 (Me). GC-MS m/z (rel intensity) 134 ([M − AcOH]$^+$, 52), 119 (100), 105 (24), 91 (54), 77 (17), 65 (6), 53 (5).

3.3.2. (S)-3,4-Dehydro-γ-cyclogeraniol Acetate (+)-**14**

The reaction sequence described above was repeated using sample of diol (−)-**13**, ([α]^{20}$_D$ = −26.8 (c 2.5, CHCl$_3$); 90% ee by chiral GC) to afford pure 3,4-dehydro-γ-cyclogeraniol acetate (+)-**14** = (S)-(6,6-dimethyl-2-methylenecyclohex-3-enyl)methyl acetate (81% yield) as a colorless oil; [α]^{20}$_D$ = +61.1 (c 3.0, CHCl$_3$); 96% of chemical purity by GC. ^{1}H-NMR, ^{13}C-NMR and GC-MS superimposable to those described for (R)-isomer.

3.3.3. (R)-γ-Cyclogeraniol Acetate (−)-**15**

A sample of diol (+)-**13**, (0.9 g, 5.3 mmol; [α]^{20}$_D$ = +29.5 (c 2.8, CHCl$_3$); 98% ee by chiral GC) was treated with pyridine (10 mL), DMAP (50 mg, 0.4 mmol) and Ac$_2$O (10 mL) and set aside at rt until acetylation was complete (8 h). The obtained diacetate was dissolved in dry THF (30 mL) and refluxed under a static nitrogen atmosphere in the presence of formic acid (0.75 g, 16.3 mmol), Et$_3$N (1.65 g, 16.3 mmol), (PPh$_3$)$_2$PdCl$_2$ (140 mg, 0.2 mmol) and triphenylphosphine (0.25 g, 0.9 mmol). After the reaction was complete (6 h, TLC analysis), the mixture was diluted with ether (100 mL) and washed with water (50 mL), 5% HCl (50 mL), satd. aq NaHCO$_3$ (50 mL), and brined. The organic phase was concentrated under reduced pressure and the residue was purified by chromatography (n-hexane/AcOEt 95:5–8:2) and bulb-to-bulb distillation to afford pure (R)-γ-cyclogeraniol acetate (−)-**15** = (R)-(2,2-dimethyl-6-methylenecyclohexyl)methyl acetate (0.81 g, 78% yield) as a colorless oil; [α]^{20}$_D$ = −10.1 (c 3.8, CHCl$_3$); 96% diastereoisomeric purity, 99% of chemical purity by GC. ^{1}H NMR (400 MHz, CDCl$_3$) δ 4.75 (s, 1H), 4.53 (s, 1H), 4.19 (dd, J = 11.0, 5.3 Hz, 1H), 4.15 (dd, J = 11.0, 9.2 Hz, 1H), 2.16–2.06 (m, 2H), 2.03–1.92 (m, 1H), 1.94 (s, 3H), 1.54–1.44 (m, 2H), 1.42–1.32 (m, 1H), 1.29–1.20 (m, 1H), 0.91 (s, 3H), 0.80 (s, 3H). ^{13}C NMR (100 MHz, CDCl$_3$) δ 171.0 (C), 147.0 (C), 109.7 (CH$_2$), 62.7 (CH$_2$), 52.1 (CH), 37.8 (CH$_2$), 34.2 (C), 33.3 (CH$_2$), 28.6 (Me), 25.0 (Me), 23.3 (CH$_2$), 20.9 (Me). Lit. for ^{1}H and ^{13}C NMR [38,39]. GC-MS m/z (rel intensity) 136 ([M − AcOH]$^+$, 80), 121 (100), 107 (43), 93 (89), 79 (33), 69 (49), 55 (9), 43 (50).

3.3.4. (S)-γ-Cyclogeraniol Acetate (+)-**15**

The reaction sequence described above was repeated using sample of diol (−)-**13**, ([α]^{20}$_D$ = −26.8 (c 2.5, CHCl$_3$); 90% ee by chiral GC) to afford pure (S)-γ-cyclogeraniol acetate (+)-**15** = (S)-(2,2-dimethyl-6-methylenecyclohexyl)methyl acetate (74% yield) as a colorless oil; [α]^{20}$_D$ = +9.1 (c 3.1, CHCl$_3$); 96% diastereoisomeric purity, 95% of chemical purity by GC. ^{1}H-NMR, ^{13}C-NMR and GC-MS superimposable to those described for (R)-isomer.

*3.4. Synthesis of the Enantiomeric Forms of the Cyclogeranylsulfonylbenzene Derivatives **11a–d***

3.4.1. General Procedure

A solution of p-toluenesulfonyl chloride (1.5 g, 7.9 mmol) in CH$_2$Cl$_2$ (4 mL) was added dropwise to a stirred solution of the suitable cyclogeraniol isomer (0.9 g, 5.8 mmol), DMAP (50 mg, 0.4 mmol) and pyridine (2 mL) in CH$_2$Cl$_2$ (4 mL). After 4 h, the mixture was diluted with ether (100 mL) and then was washed with 1 M aqueous HCl solution (50 mL), saturated NaHCO$_3$ solution (50 mL), and brined. The organic phase was dried (Na$_2$SO$_4$) and concentrated *in vacuo*. The residue was dissolved in dry DMSO (5 mL) and added dropwise to a suspension of K$_2$CO$_3$ (3.2 g, 23.1 mmol) and thiophenol (1.7 g, 15.4 mmol) in DMSO (20 mL). The resulting mixture was stirred vigorously at rt (room temperature) until the starting tosylate was no longer detectable by TLC analysis (12 h). The reaction was partitioned between water (150 mL) and ether (100 mL). The aqueous phase was extracted again with ether (100 mL) and the combined organic phases were washed with an aqueous solution of NaOH (10% w/w, 50 mL) and brined, dried (Na$_2$SO$_4$), and concentrated *in vacuo*. The residue was dissolved in methanol (50 mL) and was treated at 0 °C with (NH$_4$)$_2$MoO$_4$ (80 mg, 0.4 mmol) followed by the dropwise addition of a solution of H$_2$O$_2$ (35% wt. in water, 10 mL). The solution was then warmed to rt while stirring was continued for a further 8 h. The reaction was cooled again and a saturated solution of Na$_2$SO$_3$ was added to destroy excess oxidant. The main part of the methanol was removed under reduced pressure and the residue extracted with AcOEt (3 × 100 mL). The combined organic layers were dried (Na$_2$SO$_4$), concentrated, and the residue purified by chromatography using n-hexane/AcOEt (95:5–8:2) as eluent to afford the suitable cyclogeranylsulfonylbenzene derivative.

3.4.2. (S)-((2,6,6-Trimethylcyclohex-2-enyl)methylsulfonyl)benzene (−)-11a

According to the general procedure, (S)-α-cyclogeraniol (−)-10a = (S)-(2,6,6-trimethylcyclohex-2-en-1-yl)methanol ([α]$^{20}_D$ = −102.1 (c 2.4, EtOH); 90% ee; 97% chemical purity) was transformed into (S)-((2,6,6-trimethylcyclohex-2-enyl)methylsulfonyl)benzene (−)-11a (85% yield); [α]$^{20}_D$ = −83.9 (c 2.1, CH$_2$Cl$_2$); 96% of chemical purity by GC. ^{1}H NMR (400 MHz, CDCl$_3$) δ 7.97–7.90 (m, 2H), 7.68–7.52 (m, 3H), 5.33 (s, 1H), 3.23 (dd, J = 15.2, 4.3 Hz, 1H), 2.91 (dd, J = 15.2, 3.9 Hz, 1H), 2.25 (s, 1H), 2.06–1.84 (m, 2H), 1.62 (br s, 3H), 1.23–1.16 (m, 2H), 0.91 (s, 6H). ^{13}C NMR (100 MHz, CDCl$_3$) δ 140.4 (C), 134.8 (C), 133.5 (CH), 129.2 (CH), 128.1 (CH), 121.8 (CH), 58.6 (CH$_2$), 42.9 (CH), 32.2 (C), 31.3 (CH$_2$), 27.0 (Me), 26.2 (Me), 22.8 (CH$_2$), 22.5 (Me). Lit. for ^{1}H and ^{13}C NMR [25]. MS (ESI): 301.1 [M + Na]$^+$.

3.4.3. (R)-((2,6,6-Trimethylcyclohex-2-enyl)methylsulfonyl)benzene (+)-11a

According to the general procedure, (R)-α-cyclogeraniol (+)-10a = (R)-(2,6,6-trimethylcyclohex-2-en-1-yl)methanol, ([α]$^{20}_D$ = +96.7 (c 2.7, EtOH); 85% ee; 97% chemical purity) was transformed into (R)-((2,6,6-trimethylcyclohex-2-enyl)methylsulfonyl)benzene (+)-11a (81% yield), [α]$^{20}_D$ = +77.8 (c 2.8, CH$_2$Cl$_2$), 98% of chemical purity by GC. ^{1}H-, ^{13}C-NMR and MS superimposable to those described for (S)-isomer.

3.4.4. 2,6,6-((Trimethylcyclohex-1-enyl)methylsulfonyl)benzene 11b

According to the general procedure, β-cyclogeraniol = ((2,6,6-trimethylcyclohex-1-en-1-yl)methanol (96% chemical purity) was transformed into ((2,6,6-trimethylcyclohex-1-enyl)methylsulfonyl)benzene 11b (82% yield) as a colorless oil, 97% of chemical purity by GC. ^{1}H NMR (400 MHz, CDCl$_3$) δ 7.97–7.90 (m, 2H), 7.67–7.51 (m, 3H), 3.97 (s, 2H), 2.06 (t, J = 6.3 Hz, 2H), 1.68–1.58 (m, 2H), 1.67 (s, 3H), 1.52–1.46 (m, 2H), 1.04 (s, 6H). ^{13}C NMR (100 MHz, CDCl$_3$) δ 141.7 (C), 139.2 (C), 133.2 (CH), 129.1 (CH), 127.8 (CH), 125.9 (C), 57.7 (CH$_2$), 39.5 (CH$_2$), 34.4 (C), 33.3 (CH$_2$), 28.8 (Me), 21.8 (Me), 18.9 (CH$_2$). Lit. for ^{1}H and ^{13}C NMR [40]. GC-MS m/z (rel intensity) 278 (M$^+$, 1), 137 (100), 121 (10), 107 (6), 95 (45), 81 (28), 69 (8), 55 (6).

3.4.5. (R)-((2,2-Dimethyl-6-methylenecyclohexyl)methylsulfonyl)benzene (−)-11c

(−)-γ-3,4-dehydrocyclogeraniol acetate = (R)-(6,6-dimethyl-2-methylenecyclohex-3-en-1-yl)methyl acetate ([α]$^{20}_D$ = −69.9 (c 3.3, CHCl$_3$); 98% ee; 99% chemical purity) was hydrolyzed using NaOH in methanol, at reflux. After work-up, the obtained crude alcohol was submitted to the general procedure to give (R)-((6,6-dimethyl-2-methylenecyclohex-3-enyl)methylsulfonyl)benzene (75% yield) as a colorless oil; [α]$^{20}_D$ = −89.2 (c 3.7, CHCl$_3$); 96% of chemical purity by GC. ^{1}H NMR (400 MHz, CDCl$_3$) δ 7.92–7.86 (m, 2H), 7.66–7.60 (m, 1H), 7.58–7.51 (m, 2H), 5.96 (d, J = 9.9 Hz, 1H), 5.65–5.58 (m, 1H), 4.82 (s, 2H), 3.22 (dd, J = 14.6, 2.4 Hz, 1H), 3.04 (dd, J = 14.6, 8.1 Hz, 1H), 2.53 (dm, J = 8.1 Hz, 1H), 1.90 (dm, J = 18.7 Hz, 1H), 1.79 (dd, J = 18.7, 5.0 Hz, 1H), 0.91 (s, 3H), 0.85 (s, 3H). ^{13}C NMR (100 MHz, CDCl$_3$) δ 143.1 (C), 140.3 (C), 133.4 (CH), 129.1 (CH), 128.1 (CH), 127.4 (CH), 127.1 (CH), 115.0 (CH$_2$), 56.7 (CH$_2$), 44.8 (CH), 36.3 (CH$_2$), 32.7 (C), 27.2 (Me), 26.7 (Me). MS (ESI): 299.1 [M + Na]$^+$, 315.1 [M + K]$^+$.

3.4.6. (S)-((2,2-Dimethyl-6-methylenecyclohexyl)methylsulfonyl)benzene (+)-11c

The reaction sequence described above was repeated using (+)-γ-3,4-dehydrocyclogeraniol acetate = (S)-(6,6-dimethyl-2-methylenecyclohex-3-en-1-yl)methyl acetate ($[\alpha]^{20}_D$ = +61.1 (c 3.0, CHCl$_3$); 96% of chemical purity) to afford (S)-((6,6-dimethyl-2-methylenecyclohex-3-enyl)methylsulfonyl)benzene (74% yield), colorless oil; $[\alpha]^{20}_D$ = +78.8 (c 3.1, CHCl$_3$); 96% of chemical purity by GC. ^{1}H-NMR, ^{13}C-NMR and GC-MS superimposable to those described for (R)-isomer.

3.4.7. (R)-((2,2-Dimethyl-6-methylenecyclohexyl)methylsulfonyl)benzene (−)-11d

(−)-γ-Cyclogeraniol acetate = (R)-(2,2-dimethyl-6-methylenecyclohexyl)methyl acetate (($[\alpha]^{20}_D$ = −10.1 (c 3.8, CHCl$_3$); 96% diastereoisomeric purity; 99% chemical purity by GC) was hydrolysed using NaOH in methanol, at reflux. After work-up, the obtained crude alcohol was submitted to the general procedure to give (−)-(R)-((2,2-dimethyl-6-methylenecyclohexyl(methylsulfonyl)benzene (89% yield) as a colorless oil; $[\alpha]^{20}_D$ = −11.7 (c 3.7, CHCl$_3$); 96% diastereoisomeric purity, 95% of chemical purity by GC. ^{1}H NMR (400 MHz, CDCl$_3$) δ 7.92–7.85 (m, 2H), 7.67–7.49 (m, 3H), 4.74 (s, 1H), 4.56 (s, 1H), 3.35 (dd, J = 14.7, 9.4 Hz, 1H), 3.24 (dd, J = 14.7, 2.5 Hz, 1H), 2.44 (dm, J = 9.4 Hz, 1H), 2.07–1.93 (m, 2H), 1.55–1.44 (m, 2H), 1.35–1.28 (m, 2H), 0.90 (s, 3H), 0.78 (s, 3H). ^{13}C NMR (100 MHz, CDCl$_3$) δ 145.6 (C), 140.0 (C), 133.4 (CH), 129.0 (CH), 128.2 (CH), 110.9 (CH$_2$), 54.4 (CH$_2$), 47.8 (CH), 37.2 (CH$_2$), 35.3 (C), 32.9 (CH$_2$), 27.8 (Me), 24.9 (Me), 23.2 (CH$_2$). Lit. for ^{1}H and ^{13}C NMR [41]. MS (ESI): 301.2 [M + Na]$^+$.

3.4.8. (S)-((2,2-Dimethyl-6-methylenecyclohexyl)methylsulfonyl)benzene (+)-11d

The reaction sequence described above was repeated using (+)-γ-cyclogeraniol acetate = (S)-(2,2-dimethyl-6-methylenecyclohexyl)methyl acetate ($[\alpha]^{20}_D$ = +9.1 (c 3.1, CHCl$_3$); 96% diastereoisomeric purity, 95% of chemical purity by GC) to afford (S)-((2,2-dimethyl-6-methylenecyclohexyl)methylsulfonyl)benzene (84% yield); ($[\alpha]^{20}_D$ = +9.8 (c 2.4, CHCl$_3$); 97% of chemical purity by GC. ^{1}H-NMR, ^{13}C-NMR and GC-MS superimposable to those described for (R)-isomer.

3.5. Synthesis of the Furanosesquiterpenes (−)-Pallescensin-1 (2), Isomicrocionin-3 (3), (−)-Pallescensin-2 (4), and (−)-Dihydropallescensis-2 (5)

3.5.1. General Procedure

nBuLi (1 mL of a 2.5 M solution in hexane) was added dropwise under nitrogen to a cooled (−60 °C) solution of the suitable cyclogeranylsulfonylbenzene derivative (2.2 mmol) in dry THF (10 mL). The resulting orange solution was stirred at this temperature for 15 min and then a solution of 3-(chloromethyl)furan (260 mg, 2.23 mmol) in dry DMPU (1 mL) was added dropwise. The reaction was allowed to reach room temperature and after two hours at this temperature, and it was quenched by the addition of a saturated solution of NH$_4$Cl aqueous (50 mL). The resulting mixture was extracted with diethyl ether (3 × 50 mL) and the combined organic phases was dried (Na$_2$SO$_4$) and concentrated *in vacuo*. The crude product was dissolved in dry THF (15 mL) containing dry Et$_2$NH (1 mL). The mixture was cooled (−75 °C) and was treated under nitrogen with freshly prepared lithium naphthalenide (8 mL of a 0.72 M solution). When the staring material could no longer be detected by TLC analysis (1 h), the reaction was quenched by the addition of a saturated solution of NH$_4$Cl aqueous (50 mL) and diluted with diethyl ether (80 mL). The organic phase was separated and the aqueous phase was extracted with ethyl ether (50 mL). The combined organic layers were washed with brine, dried (Na$_2$SO$_4$) and concentrated under reduced pressure. A large part of the naphthalene content was removed by crystallization from hexane. The liquid phase was then purified by chromatography (hexane/diethyl ether 99:1–95:5) to afford the desired furanosesquiterpene.

3.5.2. Synthesis of (−)-Pallescensin-1 (2)

According to the general procedure, the alkylation/reduction of ((2,6,6-trimethylcyclohex-2-enyl)methylsulfonyl)benzene ($[\alpha]^{20}_D$ = −83.9 (c 2.1, CH$_2$Cl$_2$); 90% ee, 96% of chemical purity by GC) afforded (−)-pallescensin-1 (2) = 3-(2-(2,6,6-trimethylcyclohex-2-enyl)ethyl)furan (73% yield) as a colorless oil; $[\alpha]^{20}_D$ = −93.2 (c 3.2, CHCl$_3$); 94% of chemical purity by GC; Lit. [10] for synthetic 2: $[\alpha]^{20}_D$ = −89.5 (CHCl$_3$); Lit. [3] for natural 2: $[\alpha]^{20}_D$ = −23.5 (c 0.07, CHCl$_3$). ^{1}H NMR (400 MHz, CDCl$_3$) δ 7.34 (t, J = 1.7 Hz, 1H), 7.23–7.20 (m, 1H), 6.27 (br s, 1H), 5.31 (br s, 1H), 2.50–2.40 (m, 2H), 2.01–1.91 (m, 2H), 1.76–1.63 (m, 1H), 1.69–1.66 (m, 3H), 1.62–1.39 (m, 3H), 1.19–1.10 (m, 1H), 0.95 (s, 3H), 0.88 (s, 3H). ^{13}C NMR (100 MHz, CDCl$_3$) δ 142.6 (CH), 138.6 (CH), 136.5 (C), 125.6 (C), 120.2 (CH), 111.0 (CH), 49.0 (CH), 32.6 (C), 31.6 (CH$_2$), 31.6 (CH$_2$), 27.52 (Me), 27.46 (Me), 25.5 (CH$_2$), 23.5 (Me), 23.0 (CH$_2$). Lit. for ^{1}H and ^{13}C NMR [3]. GC-MS m/z (rel intensity) 218 (M$^+$, 8), 203 (2), 162 (3), 147 (15), 133 (13), 121 (14), 109 (26), 95 (41), 81 (100), 67 (7), 53 (13).

3.5.3. Synthesis of Isomicrocionin-3 (3)

According to the general procedure, the alkylation/reduction of ((2,6,6-trimethylcyclohex-1-enyl)methylsulfonyl)benzene (97% of chemical purity by GC) afforded isomicrocionin-3 = 3-(2-(2,6,6-trimethylcyclohex-1-enyl)ethyl)furan 3 (78% yield) as a colorless oil; 99% of chemical purity by GC. ^{1}H NMR (400 MHz, CDCl$_3$) δ 7.34 (t, J = 1.7 Hz, 1H), 7.24–7.22 (m, 1H), 6.30 (br s, 1H), 2.50–2.42 (m, 2H), 2.27–2.19 (m, 2H), 1.93 (t, J = 6.2 Hz, 2H), 1.64 (s, 3H), 1.63–1.55 (m, 2H), 1.47–1.41 (m, 2H), 1.02 (s, 6H). ^{13}C NMR (100 MHz, CDCl$_3$) δ 142.6 (CH), 138.4 (CH), 136.9 (C), 127.6 (C), 125.7 (C), 110.9 (CH), 39.8 (CH$_2$), 34.9 (C), 32.8 (CH$_2$), 29.5 (CH$_2$), 28.6 (Me), 25.6 (CH$_2$), 19.8 (Me), 19.5 (CH$_2$). Lit. for ^{1}H and ^{13}C NMR [3]. GC-MS m/z (rel intensity) 218 (M$^+$, 64), 203 ([M − Me]$^+$, 47), 185 (4), 175 (10), 162 (18), 149 (25) 137 (77), 121 (18), 109 (20), 95 (100), 81 (85), 67 (15), 53 (16).

3.5.4. Synthesis of (−)-Pallescensin-2 (4)

According to the general procedure, the alkylation/reduction of (R)-((6,6-dimethyl-2-methylenecyclohex-3-enyl)methylsulfonyl)benzene ($[\alpha]^{20}_D$ = −89.2 (c 3.7, CHCl$_3$); 96% of chemical purity by GC) afforded (−)-pallescensin-2 (4) = (R)-3-(2-(6,6-dimethyl-2-methylenecyclohex-3-enyl)ethyl)furan (79% yield) as a colorless oil; $[\alpha]^{20}_D$ = −65.1 (c 2.9, CHCl$_3$); 96% of chemical purity by GC; Lit. [1] for natural 4: $[\alpha]^{20}_D$ = +39.5.

^{1}H NMR (400 MHz, CDCl$_3$) δ 7.33 (m, 1H), 7.19 (s, 1H), 6.25 (m, 1H), 6.03 (dd, J = 9.8, 1.8 Hz, 1H), 5.69–5.59 (m, 1H), 4.91 (s, 1H), 4.74 (s, 1H), 2.53–2.42 (m, 1H), 2.33–2.22 (m, 1H), 2.05 (d, J = 18.5 Hz, 1H), 1.81–1.67 (m, 3H), 1.35–1.23 (m, 1H), 0.96 (s, 3H), 0.86 (s, 3H). ^{13}C NMR (100 MHz, CDCl$_3$) δ 145.6 (C), 142.6 (CH), 138.8 (CH), 127.8 (CH), 127.3 (CH), 125.4 (C), 112.8 (CH$_2$), 111.0 (CH), 51.1 (CH), 36.4 (CH$_2$), 32.6 (C), 28.3 (CH$_2$), 28.2 (Me), 27.6 (Me), 23.0 (CH$_2$). Lit. for ^{1}H NMR [13]. GC-MS m/z (rel intensity) 216 (M$^+$, 8), 201 ([M − Me]$^+$, 2), 173 (2), 157 (2), 145 (2), 131 (2), 122 (55), 107 (100), 91 (17), 81 (10), 65 (4), 53 (5).

3.5.5. Synthesis of (−)-Dihydropallescensis-2 (5)

According to the general procedure, the alkylation/reduction of (−)-(R)-((2,2-dimethyl-6-methylenecyclohexyl)methylsulfonyl)benzene ($[\alpha]^{20}_D$ = −11.7 (c 3.7, CHCl$_3$); 95% of chemical purity by GC) afforded (−)-dihydropallescensis-2 (5) = (R)-3-(2-(2,2-dimethyl-6-methylenecyclohexyl)ethyl)furan (71% yield) as a colorless oil; $[\alpha]^{20}_D$ = −7.1 (c 2.5, CHCl$_3$); 94% of chemical purity by GC; Lit. [15] for synthetic dextrorotatory isomer: $[\alpha]^{20}_D$ = +4.55 (c 0.1, CHCl$_3$); Lit. [2] for natural 5: $[\alpha]^{20}_D$ = +6.0 (c 0.3, CHCl$_3$). ^{1}H NMR (400 MHz, CDCl$_3$) δ 7.34 (m, 1H), 7.19 (s, 1H), 6.26 (m, 1H), 4.80 (s, 1H), 4.57 (d, J = 1.9 Hz, 1H), 2.45–2.34 (m, 1H), 2.25–1.92 (m, 3H), 1.81–1.40 (m, 6H), 1.30–1.17 (m, 1H), 0.91 (s, 3H), 0.84 (s, 3H). ^{13}C NMR (100 MHz, CDCl$_3$) δ 149.1 (C), 142.6 (CH), 138.7 (CH), 125.5 (C), 111.0 (CH), 109.1 (CH$_2$), 53.5 (CH), 36.2 (CH$_2$),

34.8 (C), 32.4 (CH$_2$), 28.3 (Me), 26.7 (CH$_2$), 26.3 (Me), 23.7 (CH$_2$), 23.3 (CH$_2$). Lit. for ^{1}H and ^{13}C NMR [15]. GC-MS m/z (rel intensity) 218 (M$^+$, 72), 203 ([M − Me]$^+$, 14), 189 (6), 175 (10), 162 (5), 147 (12) 133 (13), 124 (13), 109 (85), 95 (65), 81 (100), 69 (49), 53 (21).

3.6. Synthesis of (−)-Pallescensone (6) Starting from (R)-γ-Cyclogeraniol Acetate

3.6.1. Synthesis of (R)-2-(2,2-Dimethyl-6-methylenecyclohexyl)acetonitrile (+)-16

(−)-γ-Cyclogeraniol acetate = (R)-(2,2-dimethyl-6-methylenecyclohexyl)methyl acetate 380 mg, 1.94 mmol, ([α]$^{20}_D$ = −10.1 (c 3.8, CHCl$_3$); 98% ee; 99% chemical purity) was hydrolysed using NaOH in methanol, at reflux. After work-up, a solution of p-toluenesulphonyl chloride (570 mg, 3 mmol) in CH$_2$Cl$_2$ (3 mL) was added dropwise to a stirred solution of the obtained crude alcohol and DMAP (20 mg, 0.16 mmol) in pyridine (2 mL). After 4 h, the mixture was diluted with ether (60 mL) and washed in turn with a 1 M aqueous HCl solution (50 mL), saturated NaHCO$_3$ solution (30 mL), and brined. The organic phase was dried (Na$_2$SO$_4$) and concentrated *in vacuo*. The residue was dissolved in dry DMSO (20 mL) and treated with NaCN (1 g, 20 mmol) stirring at 80–90 °C until the starting tosylate could no longer be detected by TLC analysis (5 h). The mixture was diluted with ether (80 mL) and was washed in turn with water and brine. The organic phase was dried (Na$_2$SO$_4$) and concentrated *in vacuo*. The residue was then purified by chromatography eluting with hexane/ethyl acetate (95:5–8:2) as eluent to afford pure (R)-2-(2,2-dimethyl-6-methylenecyclohexyl)acetonitrile (+)-16 (270 mg, 85% yield) as a colorless oil; [α]$^{20}_D$ = +12.1 (c 2.2, CH$_2$Cl$_2$); 96% diastereoisomeric purity, 92% of chemical purity by GC. ^{1}H NMR (400 MHz, CDCl$_3$) δ 4.96 (s, 1H), 4.75 (s, 1H), 2.56 (dd, J = 16.7, 4.4 Hz, 1H), 2.41 (dd, J = 16.7, 10.8 Hz, 1H), 2.26–2.15 (m, 2H), 2.14–2.02 (m, 1H), 1.70–1.50 (m, 2H), 1.50–1.31 (m, 2H), 1.00 (s, 3H), 0.81 (s, 3H). ^{13}C NMR (100 MHz, CDCl$_3$) δ 146.2 (C), 119.7 (C), 110.4 (CH$_2$), 50.3 (CH), 37.7 (CH$_2$), 35.0 (C), 33.5 (CH$_2$), 28.6 (Me), 23.5 (Me), 23.2 (CH$_2$), 16.4 (CH$_2$). GC-MS m/z (rel intensity) 163 (M$^+$, 3), 148 (7), 134 (1), 120 (21), 107 (9), 91 (11), 79 (18), 69 (100), 53 (11).

3.6.2. Synthesis of (−)-Pallescensone (6)

DIBAL (0.9 mL of a 25% wt. solution in toluene, 1.34 mmol) was added dropwise under nitrogen to a cooled (−70 °C) solution of nitrile (+)-16 (200 mg, 1.23 mmol) in dry toluene (10 mL). The resulting solution was stirred at this temperature for half an hour and then was allowed to reach rt. The reaction was quenched by the carefully addition of diluted HCl aqueous (50 mL), followed by extraction with diethyl ether (2 × 50 mL). The combined organic phases were dried (Na$_2$SO$_4$) and concentrated under reduced pressure to a final volume of about 4 mL. The resulting solution was added under nitrogen to a cooled (−70 °C) solution of 3-furyllithium (10 mL of a 0.25 M solution in THF), which was previously prepared in situ by addition of *n*BuLi (2.5 M solution in hexane) to a solution of 3-bromofuran in dry THF. The resulting mixture was stirred at this temperature for 20 min, then was quenched by adding saturated aqueous NH$_4$Cl (20 mL) and was extracted with ether (2 × 60 mL). The combined organic phases were dried (Na$_2$SO$_4$) and concentrated under reduced pressure. The residue was dissolved in dry DMSO (2 mL) and was added to a stirred solution of IBX (1 g, 3.5 mmol) in dry DMSO (6 mL). The reaction was warmed at 40 °C for 4 h and then was diluted with diethyl ether (80 mL) and washed with water (2 × 50 mL) and brine. The organic phase was concentrated *in vacuo* and the residue was then purified by chromatography eluting with hexane/ethyl acetate (99:1–9:1) as eluent to afford pure (−)-pallescensone 6 = (R)-2-(2,2-dimethyl-6-methylenecyclohexyl)-1-(furan-3-yl)ethan-1-one (145 mg, 51% yield) as a pale yellow oil that solidified on standing; [α]$^{20}_D$ = −34.4 (c 1.1, CH$_2$Cl$_2$); 97% of chemical purity by GC; Lit. [18] for synthetic 6: [α]$^{20}_D$ = −31.8 (c 0.57, CH$_2$Cl$_2$); Lit. [8] for natural 6: [α]$^{20}_D$ = +36 (c 1, CHCl$_3$). ^{1}H NMR (400 MHz, CDCl$_3$) δ 8.05 (s, 1H), 7.44–7.42 (m, 1H), 6.77–6.75 (s, 1H), 4.71 (s, 1H), 4.44 (s, 1H), 2.91 (dd, J = 15.8, 9.8 Hz, 1H), 2.81 (dd, J = 15.8, 4.2 Hz, 1H), 2.66 (dd, J = 9.8, 4.2 Hz, 1H), 2.28–2.17 (m, 1H), 2.13–2.01 (m, 1H), 1.65–1.34 (m, 4H), 0.98 (s, 3H), 0.84 (s, 3H). ^{13}C NMR (100 MHz, CDCl$_3$) δ 194.5 (C), 148.9 (C), 146.7 (CH), 144.1 (CH), 128.1 (C), 108.8 (CH), 108.5 (CH$_2$), 48.7 (CH), 38.8 (CH$_2$), 38.6 (CH$_2$), 35.0 (C), 34.4 (CH$_2$), 28.9 (Me), 23.8 (Me), 23.6 (CH$_2$). Lit.

for ^{1}H and ^{13}C NMR [14,16,18]. GC-MS m/z (rel intensity) 232 (M$^+$, 5), 217 (5), 199 (2), 189 (3), 176 (3), 163 (3), 137 (3), 122 (22), 107 (24), 95 (100), 81 (12), 69 (13), 55 (6).

Funding: This research received no external funding.

Conflicts of Interest: The author declare no conflict of interest.

References

1. Cimino, G.; De Stefano, S.; Guerriero, A.; Minale, L. Furanosesquiterpenoids in sponges—I: Pallescensin-1, -2 and -3 from *Disidea pallescens*. *Tetrahedron Lett.* **1975**, *16*, 1417–1420. [CrossRef]
2. Guella, G.; Guerriero, A.; Pietra, F. Sesquiterpenoids of the sponge *Dysidea fragilis* of the north-brittany sea. *Helv. Chim. Acta* **1985**, *68*, 39–48. [CrossRef]
3. Gaspar, H.; Santos, S.; Carbone, M.; Rodrigues, A.S.; Rodrigues, A.I.; Uriz, M.J.; Savluchinske Feio, S.M.; Melck, D.; Humanes, M.; Gavagnin, M. Isomeric furanosesquiterpenes from the portuguese marine sponge *Fasciospongia* sp. *J. Nat. Prod.* **2008**, *71*, 2049–2052. [CrossRef] [PubMed]
4. Thompson, J.E.; Walker, R.P.; Wratten, S.J.; Faulkner, D.J. A chemical defense mechanism for the nudibranch *Cadlina luteomarginata*. *Tetrahedron* **1982**, *38*, 1865–1873. [CrossRef]
5. Butler, M.; Capon, R. Beyond polygodial: New drimane sesquiterpenes from a southern Australian marine sponge, *Dysidea* sp. *Aust. J. Chem.* **1993**, *46*, 1255–1267. [CrossRef]
6. Fontana, A.; Muniaín, C.; Cimino, G. First chemical study of patagonian nudibranchs: A new seco-11,12-spongiane, tyrinnal, from the defensive organs of *Tyrinna nobilis*. *J. Nat. Prod.* **1998**, *61*, 1027–1029. [CrossRef] [PubMed]
7. Huang, X.-C.; Li, J.; Li, Z.-Y.; Shi, L.; Guo, Y.-W. Sesquiterpenes from the Hainan sponge *Dysidea septosa*. *J. Nat. Prod.* **2008**, *71*, 1399–1403. [CrossRef]
8. Cambie, R.C.; Craw, P.A.; Bergquist, P.R.; Karuso, P. Chemistry of sponges, II. Pallescensone, a furanosesquiterpenoid from *Dictyodendrilla cavernosa*. *J. Nat. Prod.* **1987**, *50*, 948–949. [CrossRef]
9. Mudianta, I.W.; Challinor, V.L.; Winters, A.E.; Cheney, K.L.; De Voss, J.J.; Garson, M.J. Synthesis and determination of the absolute configuration of (−)-(5R,6Z)-dendrolasin-5-acetate from the nudibranch *Hypselodoris jacksoni*. *Beilstein J. Org. Chem.* **2013**, *9*, 2925–2933. [CrossRef] [PubMed]
10. Winters, A.E.; White, A.M.; Dewi, A.S.; Mudianta, I.W.; Wilson, N.G.; Forster, L.C.; Garson, M.J.; Cheney, K.L. Distribution of defensive metabolites in nudibranch molluscs. *J. Chem. Ecol.* **2018**, *44*, 384–396. [CrossRef]
11. Matsumoto, T.; Usui, S. Furanosesquiterpenoids absolute configuration of pallescensin-1, -2, and -A. *Chem. Lett.* **1978**, *7*, 105–108. [CrossRef]
12. Tius, M.A.; Takaki, K.S. Biomimetic synthesis of (+/−)-pallescensin 1. *J. Org. Chem.* **1982**, *47*, 3166–3168. [CrossRef]
13. Matsumoto, T.; Usui, S. Furanosesquiterpenoids: Total synthesis of pallescensins 2, F, and G. *Bull. Chem. Soc. Jpn.* **1983**, *56*, 491–493. [CrossRef]
14. Baker, R.; Cottrell, I.F.; Ravenscroft, P.D.; Swain, C.J. Stereoselective synthesis of (+/−)-ancistrofuran and its stereoisomers. *J. Chem. Soc. Perkin Trans. 1* **1985**, 2463–2468. [CrossRef]
15. Kurth, M.J.; Soares, C.J. Asymmetric aza-Claisen rearrangement: Synthesis of (+)-dihydropallescensin-2 [(+)-penlanpallescensin]. *Tetrahedron Lett.* **1987**, *28*, 1031–1034. [CrossRef]
16. Eicher, T.; Massonne, K.; Herrmann, M. Synthese von bryophyten-inhaltsstoffen 4. Synthesen des ricciocarpins A. *Synthesis* **1991**, 1173–1176. [CrossRef]
17. Cruz Almanza, R.; Hinojosa Reyes, A. A simple synthesis of γ-cyclohomocitral. *Synthetic Commun.* **1993**, *23*, 867–874. [CrossRef]
18. Vidari, G.; Lanfranchi, G.; Masciaga, F.; Moriggi, J.-D. Enantioselective synthesis of γ-cyclohomocitral, pallescensone, and ancistrodial. *Tetrahedron Asymmetry* **1996**, *7*, 3009–3020. [CrossRef]
19. Palombo, E.; Audran, G.; Monti, H. First enantioselective synthesis and determination of the absolute configuration of natural (+)-dehydro-β-monocyclonerolidol. *Tetrahedron Lett.* **2003**, *44*, 6463–6464. [CrossRef]
20. Serra, S. A practical, enantiospecific synthesis of (S)-trans-γ-monocyclofarnesol. *Nat. Prod. Commun.* **2012**, *7*, 1569–1572. [CrossRef]

21. Serra, S.; Cominetti, A.A.; Lissoni, V. A general synthetic approach to hydroquinone meroterpenoids: Stereoselective synthesis of (+)-(S)-metachromin V and alliodorol. *Nat. Prod. Commun.* **2014**, *9*, 303–308. [CrossRef]
22. Serra, S.; Cominetti, A.A.; Lissoni, V. Use of (S)-*trans*-γ-monocyclofarnesol as a useful chiral building block for the stereoselective synthesis of diterpenic natural products. *Nat. Prod. Commun.* **2014**, *9*, 329–335. [CrossRef]
23. Serra, S.; Lissoni, V. First enantioselective synthesis of marine diterpene ambliol-A. *Eur. J. Org. Chem.* **2015**, 2226–2234. [CrossRef]
24. Serra, S.; Gatti, F.G.; Fuganti, C. Lipase-mediated resolution of the hydroxy-cyclogeraniol isomers: Application to the synthesis of the enantiomers of karahana lactone, karahana ether, crocusatin C and γ-cyclogeraniol. *Tetrahedron Asymmetry* **2009**, *20*, 1319–1329. [CrossRef]
25. Bovolenta, M.; Castronovo, F.; Vadalà, A.; Zanoni, G.; Vidari, G. A simple and efficient highly enantioselective synthesis of α-ionone and α-damascone. *J. Org. Chem.* **2004**, *69*, 8959–8962. [CrossRef]
26. Luparia, M.; Boschetti, P.; Piccinini, F.; Porta, A.; Zanoni, G.; Vidari, G. Enantioselective synthesis and olfactory evaluation of 13-alkyl-substituted α-ionones. *Chem. Biodivers.* **2008**, *5*, 1045–1057. [CrossRef]
27. Serra, S. Preparation and use of enantioenriched 2-aryl-propylsulfonylbenzene derivatives as valuable building blocks for the enantioselective synthesis of bisabolane sesquiterpenes. *Tetrahedron Asymmetry* **2014**, *25*, 1561–1572. [CrossRef]
28. Nakagawa, I.; Aki, K.; Hata, T. Synthesis of 5'-alkylthio-5'-deoxynucleosides from nucleosides in a one-pot reaction. *J. Chem. Soc. Perkin Trans. 1* **1983**, 1315–1318. [CrossRef]
29. Surburg, H.; Panten, J. *Common Fragrance and Flavor Materials: Preparation, Properties and Uses*, 6th ed.; Wiley-VCH Verlag GmbH & Co. KGaA: Weinheim, Germany, 2016; ISBN 9783527331604.
30. Serra, S. Recent advances in the synthesis of carotenoid-derived flavours and fragrances. *Molecules* **2015**, *20*, 12817–12840. [CrossRef]
31. Serra, S.; Fuganti, C.; Brenna, E. Synthesis, olfactory evaluation, and determination of the absolute configuration of the 3,4-didehydroionone stereoisomers. *Helv. Chim. Acta* **2006**, *89*, 1110–1122. [CrossRef]
32. Smith, P.M.; Thomas, E.J. Approaches to a synthesis of galbonolide B. *J. Chem. Soc. Perkin Trans. 1* **1998**, 3541–3556. [CrossRef]
33. Frigerio, M.; Santagostino, M. A mild oxidizing reagent for alcohols and 1,2-diols: O-iodoxybenzoic acid (IBX) in DMSO. *Tetrahedron Lett.* **1994**, *35*, 8019–8022. [CrossRef]
34. Bourdron, J.; Commeiras, L.; Audran, G.; Vanthuyne, N.; Hubaud, J.C.; Parrain, J.-L. First total synthesis and assignment of the stereochemistry of crispatenine. *J. Org. Chem.* **2007**, *72*, 3770–3775. [CrossRef]
35. Vidari, G.; Lanfranchi, G.; Sartori, P.; Serra, S. Saponaceolides: Differential cytotoxicity and enantioselective synthesis of the right-hand lactone moiety. *Tetrahedron Asymmetry* **1995**, *6*, 2977–2990. [CrossRef]
36. Tanis, S.P. A simple synthesis of 3-substituted furans. The preparations of dendrolasin, perillene and congeners. *Tetrahedron Lett.* **1982**, *23*, 3115–3118. [CrossRef]
37. Meyers, A.I.; Collington, E.W. Facile and specific conversion of allylic alcohols to allylic chlorides without rearrangement. *J. Org. Chem.* **1971**, *36*, 3044–3045. [CrossRef]
38. Fujii, M.; Morimoto, Y.; Ono, M.; Akita, H. Preparation of (S)-γ-cyclogeraniol by lipase-catalyzed transesterification and synthesis of (+)-trixagol and (+)-luffarin-P. *J. Mol. Catal. B Enzym.* **2016**, *123*, 160–166. [CrossRef]
39. Tsangarakis, C.; Stratakis, M. Biomimetic cyclization of small terpenoids promoted by zeolite NaY: Tandem formation of α-ambrinol from geranyl acetone. *Adv. Synth. Catal.* **2005**, *347*, 1280–1284. [CrossRef]
40. Proszenyák, Á.; Charnock, C.; Hedner, E.; Larsson, R.; Bohlin, L.; Gundersen, L.-L. Synthesis, antimicrobial and antineoplastic activities for agelasine and agelasimine analogs with a β-cyclocitral derived substituent. *Arch. Pharm.* **2007**, *340*, 625–634. [CrossRef]
41. Trost, B.M.; Shen, H.C.; Surivet, J.-P. Biomimetic enantioselective total synthesis of (−)-siccanin via the Pd-catalyzed asymmetric allylic alkylation (AAA) and sequential radical cyclizations. *J. Am. Chem. Soc.* **2004**, *126*, 12565–12579. [CrossRef]

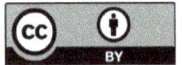

© 2019 by the author. Licensee MDPI, Basel, Switzerland. This article is an open access article distributed under the terms and conditions of the Creative Commons Attribution (CC BY) license (http://creativecommons.org/licenses/by/4.0/).

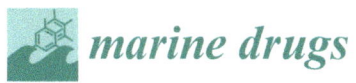

Article

Syntheses of Benzo[*d*]Thiazol-2(3*H*)-One Derivatives and Their Antidepressant and Anticonvulsant Effects

Qinghao Jin [1], Zhiyang Fu [2], Liping Guan [2,*] and Haiying Jiang [3,*]

1. Donghai Science and Technology College, Zhejiang Ocean University, Zhoushan 316000, China
2. Food and Pharmacy College, Zhejiang Ocean University, Zhoushan 316022, China
3. College of Medicine, Jiaxing University, Jiaxing 314001, China
* Correspondence: glp730@163.com (L.G.); jiangyang7689@aliyun.com (H.J.); Tel.: +86-580-2555280 (L.G.); +86-573-83643808 (H.J.)

Received: 4 July 2019; Accepted: 19 July 2019; Published: 23 July 2019

Abstract: Thirty-four new benzo[*d*]thiazol derivatives **2a–2i**, **3a–3r**, and **4a–4g** were synthesized and investigated for their potential antidepressant and anticonvulsant effects. In a forced swimming test, **2c** and **2d** showed the highest antidepressant and anticonvulsant effects. **2c** and **2d** displayed a higher percentage decrease in immobility duration (89.96% and 89.62%, respectively) than that of fluoxetine (83.62%). In the maximal electroshock seizure test, **3n** and **3q** showed the highest anticonvulsant effect, with ED_{50} values of 46.1 and 64.3 mg kg^{-1}, and protective indices of 6.34 and 4.11, respectively, which were similar to those of phenobarbital or valproate. We also found that the mechanism for the antidepressant activity of **2c** and **2d** may be via increasing the concentrations of serotonin and norepinephrine.

Keywords: benzo[*d*]thiazol; synthesis; antarctic-derived fungus; antidepressant; anticonvulsant

1. Introduction

During selective evolution, microorganisms in the polar region are distinct from other microorganisms with respect to genomic composition and have unique molecular–biological mechanisms, including metabolic regulation. Tan et al. reported very rich microbial resources in the Arctic and Antarctic [1]. In addition to extremely high species diversity [2], the structures of secondary metabolites of polar microbes also show diversity. Therefore, the Arctic and Antarctic regions are considered to be valuable natural products pools.

In an investigation of the secondary metabolites of the Antarctic-derived fungus *Penicillium sp.* 44.42 °W, 60.54 °S, 239 m underwater, water temperature of −1.16 °C), Jiao et al. reported the isolation of nine compounds from the fermentation broth of *Penicillium sp.* [3], including benzo[*d*]thiazol-2(3*H*)-one (Figure 1). Benzothiazoles are heterocyclic aromatic hydrocarbons containing phenyl and thiazole rings, as well as sulfur and nitrogen atoms in their structures. Benzothiazole derivatives display a wide spectrum of pharmacologic effects, including anti-inflammatory [4], antibacterial [5], antiviral [6], antioxidant [7], and immunomodulatory properties [8]. In addition to the central nervous system (CNS)-related pharmacologic effects, benzothiazole compounds have been reported to display selective inhibitory effects against monoamine oxidase [9–12], as well as anti-Alzheimer's disease [13] and convulsions [14]. The antidepressant effect of a series of benzothiazole derivatives has been demonstrated through animal models such as the tail suspension test (TST) and forced swimming test (FST) [15,16].

Several reports have described the antidepressant and anticonvulsant activities of benzothiazole derivatives [15,16]. For this reason, we synthesized thirty-four new benzo[*d*]thiazole derivatives **2a–2i**, **3a–3r** and **4a–4g** (Schemes 1 and 2) and investigated their potential antidepressant activity using the FST and their potential anticonvulsant effect using the maximal electroshock seizure (MES) test as well as their toxicity.

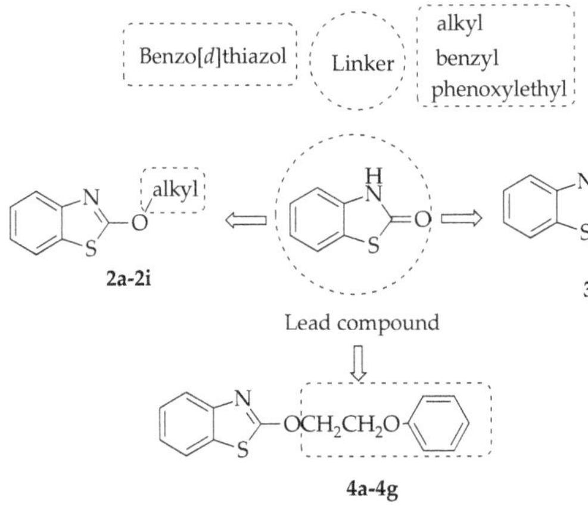

Figure 1. Structures of the lead compounds and derivatives **2a–2i**, **3a–3r**, and **4a–4g**.

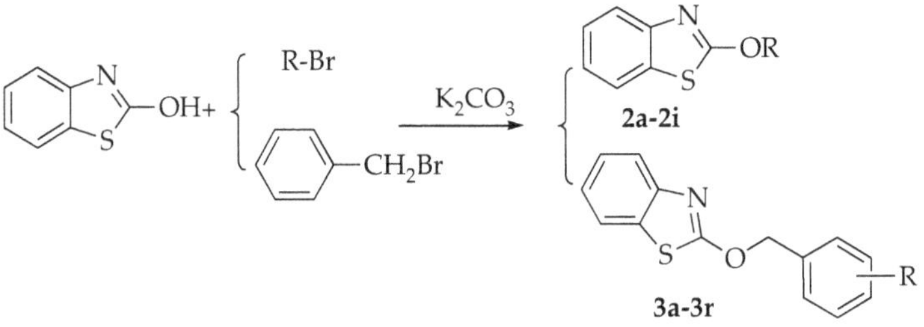

R:

2a = -CH$_2$CH$_3$	**2b** = -(CH$_2$)$_2$CH$_3$	**2c** = -(CH$_2$)$_3$CH$_3$	**2d** = -(CH$_2$)$_4$CH$_3$	**2e** = -(CH$_2$)$_5$CH$_3$
2f = -(CH$_2$)$_6$CH$_3$	**2g** = -(CH$_2$)$_7$CH$_3$	**2h** = -(CH$_2$)$_8$CH$_3$	**2i** = -(CH$_2$)$_9$CH$_3$	
3a = -H	**3b** = 2-F	**3c** = 3-F	**3d** = 4-F	**3e** = 2-Cl
3f = 3-Cl	**3g** = 4-Cl	**3h** = 2-Br	**3i** = 3-Br	**3j** = 4-Br
3k = 4-NO$_2$	**3l** = 4-CN	**3m** = 2-CF$_3$	**3n** = 4-CF$_3$	**3o** = 4-CH$_3$
3p = 4-OCH$_3$	**3q** = 3,5-(CH$_3$)$_2$	**3r** = 3,5-(OCH$_3$)$_2$		

Scheme 1. Synthesis of **2a–2i** and **3a–3r**.

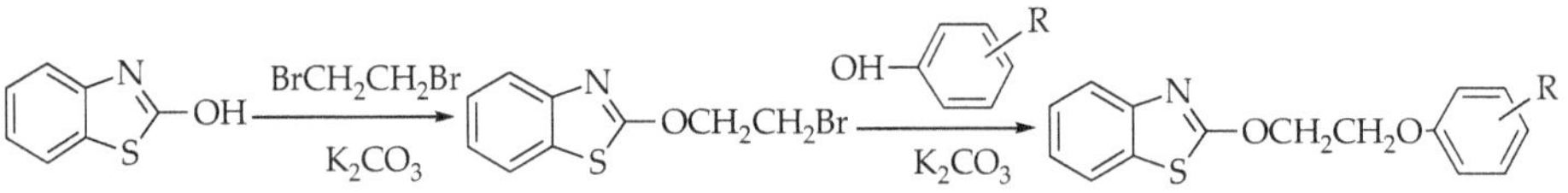

R:

4a = -H   **4b** = 4-F   **4c** = 4-Cl   **4d** = 4-Br   **4e** = 2,4-2F   **4f** = 2,4-2Cl   **4g** = 2,4-2Br

Scheme 2. The synthetic route of derivatives **4a–4g**.

2. Results

2.1. Synthesis

Target compounds **2a–2i**, **3a–3r**, and **4a–4g** were prepared as shown in Schemes 1 and 2. Commercially available benzo[*d*]thiazol-2-ol was the starting material; the derivatives **2a–2i** and **3a–3r** were obtained through the introduction of an alkyl group or benzyl group by a one-step nucleophilic substitution reaction. Compounds **4a–4g** were obtained through a two-step reaction. The intermediate 2-(2-bromoethoxy)benzo[*d*]thiazole was synthesized and underwent a nucleophilic substitution reaction with 1,2-dibromoethane, then the 2-(2-bromoethoxy) benzo[*d*] thiazole formed was reacted with substituted phenols. The structures of **2a–2i**, **3a–3r**, and **4a–4g** were determined by infrared spectrophotometry, ^{1}H and ^{13}C NMR spectroscopy, as well as mass spectrometry.

2.2. Antidepressant Activity of **2a–2i**, **3a–3r**, and **4a–4g** in the FST

The antidepressant activity of fluoxetine, **2a–2i**, **3a–3r**, and **4a–4g**, as indicated by the immobility time in the FST, is displayed in Table 1. Most of the compounds, except for **3h**, **3k**, **3l**, **3r**, **4c**, and **4e**, induced a significant decrease in the immobility time at 30 mg kg^{-1} and showed a marked antidepressant effect (Table 1). In particular, **2b–2d**, **2f**, and **3q** possessed the highest antidepressant effect and induced a significant decrease in the immobility time compared with that of the control group ($p < 0.001$).

Table 1. Antidepressant effect of **2a–2i**, **3a–3r**, and **4a–4g**.

Compounds	Antidepressant Effect	
	Duration of Immobility (s)	TID ^{a} (%)
2a	122.5 ± 9.2 *	31.64
2b	59.3 ± 8.8 ***	66.91
2c	18.0 ± 2.4 ***	89.96
2d	18.6 ± 6.8 ***	89.62
2e	104.2 + 9.7 *	46.32
2f	26.7 ± 7.4 ***	85.10
2g	67.7 ± 10.7 **	62.22
2h	76.0 ± 13.2 **	57.59
2i	93.0 ± 9.0 **	48.10
3a	81.2 ± 9.4 **	54.69
3b	84.8 ± 5.6 **	52.68
3c	61.5 ± 3.3 **	65.68
3d	75.2 ± 8.2 **	58.04
3e	132.2 ± 8.5 *	26.23
3f	68.2 ± 11.5 **	61.94
3g	80.3 ± 11.9 **	55.19
3h	141.3 ± 8.5	21.15
3i	66.0 ± 8.1 **	63.17
3j	99.3 ± 8.7 **	44.59
3k	153.8 ± 11.0	14.17
3l	172.5 ± 5.4	3.74
3m	125.8 ± 13.6 *	29.80
3n	124.5 ± 14.3 *	30.52
3o	130.6 ± 5.4 *	27.12
3p	71.2 ± 7.0 **	60.27
3q	26.3 ± 10.3 ***	85.32
3r	143.2 ± 11.4	20.09
4a	67.5 ± 7.3 **	62.33
4b	130.5 ± 7.9 *	37.56
4c	141.7 ± 9.1	32.20
4d	116.2 ± 7.0 *	44.40
4e	151.7 ± 14.1	27.42
4f	129.5 ± 5.4 *	38.04
4g	124.2 ± 8.1 *	40.57
control	194.1 ± 11.1	-
fluoxetine	31.8 ± 7.7 ***	83.62

^{a} TID: percentage decrease in immobility duration. Significant differences versus control values. * $p < 0.05$, ** $p < 0.01$, *** $p < 0.001$.

To better understand the antidepressant effect of **2a–2i**, **3a–3r**, and **4a–4g**, the percentage reduction in the time of immobility (% TID) was calculated using the formula

$$\% \text{ TID} = [(X - Y)/X] \times 100$$

where X is the immobility time (s) for the control group and Y is the immobility time (s) for the test group. **2c**, **2d**, **2f**, and **3q** reduced the immobility time and showed higher TID values than the other tested compounds (Table 1). The % TID values for **2f** (85.10%) and **3q** (85.32%) were similar to that of fluoxetine at a concentration of 30 mg kg^{-1} in the FST. However, **2c** and **2d** showed higher % TID values (89.96% and 89.62%, respectively) than that of fluoxetine (83.62%), suggesting that these compounds may have superior antidepressant effects compared with that of fluoxetine (duration of immobility (s): **2c** = 18.0 ± 2.4; **2d** = 18.6 ± 6.8; fluoxetine = 31.8 ± 7.7).

2.3. Anticonvulsant Activity of **2a–2i**, **3a–3r**, and **4a–4g** in the MSE Test

The phase-I test study comprised two parts: MES and toxicity. The toxicity was measured by the rotorod toxicity experiment. Compounds **2a–2i**, **3a–3r**, and **4a–4g** were assessed for their anticonvulsant activity. The phase-I test was a qualitative analysis, with three doses of the test compounds administered (30, 100, and 300 mg kg^{-1}). A protective effect was observed in mice through intraperitoneal administration of **2a–2i**, **3a–3r**, and **4a–4g** in the MES test (Table 2). Except for **2f–2i**, **3h**, **3j**, **3k**, **4a** and **4f**, other derivatives displayed an anticonvulsant effect. Compounds **2a**, **3a**, **3l**, **3n–3q**, and **4b** displayed the highest anticonvulsant effect at 30 mg kg^{-1} in an MES test. Compounds **2c–2e**, **3b**, **3e–3g**, **3i**, **3m**, **3r**, **4d**, **4e** and **4g** were active at 100 mg kg^{-1}. While **2b**, **3c**, **3d**, and **4c** showed the anticonvulsant activity at 300 mg kg^{-1}. The rotorod toxicity experiment indicated that **2a–2i**, **3a–3r**, and **4a–4g** did not display toxicity at the test doses. In addition, all compounds were excreted or metabolized in ~4 h.

Table 2. Anticonvulsant activity of **2a–2i**, **3a–3r**, and **4a–4g** in a phase-I study.

Compounds	Dosage (mg·kg^{-1})	MES [a]		Rotorod [b]	
		0.5 h	4 h	0.5 h	4 h
2a	30	1/3	0/3	0/3	0/3
2b	300	1/3	0/3	0/3	0/3
2c	100	1/3	0/3	0/3	0/3
2d	100	1/3	0/3	0/3	0/3
2e	100	1/3	0/3	0/3	0/3
2f	300	0/3	0/3	0/3	0/3
2g	300	0/3	0/3	0/3	0/3
2h	300	0/3	0/3	0/3	0/3
2i	300	0/3	0/3	0/3	0/3
3a	30	1/3	0/3	0/3	0/3
3b	100	3/3	0/3	0/3	0/3
3c	300	1/3	0/3	0/3	0/3
3d	300	1/3	0/3	0/3	0/3
3e	100	3/3	0/3	0/3	0/3
3f	100	1/3	0/3	0/3	0/3
3g	100	1/3	0/3	0/3	0/3
3h	300	0/3	0/3	0/3	0/3
3i	100	1/3	0/3	0/3	0/3
3j	300	0/3	0/3	0/3	0/3
3k	300	0/3	0/3	0/3	0/3
3l	30	2/3	0/3	0/3	0/3
3m	100	2/3	0/3	0/3	0/3
3n	30	3/3	0/3	0/3	0/3
3o	30	1/3	0/3	0/3	0/3

Table 2. Cont.

Compounds	Dosage (mg·kg^{-1})	MES [a]		Rotorod [b]	
		0.5 h	4 h	0.5 h	4 h
3p	30	2/3	0/3	0/3	0/3
3q	30	3/3	0/3	0/3	0/3
3r	100	2/3	0/3	0/3	0/3
4a	300	0/3	0/3	0/3	0/3
4b	30	1/3	0/3	0/3	0/3
4c	300	1/3	0/3	0/3	0/3
4d	100	1/3	0/3	0/3	0/3
4e	100	1/3	0/3	0/3	0/3
4f	300	0/3	0/3	0/3	0/3
4g	100	1/3	0/3	0/3	0/3
Valproate	100	3/3	0/3	0/3	0/3

[a] MES test (numbers of mice defended/numbers of mice detected); [b] Toxicity: rotorod test (numbers of mice showing toxicity/numbers of mice detected).

Next, the effect of **2a, 3a, 3b, 3e, 3l, 3n–3q,** and **4b** were evaluated quantitatively for their anticonvulsant activity median effective dose (ED_{50}) and neurotoxicity median toxicity dose (TD_{50}) (Table 3) in a phase-II experiment. **3n** and **3q** showed the greatest effect, with ED_{50} values of 46.1 and 64.3 mg kg^{-1}, and protective index (PI) of 6.34 and 4.11, respectively, which were higher than those of phenobarbital and valproate.

Table 3. Anticonvulsant activity of **2a, 3a, 3b, 3e, 3l, 3n–3q** and **4b** in a phase-II study.

Compounds	ED_{50} [a] (mg/kg)	TD_{50} [b] (mg/kg)	PI (TD_{50}/ED_{50})
2a	90.8	>200	3.20
3a	105.9	>200	2.89
3b	>300	>200	1.89
3e	147.2	>200	2.36
3l	>300	>200	2.04
3n	46.1	>200	6.34
3o	84.3	>200	3.37
3p	>300	>200	1.13
3q	64.3	>200	4.11
4b	74.5	>200	3.69
Phenobarbital [c]	21.8	69.0	3.2
Valproate	247	>200	1.6

[a] ED_{50}: Median effective dose affording anticonvulsant defense for 50% animals; [b] TD_{50}: Median toxic dose eliciting minimal neurological toxicity for 50% animals; [c] data from Krall et al. 1978 [17].

2.4. Effects of 2c and 2d on Monoamine Levels

Monoamine concentrations in the mouse brain are shown in Table 4. The concentration of **2c, 2d,** and fluoxetine was 30 mg kg^{-1}. The neurotransmitter concentration was calculated as ng g per brain region wet weight. **2c** and **2d** did not alter the dopamine concentration, but increased the concentrations of serotonin and norepinephrine in mouse brain significantly in the FST, and these effects were similar to those of the positive control fluoxetine.

Table 4. Effect of 2c and 2d on monoamine concentrations in mouse brain.

Groups	Serotonin	Norepinephrine	Dopamine
Normal Vehicle	325.1 ± 28.3	298.4 ± 22.4	357.4 ± 29.8
Stress Vehicle	202.4 ± 38.4 [c]	207.3 ± 25.7 [c]	218.7 ± 20.0
2c	334.5 ± 31.9 [b,c]	309.5 ± 20.6 [a,c]	201.5 ± 19.2
2d	329.0 ± 27.8 [b,c]	310.7 ± 24.9 [a,c]	206.0 ± 18.7
Fluoxetine	340.3 ± 32.5 [b,c]	321.8 ± 29.1 [a,c]	202.6 ± 17.8

Values are given as mean ± SEM (n = 8). [a] $P < 0.05$, [b] $P < 0.01$ vs. stress vehicle; [c] $P < 0.05$ vs. normal vehicle.

3. Discussion

The FST is a model of depression. It mimics the condition of hopelessness and has a good predictive validity in mice. In this model, mice are limited in movement and cannot abscond, which results in motionlessness [18]. The immobility displayed in this model has been assumed to correspond to a behavioral response to hopelessness which, in turn, might correspond to a depressive disorder in humans [19].

Nine benzo[d]thiazole derivatives (2a–2i) containing an alkyl group with 2–10 carbons displayed antidepressant activity. Among them, 2c (n-butyl group) and 2d (n-pentyl group) exhibited the highest antidepressant activity. Although alkyl groups are not a functional group, they can play an important role in the binding interactions of a drug with its target. Alkyl chains are hydrophobic and can interact with the hydrophobic region of a receptor through Van der Waals interaction in the binding site. Varying the size of the group allows exploration of the hydrophobic region [20].

Among 18 benzyloxybenzo[d]thiazole derivatives 3a–3r, most of the compounds, except for 3h, 3k, 3l and 3r, induced a significant decrease in the immobility time at 30 mg kg^{-1} and showed marked antidepressant effect. Interestingly, 3q, which has two methyl substituents on the phenyl ring, displayed the highest antidepressant effect.

However, the reduction conditions needed would be quite harsh and might not be feasible without causing drug degradation [20]. The position of halogen atoms affects antidepressant activity on the phenyl ring.

Comparing the F-substituted compounds 3b, 3c and 3d at different positions on the phenyl ring, the sequence of effect was 3-F > 4-F > 2-F, and the sequence of effect for Cl-substituted compounds 3e, 3f, and 3g was 3-Cl > 4-Cl > 2-Cl. The sequence of effect for different Br-substituted compounds 3h, 3i, and 3j was 3-Br > 4-Br > 2-Br. In addition, among the compounds with electron-withdrawing groups (i.e., 3k, 3l, 3m, and 3n), only 3m and 3n (with a –CF$_3$ group) exhibited the antidepressant activities. For compounds with electron-donating groups, 3o–3r, the sequence of activity was 3,5-(CH$_3$)$_2$ > 4-OCH$_3$ > 4-CH$_3$ > 3,5-(OCH$_3$)$_2$. Of seven phenoxyethoxybenzo[d]thiazole compounds 4a–4g, except for 4c and 4e, the remaining five compounds 4a, 4b, 4d, 4f, and 4g induced a significant decrease in the immobility time at 30 mg kg^{-1} and exhibited antidepressant effects. Among them, 4a displayed the highest antidepressant activity.

Nervous stress can cause impressionable individuals to develop epilepsy, and depressive illness is a general comorbidity related to epilepsy [21]. Nevertheless, understanding the heterogeneity of depression and epilepsy is difficult [22] Antiepileptic drugs might ameliorate the symptoms of depression, as indicated in clinical studies. Curing depression will have positive effects on epilepsy and quality of life.

The anticonvulsant effects of 2a–2i, 3a–3r, and 4a–4g were evaluated using the MES test. The most efficacious compounds, 3n and 3q, exhibited ED$_{50}$ values of 46.1 and 64.3 mg kg^{-1} and had PI values of 6.34 and 4.11, respectively, which were greater than those of phenobarbital or valproate. Therefore, 3n and 3q might be useful candidates as antidepressant drugs for curing depression in patients with epilepsy.

A disruption in the release of neurotransmitters in the CNS, such as serotonin, norepinephrine, and dopamine, has been proposed to be a characteristic of depression. The metabolic imbalance of monoamine transmitters is considered to be a fundamental neurochemical feature in patients with depression. Hence, patients could be treated by increasing monoamine concentrations in the CNS [23]. We found that **2c** and **2d** increased concentrations of serotonin and norepinephrine markedly without altering dopamine concentrations in mouse brains, in a similar manner to that seen with the positive control fluoxetine in the FST. A cure for patients with major depression is deemed to include an increase in levels of serotonin or norepinephrine [24,25]. Thus, the antidepressant activities of **2c** and **2d** could be reflected by measuring levels of serotonin and norepinephrine in the CNS.

4. Method and Material

4.1. Reagents and Instruments

Positive drug: fluoxetine (purity > 99%) was purchased from Sigma. Melting points were measured by the melting point apparatus (WRS-1B, Shanghai, China). Infrared spectra (IR in KBr) were recorded using FT-IR1730 (Bruker, Switzerland). ^{1}H and ^{13}C NMR spectra were recorded on an AV-300 (Bruker, Switzerland), and the chemical shift values are in ppm relative to the TMS or solvent peaks. Mass spectra were recorded on MALDI-TOF/TOF mass spectrometer (Bruker Daltonik, Bremen, Germany). Main reagents were purchased from Aldrich Chemical Corporation (Shanghai, China).

*4.2. Synthesis of Benzo[d]thiazol and Benzyloxybenzo[d]thiazole Derivatives **2a–2i**, **3a–3r***

A solution of benzo[*d*]thiazol-2-ol (3.0 mmol), anhydrous K$_2$CO$_3$ (3.0 mmol) and 5 mL DMF was stirred in a round-bottomed flask for 1 h at 60 °C, then, 1.2 mmol of alkyl bromide or substituted brominated benzyl compound was added slowly to the reaction solution. The reaction solution was refluxed for 5 h, the reaction was monitored by TLC. DMF was evaporated under reduced pressure, the residue was washed with water, filtered, dried and the crude product was crystallized from MeOH. The yield, melting point, and spectral data of each compound are given below.

*4.3. Synthesis of Ethoxylbenzo[d]thiazole Derivatives **4a–4g***

A mixture of benzo[*d*]thiazol-2-ol (3.0 mmol, 0.5 g), 1,2-dibromoethane (3.0 mmol, 0.6 g) and anhydrous K$_2$CO$_3$ (3.0 mmol, 0.4 g) was refluxed in DMF for 1 h, after the completion of the reaction (as monitored by TLC), DMF was evaporated and the precipitated product was washed with deionized water, dried. Then, 2-(2-bromoethoxy)benzo[*d*]thiazole (3.0 mmol, 0.8 g), 10 mL of a mixture of NaOH and substituted phenol was refluxed in EtOH for 2–5 h. After the completion of the reaction (as monitored by TLC), the solution was filtered and washed with 10% HCl and water. The crude product was recrystallized from MeOH. The melting points, yields, and spectral data of **4a–4g** are given below.

4.4. Experimental Animal and Compounds Treatment

Male ICR mice (20 ± 2 g) were purchased from the laboratory of animal study of Zhejiang Academy of medical sciences. Before the experiment started, mice were tamed for 1 week. During and before the test, mice were kept at 23 ± 2 °C for 12 h, at day and night circle, and tap water and standard food granules were provided. The procedures were adopted according to the National Institute of Health Guide for the Care and Use of Laboratory Animals and approved by the Ethics Committee of our Institution in this study. All the test compounds were dissolved in PEG-400 (polyethylene glycol-400). Other drugs were dissolved in 0.9% NaCl (isotonic saline solution). Fluoxetine, phenobarbital, and valproate were used as positive controls and the vehicle as the negative control. All the test compounds and other drugs were administered intraperitoneally for 30 min in the FST, the volume of the drug solution and vehicle was 0.1 mL/20 g of mice.

4.5. In the FST

Male ICR mice were randomized into groups. On the day of the experiment, mice were placed one at a time into a Perspex barrel (elevation 20 cm, 10 cm diameter) including 10 cm water about

22 °C. Mice were arranged into different groups ($n = 8$). Next, a mouse was placed independently into the perspex barrel and kept in the water for six minutes. After two minutes of fierce struggle, the mice were immobile. The duration of immobility was recorded during the last four min of the six min test. The immobility course was treated as the time that the mice floating on the water without struggle and maintained only the movements necessary to provide their head above the water [26,27].

4.6. In the MES Experiment

Convulsions were initiated in mice with a 60 Hz alternating current for 50 mA. The electric current was implemented via corneal electrodes for 0.3 s. Protection against the spread of the maximal electroshock seizure-induced seizures was defined as the abolition of the hind leg and tonic maximal extension component of the seizure. At 30 min after the administration of the compounds, the activity was evaluated in the maximal electroshock seizure test [28].

4.7. Experiment of Neurotoxicity

The neurotoxicity experiment of the compounds and drugs was evaluated through the rotorod experiment in mice. The mice were trained to stay on an accelerating rotorod of diameter 3.2 cm that rotated at 10 rpm. Trained animals were given an intraperitoneal injection of the test compounds. Neurotoxicity was indicated by the inability of the animal to maintain equilibrium on the rod for at least 1 min in each of the trials. The MES and rotorod tests were carried out according to the standard procedure described in the Antiepileptic Drug Development Program (ADD) of the National Institutes of Health (USA) [29].

4.8. HPLC conditions and Sample Preparation

The dosage of 30 mg kg^{-1} of **2b**, **2c** and fluoxetine was used for testing the action on MOA neurochemical levels in rat brain. Mice were randomly divided into five groups ($n = 10$). **2b**, **2c** and fluoxetine, normal vehicle, stress vehicle oral gavage once a day for seven days. After the end of the test, the mouse was immediately sacrificed by cervical dislocation, then the brain tissue was immediately removed, and quickly frozen and at −80 °C until used for neurochemical analysis. The brain tissues were sonicated in 0.1 M NaH$_2$PO$_4$ aqueous solution including 0.85 mM OSA, 0.5 mM Na$_2$·EDTA (ethylenediamine tetraacetic acid disodium), centrifuged at 13,000× g at 4 °C for 15 minutes. Then serotonin, norepinephrine and dopamine were analyzed by High-Performance Liquid chromatography coupled with an electron capture detector. The mobile phase was made up of 0.1 mol L^{-1} anhydrous sodium dihydrogen phosphate containing 0.5 mM EDTA and 0.85 mM osanetant (OSA) and 11% MeOH and regulated to pH 3.4 using phosphate acid buffer solution and filtered by the pore size ultrafiltration membrane of 0.45 µM. The external standard curves were used to quantify the amounts of serotonin, noradrenaline, and dopamine in each sample calculated by area under the curve. The injection volume dose was 20 µL. The detection limit of the analysis was 20 pg·g^{-1} sample.

4.9. Statistic Analysis

All analyses were performed using the GraphPad Prism program (GraphPad software, Inc., San Diego, CA, USA). The statistical analysis of the behavioral tests was performed by analysis of variance (ANOVA), which was followed by Tukey's post hoc comparison test. All experimental results are presented as mean (s) ± standard error of the mean (SEM), with a p-value smaller than 0.05 considered statistically significant.

5. Conclusions

Thirty-four previously unreported benzo[*d*]thiazol derivatives **2a–2i**, **3a–3r**, and **4a–4g** were prepared and assessed for their potential antidepressant and anticonvulsant effects. **2c** and **2d** decreased the immobility time markedly and displayed the highest antidepressant effects in the FST, and also showed anticonvulsant activity. **2c** and **2d** did not change the dopamine concentration but increased the concentrations of serotonin and norepinephrine significantly in the mouse brain in the FST, similar to that observed with the positive control fluoxetine. These results suggest that **2c** and **2d** may be potential leads for the development of therapeutic agents for the treatment of depression and epilepsy.

Author Contributions: L.G. and H.J. designed the research and conducted the animal experiments in the study. Q.J. and Z.F. discussed the pharmacological results in this study. The test data were gathered by Z.F. Q.J. and L.G. performed the synthetic work. The manuscript was written by L.G. and H.J. All authors discussed, edited and approved the final version.

Funding: This study was financially supported by the National Natural Science Foundation of China (No. 81560149; No. 81760207).

Acknowledgments: We thank Si-Hong Wang from Yanbian University, China, for spectral testing and spectral analysis of compounds of this manuscript. Victoria Muir and Koji Yamashita from Liwen Bianji, Edanz Group China (www.liwenbianji.cn/ac), edited the English text of a draft of this manuscript.

Conflicts of Interest: The authors declare no conflict of interest.

References

1. Tan, R.W. Marine microorganisms: An important source of new natural drugs. *Chin. J. Nat. Med.* **2006**, *4*, 2–4.
2. Shang, X.H.; Liu, X.Y.; Zhang, J.P.; Gao, Y.; Jiao, B.H.; Zheng, H.; Lu, X.L. Traditional Chinese medicine-sea urchin. *Mini Rev. Med. Chem.* **2014**, *14*, 537–542. [CrossRef] [PubMed]
3. Zhou, Y.; Li, Y.H.; Yu, H.B.; Liu, X.Y.; Lu, X.L.; Jiao, B.H. Furanone derivative and sesquiterpene from Antarctic marine-derived fungus *Penicillium* sp. S-1-18. *J. Asian Nat. Prod. Res* **2018**, *2012*, 1108–1115. [CrossRef] [PubMed]
4. Leleu-Chavain, N.; Baudelet, D.; Heloire, V.M.; Rocha, D.E.; Renault, N.; Barczyk, A.; Djouina, M.; Body-Malapel, M.; Carato, P.; Millet, R. Benzo[*d*]thiazol-2(3*H*)-ones as new potent selective CB$_2$ agonists with anti-inflammatory properties. *Eur. J. Med. Chem.* **2019**, *165*, 347–362. [CrossRef] [PubMed]
5. Cindrić, M.; Perić, M.; Kralj, M.; Martin-Kleiner, I.; David-Cordonnier, M.H.; Paljetak, H.Č.; Matijašić, M.; Verbanac, D.; Karminski-Zamola, G.; Hranjec, M. Antibacterial and antiproliferative activity of novel 2-benzimidazolyl-and 2-benzothiazolyl-substitutedbenzo[*b*]thieno-2-carboxamides. *Mol. Div.* **2018**, *22*, 637–646. [CrossRef] [PubMed]
6. Akhtar, T.; Hameed, S.; Al-Masoudi, N.A.; Loddo, R.; La Colla, P. In vitro antitumor and antiviral activities of new benzothiazole and 1,3,4-oxadiazole-2-thione derivatives. *Acta Pharm.* **2008**, *58*, 135–149. [CrossRef] [PubMed]
7. Nagararaju, G.; Sai, K.B.; Chandana, K.; Guldipati, M.; Suresh, P.V.; Ramarao, N. Synthesis, evaluation of antioxidant and antimicrobial study of 2-substituted benzothiazole derivatives. *Indo Am. J. Pharm. Res.* **2015**, *5*, 1288–1296.
8. Khan, K.M.; Mesaik, M.A.; Abdalla, O.M.; Rahim, F.; Soomro, S.; Halim, S.A.; Mustafa, G.; Ambreen, N.; Khalid, A.S.; Taha, M. The immunomodulation potential of the synthetic derivatives of benzothiazoles: Implications in immune system disorders through in vitro and in silico studies. *Bioorg. Chem.* **2016**, *64*, 21–28. [CrossRef]
9. Tripathi, R.K.; Ayyannan, S.R. Design, Synthesis, and evaluation of 2-amino-6-nitrobenzothiazole-derived hydrazones as MAO inhibitors: Role of the methylene spacer group. *ChemMedChem* **2016**, *11*, 1551–1567. [CrossRef]
10. Tripathi, R.K.; Goshain, O.; Ayyannan, S.R. Design, synthesis, in vitro MAO-B inhibitory evaluation, and computational studies of some 6-nitrobenzothiazole-derived semicarbazones. *ChemMedChem* **2013**, *8*, 462–474. [CrossRef]
11. Kaya, B.; Sağlık, B.N.; Levent, S.; Özkay, Y.; Kaplancıklı, Z.A. Synthesis of some novel 2-substituted benzothiazole derivatives containing benzylamine moiety as monoamine oxidase inhibitory agents. *J. Enzym. Inhib. Med. Chem.* **2016**, *31*, 1654–1661. [CrossRef] [PubMed]
12. Demir Özkay, Ü.; Kaya, C.; Acar Çevik, U.; Devrim Can, Ö. Synthesis and antidepressant activity profile of some novel benzothiazole derivatives. *Molecules* **2017**, *22*, 1490–1504. [CrossRef] [PubMed]
13. Keri, R.S.; Quintanova, C.; Marques, S.M.; Esteves, A.R.; Cardoso, S.M.; Santos, M.A. Design, synthesis and neuroprotective evaluation of novel tacrine-benzothiazole hybrids as multi-targeted compounds against Alzheimer's disease. *Bioorg. Med. Chem.* **2013**, *21*, 4559–4569. [CrossRef] [PubMed]

14. Liu, D.C.; Zhang, H.J.; Jin, C.M.; Quan, Z.S. Synthesis and biological evaluation of novel benzothiazole derivatives as potential anticonvulsant agents. *Molecules* **2016**, *21*, 1635–1652.
15. Wang, S.; Chen, Y.; Zhao, S.; Xu, X.; Liu, X.; Liu, B.F.; Zhang, G. Synthesis and biological evaluation of a series of benzoxazole/benzothiazole-containing 2,3-dihydrobenzo[*b*][1,4] dioxine derivatives as potential antidepressants. *Bioorg. Med. Chem. Lett.* **2014**, *24*, 1766–1770. [CrossRef] [PubMed]
16. Siddiqui, N.; Rana, A.; Khan, S.A.; Ahsan, W.; Alam, M.S.; Ahmed, S. Analgesic and antidepressant activities of benzothiazole-benzamides. *Biomed. Pharm. J.* **2008**, *1*, 297–300.
17. Krall, R.L.; Penry, J.K.; White, B.G.; Kupferberg, H.J.; Swinyard, E.A. Antiepileptic drug development: II. Anticonvulsant drug screening. *Epilepsia* **1978**, *19*, 409–428. [CrossRef] [PubMed]
18. Borsini, F.; Voltera, G.; Meli, A. A dose the behavioral 'despair' test measure 'despair'. *Physiol. Behav.* **1986**, *38*, 385–389. [CrossRef]
19. Zhen, X.H.; Quan, Y.C.; Jiang, H.Y.; Wen, Z.S.; Qu, Y.L.; Guan, L.P. Fucosterol, a sterol extracted from *Sargassum fusiforme*, shows antidepressant and anticonvulsant effects. *Eur. J. Pharmacol.* **2015**, *768*, 131–138. [CrossRef] [PubMed]
20. Patrick, G. *Instant Notes in Medicinal Chemistry*; The United Kingdom BIOS Scientific Publishers Limited: Cambridge, UK, 2001; Volume 3, p. 119.
21. Drinovac, M.; Wagner, H.; Agrawal, N.; Cock, H.R.; Mitchell, A.J.; von Oertzen, T.J. Screening for depression in epilepsy: A model of an enhanced screening tool. *Epilepsy Behav.* **2015**, *44*, 67–72. [CrossRef]
22. Fiest, K.M.; Patten, S.B.; Altura, K.C.; Bulloch, A.G.; Maxwell, C.J.; Wiebe, S.; Macrodimitris, S.; Jetté, N. Patterns and frequency of the treatment of depression in persons with epilepsy. *Epilepsy Behav.* **2014**, *39*, 59–64. [CrossRef] [PubMed]
23. Hao, C.W.; Lai, W.S.; Ho, C.T.; Sheen, L.Y. Antidepressant-like effect of lemon essential oil is through a modulation in the levels of norepinephrine, dopamine, and serotonin in mice: Use of the tail suspension test. *J. Funct. Foods* **2013**, *5*, 370–379. [CrossRef]
24. Xu, J.; Xu, H.; Liu, Y.; He, H.; Li, G. Vanillin-induced amelioration of depression-like behaviors in rats by modulating monoamine neurotransmitters in the brain. *Psychiatry Res.* **2015**, *225*, 509–514. [CrossRef] [PubMed]
25. Guan, L.P.; Liu, B.Y. Antidepressant-like effects and mechanisms of flavonoids and related analogues. *Eur. J. Med. Chem.* **2016**, *121*, 47–57. [CrossRef] [PubMed]
26. Porsolt, R.D.; Bertin, A.; Jalfre, M. Behavioural despair in mice: A primary screening test for antidepressants. *Arch. Int. Pharmacodyn.* **1997**, *229*, 327–336.
27. Zhao, D.H.; Wang, Y.C.; Zheng, L.W.; Liu, B.Y.; Guan, L.P. Antidepressant-like effect of a chalcone compound, DHIPC and its possible mechanism. *Iran. J. Pharm. Res.* **2018**, *17*, 193–201.
28. Porter, R.J.; Cereghino, J.J.; Gladding, G.D.; Hessie, B.J.; Kupferberg, H.J.; Scoville, B.; White, B.G. Antiepileptic drug development program. *Cleve Clin. Q.* **1984**, *51*, 293–305. [CrossRef]
29. Guan, L.P.; Quan, Z.S. 3,4-DHQLO and triazole and its related analogues with anticonvulsant effects. *Mini Rev. Med. Chem.* **2016**, *16*, 323–342. [CrossRef]

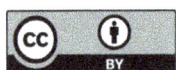

© 2019 by the authors. Licensee MDPI, Basel, Switzerland. This article is an open access article distributed under the terms and conditions of the Creative Commons Attribution (CC BY) license (http://creativecommons.org/licenses/by/4.0/).

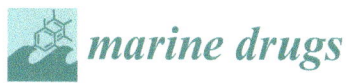

Article

Discovery of Geranylgeranyl Pyrophosphate Synthase (GGPPS) Paralogs from *Haematococcus pluvialis* Based on Iso-Seq Analysis and Their Function on Astaxanthin Biosynthesis

Danqiong Huang [1,2], Wenfu Liu [1], Anguo Li [1], Chaogang Wang [1,*] and Zhangli Hu [1,*]

[1] Shenzhen Key Laboratory of Marine Bioresource and Eco-environmental Science, Shenzhen Engineering Laboratory for Marine Algal Biotechnology, Guangdong Provincial Key Laboratory for Plant Epigenetics, College of Life Sciences and Oceanography, Shenzhen University, Shenzhen 518060, China; dqhuang@szu.edu.cn (D.H.); liuwenfu2017@email.szu.edu.cn (W.L.); 1800251012@email.szu.edu.cn (A.L.)

[2] Key Laboratory of Optoelectronic Devices and Systems of Ministry of Education and Guangdong Province, College of Optoelectronic Engineering, Shenzhen University, Shenzhen 518060, China

* Correspondence: charlesw@szu.edu.cn (C.W.); huzl@szu.edu.cn (Z.H.); Tel.: +86-755-2655-8081 (C.W.); +86-755-2653-6629 (Z.H.)

Received: 20 November 2019; Accepted: 10 December 2019; Published: 12 December 2019

Abstract: *Haematococcus pluvialis* is widely distributed in the world and well known as the richest natural source of astaxanthin that is a strong antioxidant with excellent commercial value. The pathway of astaxanthin biosynthesis in *H. pluvialis* has been documented as an enzymatic reaction. Several enzymes have been reported, but their isoforms or homologs have not been investigated genome-wide. To better understand the astaxanthin biosynthesis pathway in *H. pluvialis*, eight candidates of the geranylgeranyl pyrophosphate synthase gene (*HpGGPPS*) predicted from Iso-seq data were isolated in this study. The length of coding region of these candidates varied from 960 bp to 1272 bp, composing of 7–9 exons. The putative amino acids of all candidates composed the signature domain of *GGPPS* gene. However, the motifs in the domain region are varied, indicating different bio-functions. Phylogenetic analysis revealed eight candidates can be clustered into three groups. Only two candidates in Group1 encode the synthase participating in the astaxanthin formation. The yield of astaxanthin from these two candidates, 7.1 mg/g (DW) and 6.5 mg/g (DW) respectively, is significant higher than that from *CrtE* (2.4 mg/g DW), a *GGPPS* gene from *Pantoea ananatis*. This study provides a potential productive pathway for astaxanthin synthesis.

Keywords: *GGPPS*; *Haematococcus pluvialis*; astaxanthin; Iso-Seq

---

1. Introduction

Astaxanthin ($C_{40}H_{52}O_4$), a keto-carotenoid, has been well known as super vitamin E due to its hydroxyl and ketone functional groups and multiple conjugated double bonds that can reduce the reactive oxidizing molecule. Thus, astaxanthin can be consumed as a dietary supplement or aging related-cosmetics. Meanwhile, astaxanthin also has been used as an aquaculture consumption due to its additive of the blood-red color, contributing to over $500 million a year in the market [1]. Astaxanthin can be produced chemically in the factory or naturally from organisms such as the microalga *Haematococcus pluvialis* and the yeast fungus *Xanthophyllomyces dendrorhous* [2]. Compared with chemically synthetic astaxanthin from the Wittig reaction using asta-C15-triarylphosphonium salt and the C10-dialdehyde [3], the naturally isolated astaxanthin has 20-times higher antioxidant activity and is capable for human consumption [4,5].

As the most important source of natural astaxanthin, it is imperative to understand the biological process and the regulation of astaxanthin formation in *H. pluvialis* aiming to improve the productivity of astaxanthin. The pathway of astaxanthin production in *H. pluvialis* is complex but still has been described, which is originally started from pyruvate and glyceraldehyde-3-phosphate (GA-3P) followed by a series of enzymatic reactions [6,7]. Briefly, isopentenyl diphosphate (IPP), the precursor of carotenoids, was synthesized through methyl-D-erythritol 4-phosphate (MEP) pathway using pyruvate, GA-3P, and enzymes of DXS and IspC-IspH [8,9]. Subsequently, IPP and dimethylallyl diphosphate (DMAPP, an isomer of IPP that was formed by isopentenyl pyrophosphate isomerase (IPI) or 4-hydroxy-3-methylbut-2-enyl diphosphate reductase (HDR)), were used to form a C20 compound, geranylgeranyl pyrophosphate (GGPP), with the help of geranylgeranyl pyrophosphate synthase (GGPPS) [10–13]. Carotenoids were then initialized using GGPP, in the main order of phytoene, ζ-carotene, lycopene, β-carotene, cathaxanthin, and astaxanthin, with cooperation of enzymes of phytoenesysthase (PSY), phytoenedesaturase (PDS), ζ-carotenedesaturase (ZDS), lycopene β-cyclase (LCY-b), β-carotene ketolase (BKT), and β-carotene 3,3′-hydroxylase (CrtR-b) [2,7,13]. Thereby, the GGPPS, a key enzyme defining the initial GGPP availability, is crucial for the subsequent flux of carotenoids biosynthesis, theoretically. It has been reported that the mechanism of the enzymatic reaction converting IPP to GGPP is conserved among organisms from bacteria to human [14,15]. However, the number of *GGPPS* paralogs were varied within species, as high as 12 in *Arabidopsis* [16] and as low as one in *Chlamydomonas reinhardtii* [17]. Specifically, three *GGPPS* genes were found in *H. pluvialis* based on a RNA-Seq transcriptome analysis (Genbank accessions: KX236181–KX236183). With the advantage of obtaining the full-length of transcripts to identify isoforms, alternative splicing, fusion transcripts, LncRNA, and new homologous genes, the single-molecule real-time (SMRT) long-read isoform sequencing (Iso-Seq) developed by Pacific BioSciences (PaciBio) is more preferred to discover more paralogs over the RNA-Seq technology [18]. As one of successful examples, more than 113,000 novel splice isoforms were discovered in a Iso-Seq data of *Sorghum bicolor* L. Moench and some of them are functional which confirmed by additional experiments of gene cloning and RT-PCR [19].

Since the whole genome sequence of *H. pluvialis* is available [20], it is possible to discover more reliable novel *GGPPS* genes from the Iso-Seq data. The main objectives of this study were to explore more *GGPPS* paralogs in *H. pluvialis* using an Iso-Seq data, to determine their evolutionary relationship, and to characterize their performance on astaxanthin biosynthesis. By comparing the productivity of astaxanthin using different *GGPPS* genes from *H. pluvialis*, it is expected to arrange a more efficient pathway for astaxanthin biosynthesis.

2. Results

2.1. Cloning and Sequence Characterization of HpGGPPS Genes

Using three reported *GGPPS* genes of *H. pluvialis* retrieved from Genbank (accession nos. KX236181, KX236182, and KX236183), eight candidates were carried out from the Iso-Seq data by BlastN analysis with e-value of 0. Using designated gene-specific primers, the full-length coding sequences (CDS) of eight putative *HpGGPPS* genes (*HpGGPPS1-1*, *HpGGPPS1-2*, *HpGGPPS2-1*, *HpGGPPS2-1*, *HpGGPPS3-1*, *HpGGPPS3-2*, *HpGGPPS3-3*, and *HpGGPPS3-4*) were successfully isolated. Sequences were submitted to Genbank with accession numbers MN689792–MN689799.

The nucleotide sequence analysis revealed that eight putative *HpGGPPS* genes are ranging 1011–1455 bp in length and varied from 960 bp to 1272 bp in CDS region (Supplemental Table S1). Their deduced amino acids are ranging 319–423 aa with putative molecular weight of 36.27–45.75 KDa, respectively (Supplemental Table S1). The alignment of nucleotide sequences of eight *HpGGPPS* genes suggested 39.9–100% similarity in the CDS region (Supplemental Figure S1). Clearly, three classes were presented according to the similarity. High nucleotide sequence similarity was found within classes, including 98.6% identity between *HpGGPPS1-1* and *HpGGPPS1-2*, 97.4% identity between *HpGGPPS2-1* and *HpGGPPS2-2*, and 99.1–100% identity among *HpGGPPS3-1*, *HpGGPPS3-2*, *HpGGPPS3-3*, and

HpGGPPS3-4. It is noted that In-Del variation was found between sequences of *HpGGPPS3-1* and *HpGGPPS3-2* (sharing 100% similarity with each other), and between sequences of *HpGGPPS3-3* and *HpGGPPS3-4* (sharing 100% similarity with each other). By contrast, low percentage of nucleotides identity was found among classes, which was lower than 49%.

By the local BlastN against *H. pluvialis* genome sequences, *HpGGPPS1-1*, *HpGGPPS1-2*, *HpGGPPS2-1*, and *HpGGPPS2-2* hit different scaffolds, revealing different genome region. Differently, *HpGGPPS3-1* and *HpGGPPS3-2* hit the same scaffold, as well as *HpGGPPS3-3* and *HpGGPPS3-4*. By considering their 100% sequence identity, they might be isoforms from alternative splicing. Further sequences alignment of *HpGGPPS* genes with corresponding genome scaffolds confirmed that *HpGGPP3-1* and *HpGGPP3-2* were isoforms from modified splicing of intron, while *HpGGPPS3-3* and *HpGGPPS3-4* were isoforms from exon exclusion (Figure 1). Gene structure analysis suggested that *HpGGPPS1-1* and *HpGGPPS1-2* were composed from nine exons, as well as *HpGGPPS3-1*, and *HpGGPPS3-2*. Diversely, *HpGGPPS2-1* and *HpGGPPS2-2* were from seven and eight exons, respectively (Figure 1). Due to the missing nucleotide information in the scaffold, the gene structure of *HpGGPPS3-3* and *HpGGPPS3-4* is not complete.

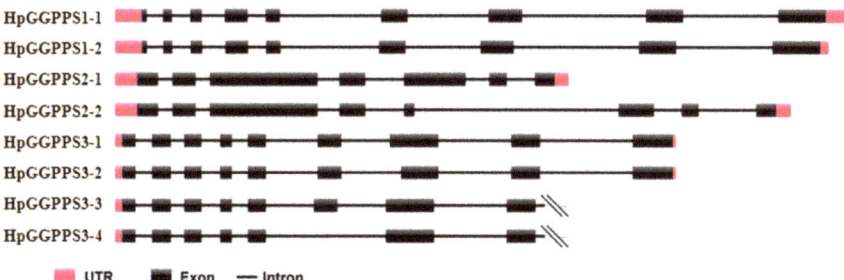

Figure 1. Schematic diagram of *HpGGPPS* gene structure, which was predicted by aligning with corresponding genome sequences. The slash indicates incomplete genome sequences resulting partial gene structure.

2.2. Molecular Evolution of HpGGPPS Genes

To predict the function of isolated *HpGGPPS* candidates, the domain of their putative amino acids was analyzed. According to SMART online prediction, the deduced amino acids of seven out of eight candidates contained the full domain of Polyprenyl_syn (Pfam accession: PF00348), which is associated with isoprenoid compounds synthesis. The excluded candidate, *HpGGPPS3-4*, has incomplete Polyprenyl_syn domain, because of the missing exon in comparison with *HpGGPPS3-3*. By aligning the deduced amino acids of eight *HpGGPPS* candidates from this study and four from Genbank (KX236181, KX236182, and KX236183 from *H. pluvialis*; XM001703117 from *Chlamydomonas reinhardtii*), motifs analysis was performed and results revealed that all 12 genes contained the signature asparate rich motifs, SARM (DDxxxD, which x refers to any amino acids) and FARM (DDxxxxD, which x refers to any amino acids), commonly found in *GGPPS* gene (Figure 2). Unlike the SARM domain conserved among aligned genes, the variation was found in the FARM motifs. In detailed, *HpGGPPS1-1*, *HpGGPPS2-1*, KX236181, and XM_001703117 have the traditional motifs of DDxxxxD, while rest genes have a modified motifs of DDxx–D. Moreover, *HpGGPPS1-1*, *HpGGPPS2-1*, KX236181, and XM_001703117 have the additional CxxxC motifs, indicating they might have different bio-functions from the rest of genes. Besides, *GGPPS* genes from *H. pluvialis* (*HpGGPPS1-1*, *HpGGPPS2-1*, and KX236181) have the modified TxxxC motifs, comparing with the *GGPPS* gene from *C. reinhardtii*.

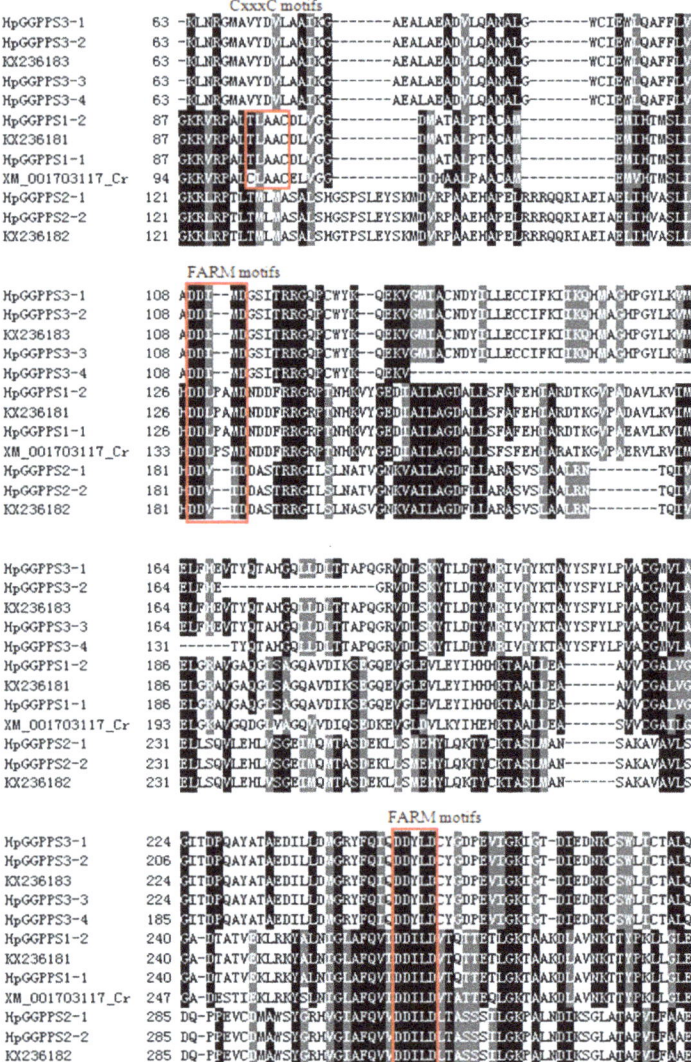

Figure 2. Alignment of Polyprenyl_syn domain region in the deduced amino acids of *GGPPS* genes. The motifs for CxxxC, FARM, and SARM are red squared. The sequence of XM_001713117 is from *Chlamydomonas reinhardtii*, while the rest of 11 sequences are from *Haematococcus pluvialis*.

To further evaluate the evolutionary pattern of *HpGGPPS* genes, a phylogenetic tree was constructed using *GGPPS* genes obtained in this study and retrieved from Genbank which originally from other species including Planta, Bacteria, Archaea, and Fungi (Figure 3). Eight *HpGGPPS* genes were clustered into three distinguish groups, paralleled with the three classes identified according to sequence similarity. The Group1 genes, composing of *HpGGPPS1-1* and *HpGGPPS1-2*, were clustered with *GGPPS* genes from Plantae and were more close to *Euglena gracillis* and *Thermosynehococcus elongatus* belonging to photosynthetic unicellular species, compared with other high plant species. The Group2 genes, composing of *HpGGPPS2-1* and *HpGGPPS2-2*, were in a distinct cluster apart from the cluster containing *HpGGPPS3-1*, *HpGGPPS3-2*, *HpGGPPS3-3*, and *HpGGPPS3-4* (Group3). It is interesting that six putative *HpGGPPS* genes from Group2 and Group3 were more likely clustered with *GGPPS* genes from Bacteria, which implied that their function might different from *HpGGPPS1-1* and *HpGGPPS1-2* that are close to Planta evolutionarily.

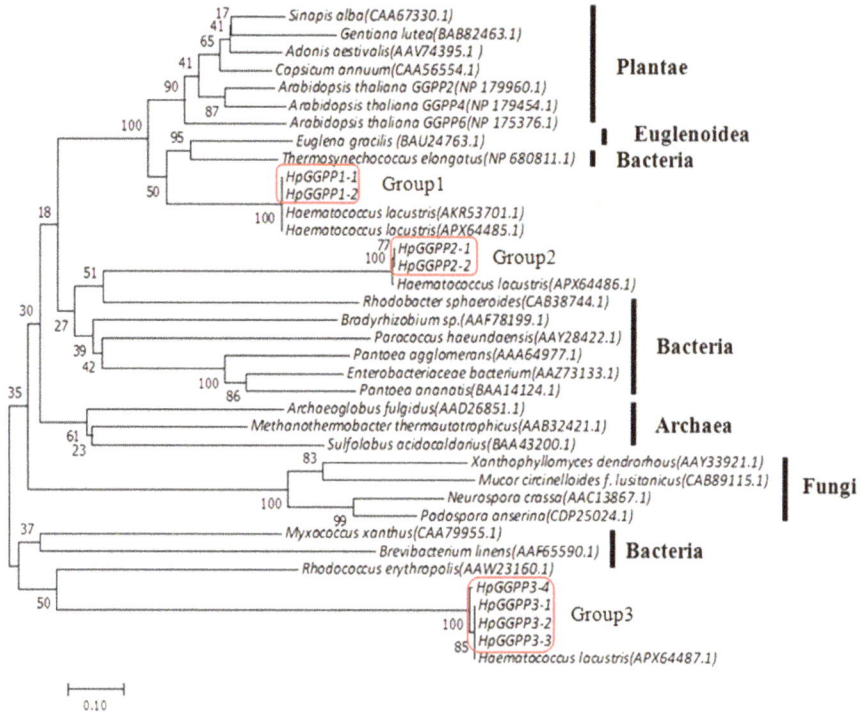

Figure 3. Phylogenetic relationships of the deduced amino acid sequences of *GGPPS* genes obtained in this study and retried from Genbank. Numbers in parentheses are accession numbers of *GGPPS* genes. The phylogenetic tree was constructed by MEGA version 7.0 using neighbor-joining method. Bootstrap values from the percentages of 1000 replications are indicated beside each node.

2.3. Functional Identification of HpGGPPS Genes in Escherichia coli

The function of isolated *HpGGPPS* genes was analyzed by hetero-expression studies in *E. coli* targeting the astaxanthin formation. The transformed *E. coli* cells with pFZ153ΔE/CrtE, a plasmid containing astaxanthin biosynthetic gene cluster originally from Bacteria as the positive control, displayed orange-red color in the cell pellet as a result of pigmentation of astaxanthin (Figure 4). Served as the negative control, *E. coli* cells harboring pFZ153ΔE (NCK), a plasmid without *GGPPS* gene but with all rest genes (CrtI, CrtB, IPI, CrtY, CrtZ, CrtW) for astaxanthin production, displayed slight yellow color in the cell pellet. Similar as the positive control, the *E. coli* transformants harboring pFZ153ΔE/GGPPS1-1 (1-1) and pFZ153ΔE/GGPPS1-2 (1-2) also displayed orange-red color, but relatively darker, which might be explained by more pigmentation. By contrast, the pigmentation was not observed in *E. coli* pellets harboring pFZ153ΔE/GGPPS2-1 (2-1), pFZ153ΔE/GGPPS2-2 (2-2), pFZ153ΔE/GGPPS3-1 (3-1), pFZ153ΔE/GGPPS3-2 (3-2), pFZ153ΔE/GGPPS3-3 (3-3), or pFZ153ΔE/GGPPS3-4 (3-4) (Figure 4), indicating that they might not encode proteins associated with pigment production. Therefore, only proteins encoded by *HpGGPPS1-1* and *HpGGPPS1-2* have GGPP synthase activity to participate pigment formation.

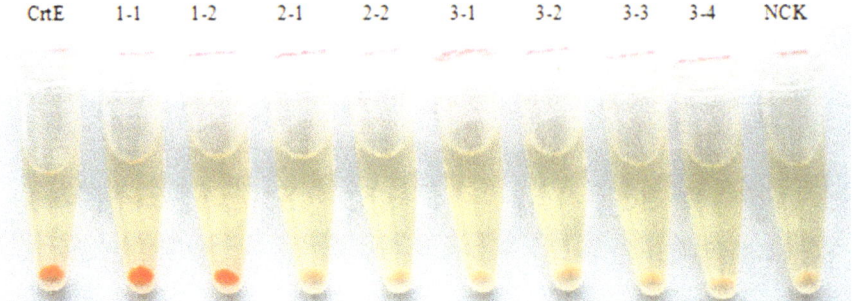

Figure 4. Hetero-expression experiments of pFZ153ΔE/GGPPS in *E. coli* targeting astaxanthin synthesis. *E. coli* strain BL21 (DE3) was used as the host. CrtE refers to the *GGPPS* gene from *Pantoea ananatis*, served as the positive control producing astaxanthin; 1-1, 1-2, 2-1, 2-2, 3-1, 3-2, 3-3, and 3-4 refers to corresponding *HpGGPPS* genes isolated in this study; NCK refers to the negative control, which is the BL21 (DE3) containing pFZ153ΔE without *GGPPS* gene for production of no astaxanthin. Colors of *E. coli* pellet are representative of at least five transformants with similar results.

To further confirm and quantify the astaxanthin production in *E. coli* cells, a HPLC analysis was successfully conducted. The chromatographic profile of astaxanthin was generated using commercial standards (Supplemental Figure S2a). As expected, an absorption peak of astaxanthin was detected in the positive control and but not detected in the negative control. Similarly, the pigment in *E. coli* cells harboring pFZ153ΔE/GGPPS1-1 and pFZ153ΔE/GGPPS1-2 have a peak at the same retention time as astaxanthin standard, indicating the existence of astaxanthin (Supplemental Figure S2b). Consisting with the color evaluation in cell pellets, astaxanthin was not detected in *E. coli* cells harboring pFZ153ΔE/GGPPS2-1, pFZ153ΔE/GGPPS2-2, pFZ153ΔE/GGPPS3-1, pFZ153ΔE/GGPPS3-2, pFZ153ΔE/GGPPS3-3, and pFZ153ΔE/GGPPS3-4. Besides, no other absorption peaks were observed in their chromatographic profile. Meanwhile, the quantity of astaxanthin was measured using a standard curve constructed from a set of astaxanthin standards. Results showed that *E. coli* cells harboring pFZ153ΔE/GGPPS1-1 produced as high as 7.1 mg astaxanthin per gram of dried cells in average from three independent pigment extraction, which is slight more (but not significant at the level of 0.05) than *E. coli* cells harboring pFZ153ΔE/GGPPS1-2 (6.5 mg/g DW in average). Notably, the positive control has significant less yield of astaxanthin (2.4 mg/g DW in average), compared with *E. coli* cells with *HpGGPPS* genes (Figure 5).

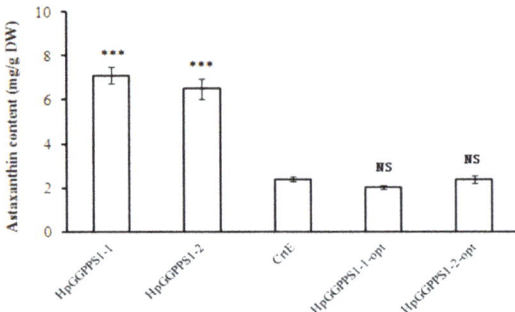

Figure 5. Astaxanthin content in *E. coli* (BL21 DE3) transformants with plasmids harboring astaxanthin synthetic gene cluster, according to HPLC analysis. Specifically, HpGGPPS1-1-opt and HpGGPPS1-2-opt refers to the bacteria codon optimized *HpGGPPS1-1* and *HpGGPPS1-2* gene, respectively. Data were the mean from at least three replicates and the standard error was presented as the bar. *** indicates the significant differences at the level of 0.001. NS indicates no significant differences at the level of 0.05.

3. Discussion

Astaxanthin is one of the strongest antioxidants and its natural format is being demanded by increasing market looking for natural products [1]. Thereby, the topic of improving astaxanthin production from natural sources is attractive for the industry. Lots of effort has been made by scientists trying to design an efficient protocol for astaxanthin production using natural source [7]. As a major natural source of astaxanthin, *Haematococcus pluvialis* accumulated as high as 5% dry weight of astaxanthin [21] and its dairy supplements can be used human-friendly [22]. It was found that two specific enzymes, β-carotene hydroxylase (CrtR-b) and ketolase (BKT), are crucial for astaxanthin formation [23–26] and many researches were focused on aiming to improve astaxanthin content [27–29]. However, as the important precursor to initial the carotenoids synthesis in *H. pluvialis*, limited research was conducted for the regulation of geranylgeranyl pyrophosphate (GGPP) on astaxanthin production. It was recorded that GGPP synthase (GGPPS) plays an important role on GGPP formation [6]. In *Arabidopsis*, a well-studied species, 12 *GGPPS* genes were found and 10 of them have the ability to produce GGPP [30]. Research suggested that GGPP formation was regulated with different pattern in *Arabidopsis* [30].

Previously, there are three *GGPPS* genes from *H. pluvialis* in Genbank and one (Genbank accession no. KX236181) have the activity to catalyze GGPP formation [31]. Unfortunately, no further information was reported regarding the other two *GGPPS* genes (Genbank accession nos. KX236182, KX236183). With the expectation of discovering more paralogs having enzymatic activity, this study screened an Iso-Seq data covering transcripts from the control and stressed *H. pluvialis* cells. The stress condition was high light and salt which was normally used to induce the astaxanthin formation [20]. Eight candidates were found and their gene structures were illustrated in this study (Figure 1), using the available genome sequences (BIG Data Center GSA Database accession no. PRJCA000614) [20]. Generally, two conserved aspartate rich motifs, FARM and SARM, and flexible CxxxC motifs are presented in the domain of amino acids of *GGPPS* genes [16,31,32]. Based on the domain analysis, FARM and SARM motifs were presented in all eight *HpGGPPS* genes while CxxxC motifs was only found in *HpGGPPS1-1*, *HpGGPPS1-2*, KX236181, and XM_001703117 (Figure 2). It has been documented that FARM, SARM and CxxxC motifs are important for GGPP biosynthesis by affecting the IPP and DMAPP substrate binding process and by affecting the physical interaction between subunits of heteroimeric GPP, respectively [31,32]. Proteins with features of conserved FARM, SARM, and CxxxC motifs displayed the function of catalyzing GGPP formation [33], indicating similar function might be employed by *HpGGPPS1-1* and *HpGGPPS1-2*. Differently, the CxxxC motifs was not found in other six *HpGGPPS* genes (Figure 2). Such proteins with conserved FARM and SARM motifs but without CxxxC motifs was shown to be involved in the production of medium (C25) to long (C45) chain isoprenoids [34]. It is noted that six *HpGGPPS* genes isolated in this study (*HpGGPPS2-1*, *HpGGPPS2-2*, *HpGGPPS3-1*, *HpGGPPS3-2*, *HpGGPPS3-3*, and *HpGGPPS3-4*) and two previously reported *GGPPS* genes (KX236182 and KX236183) have modified FARM motifs (DDxx–D instead of DDxxxxD). The effect of this type of modification on their bio-function has not been reported. The feature of modified FARM motifs, conserved SARM motifs, and lacking CxxxC motifs was also observed in *GGPPS* genes from other species, such as *Linus usitatissimum*, *Ricinus communis*, *Physcomitrella patens*, *Zea mays*, and *Vitis vinifera* [16].

According to the nucleotide sequence similarity and phylogenetic tree analysis constructed from putative amino acids, eight candidates can be grouped into three classes with more than one member in each class (Figure 3). To directly evaluate their function on astaxanthin biosynthesis, hetero-expression in *E. coli* was performed using candidate genes together with other genes that are essential for astaxanthin biosynthesis. It is not surprised that two candidates, *HpGGPPS1-1* and *HpGGPPS1-2* that closely related to *GGPPS1* (Genbank accession no. KX236181), could promote the formation of astaxanthin in *E. coli* (Figure 4). Sequence similarity analysis showed that *HpGGPPS1-1* and *HpGGPPS1-2* shared 99% identity in nucleotides of coding region and only one amino acid differences. By contrast, big variation (90% identity) was found in the 5′UTR region of *HpGGPPS1-1* and *HpGGPPS1-2*, indicating there are two functional *HpGGPPS* in *H. pluvialis* rather than one as previously reported [35]. No astaxanthin or other visible pigments were observed in *E. coli* carrying the rest of six *HpGGPPS* candidates, indicating they might not directly associate with astaxanthin production. Similar findings were also found in other species, such as *Arabidposis* having *AtGGPPS5* and *AtGGPPS12* gene with GGPPS domain features but without the function of converting IPP and DMAPP to GGPP [30,36]. Additional in vitro studies could be conducted to investigate the potential function of these non-astaxanthin-related *HpGGPPS* genes.

Furthermore, the yield of astaxanthin in *E. coli* carrying *HpGGPPS1-1* and *HpGGPPS1-2* genes is about 271–296% increased than that carrying *CrtE* gene (the *GGPPS* gene driven from *Pantoea ananatis* as the positive control). In general, codon optimization is considered as an essential step to produce heterologous protein in *E. coli* to overcome the impairment of gene expression from the codon bias [37,38]. Followed by this conventional strategy, we expected more GGPPS proteins in *E. coli* transformants with codon-optimized genes, thereby leading to more astaxanthin production, theoretically. Nevertheless, *E. coli* with codon optimized *HpGGPPS1-1* and *HpGGPPS1-2* produced significant lower amount of astaxanthin (Figure 5), comparing with non-codon optimized corresponding genes, but produced similar amount of astaxanthin as *CrtE* (Figure 5). A possible explanation would be that excessive GGPPS might inhibit the astaxanthin biosynthesis in *E. coli*. This hypothesis is partly supported by the evidence that no change or downregulation of *GGPPS* was found in the salicylic acid and jasmonic acid stressed transcriptome analysis in *H. pluvialis* during astaxanthin formation [39]. Further research can be conducted to test the suppressive role of GGPPS during astaxanthin biosynthesis.

In conclusion, this study found two *HpGGPPS* gene having the synthase activity to participate in the astaxanthin biosynthesis. Non-codon optimized *H. pluvialis*-driven *GGPPS* genes produced significant higher amount of astaxanthin in *E. coli*, compared with bacteria-driven *GGPPS* gene. This study improves the understanding of the role of *GGPPS* in astaxanthin biosynthesis and thereby contributes to the design of efficient pathway for astaxanthin production.

4. Materials and Methods

4.1. Microalga Culture, Treatment, and Sample Collection

The microalga *Haematococcus pluvialis* strain 192.80, originally purchased from EPSAG (Experimental Phycology and Culture Collection of Algae, Goettingen University, Goettingen, Germany), was used in this study. The alga cells were grown in a 250 mL flask containing 100 mL ESP Ag medium [40] at 22 °C under continuous illumination of 25 µmol photon $m^{-2}s^{-1}$ in an incubator.

For the stress treatment to induce astaxanthin production, a final concentration of 45 mM sodium acetate was added into cultures when alga cells reached to the logarithmic phase (OD_{730} = 0.8), along with the exposure of continuous high light (irradiance at 500 µmol photon $m^{-2}s^{-1}$). To maximize the transcripts in the following SMRT sequencing, alga samples were harvested from the control (0 h) and at the time points of 1.5 h, 3 h, 6 h, 9 h, 12 h, 24 h, and 48 h after treatment. Alga cells were collected by centrifugation at 10,000× *g* for 5 min and frozen immediately by liquid nitrogen. Samples were stored at −80 °C until use.

4.2. Discovery, Isolation, and Sequencing of HpGGPPS Genes

Equal amounts of algae cells collected from different time points of stress treatment were pooled together for the total RNA extraction and sent to Gene Denovo Biotechnology Co. (Guangzhou, China) for SMRT sequencing to get the Iso-Seq data. To obtain *GGPPS* paralogs in *H. pluvialis*, a local BlastN against the Iso-Seq data was performed, using three reported *GGPPS* genes of *H. pluvialis* deposited in NCBI (Genbank accession no. KX236181, KX236182, and KX236183). To clone *HpGGPPS* candidates, PCR was performed using gene specific primers (Table 1) designed using the target nucleotide sequences from Iso-Seq data. The cDNA template for PCR was from the total RNA that was used for SMRT sequencing. The PCR reaction was carried out in a 20 µL volume containing

1 µL cDNA, 4.0 µL 5× SuperFi buffer, 4.0 µL 5× SuperFi GC Enhancer, 1.6 µL dNTP mix (2.5 mM), 1.0 µL each forward and reverse primer (10 µM), 0.2 µL SuperFi DNA polymerase (Invitrogen Life technologies, Carlsbad, CA, USA), and 7.2 µL ddH$_2$O. The PCR was implemented on the Bio-Rad T100 thermal cycler (Bio-Rad, Hercules, CA, USA) under following conditions: 98 °C for 2 min; 35 cycles of 98 °C for 10 s, 60 °C for 10 s, 72 °C for 1.5 min; and a final extension at 72 °C for 5 min. PCR products were run on 1.0% agarose gel and target fragments were purified by E.Z.N.A. Gel Extraction Kit (Omega Bio-tek Inc. Norcross, GA, USA) according to the manufacturer's instruction. Purified PCR fragments were treated by A-Tailing Kit (Takara, Japan), ligated into pGEM-T easy vector (Promega, Madison, WI, USA), and transformed into *E. coli* Top10 chemically competent cell, as described in manufacturer's instructions. Positive colonies were selected by the blue-white screening strategy on the LB agar plate containing ampicillin (50 µg/mL) and sent to Guangzhou IGE Biotechnology Ltd. (Guangzhou, China) for sequencing.

Table 1. Primers used in this study.

Primer ID	Sequences (5'–3')	Used for
GGPP1F1	CACTGCCTATCCCCGTTTCCAATC	Cloning of HpGGPPS1-1 and
GGPP1R1	GCACCTGCTGACCCGCTCTG	HpGGPPS1-2
GGPP2F1	GGCGACGCGGGCAAATCAGT	Cloning of HpGGPPS2-1 and
GGPP2R1	AAGCGCCAGGGAATACCAAACATA	HpGGPPS2-2
GGPP3F1	GCTCTCTTCGCACTTCTTGG	Cloning of HpGGPPS3-1, HpGGPPS3-2,
GGPP3R1	TGATGCCTAGACAGCTCACTT	HpGGPPS3-3 and HpGGPPS3-4
fGGPP1F2	GTATCT*GAATTC*AAAAAATGATCCGAGCGATGCACA [†]	Subcloning of HpGGPPS1-1
GGPP1R2	CATAGA*AAGCTT*TCAGTTCTTGCGGTATCCTA	
GGPP1F3	GTATCT*GAATTC*AAAAAATGATCCGAGCGATGCACA	Subcloning of HpGGPPS1-2
GGPP1R3	CATAGA*AAGCTT*TCAGTTCTTGCGGTACCCT	
GGPP2F2	GTATCT*GAATTC*AAAAAATGAGGGGCCTAGCGGGCAA	Subcloning of HpGGPPS2-1 and
GGPP2R2	CATAGA*GCGGCC*GCCTATTTCTTTCTGCTCAGGACTC	HpGGPPS2-2
GGPP3F2	GTATCT*GAATTC*AAAAAATGGTATCGGATGTGATGCAAG	Subcloning of HpGGPPS3-1
GGPP3R2	CATAGA*AAGCTT*TCACTTGCAGCGCTTGTAAATC	
GGPP3F3	GTATCT*GAATTC*AAAAAATGGTATCGGATGTGATGCAAG	Subcloning of HpGGPPS3-2,
GGPP3R3	CATAGA*AAGCTT*TCACTTGCAGCGCTTGTAAATC	HpGGPPS3-3, and HpGGPPS3-4
CrtIB-F2	GTATCT*TCTAGA*GTAAGGATCCTAACATGAAACCGACCACGGTGA	Subcloning of CrtIB
CrtIB-R2	CATAGA*GAATTC*ATGTCGACAAGTTACGCGGACGTTGCCAC	
CrtE-F1	GTATCT*GAATTC*ATACCATGACCGTGTGTGCGAA	Subcloning of CrtE
CrtE-R1	ATAGA*AAGCTT*TCCTTTACGACACCGCTGCCA	

[†] Restriction enzyme sites are formatted in italics.

4.3. Sequences Analysis and Molecular Evolution of HpGGPPS Genes

The ORFs of obtained nucleotide sequences of *HpGGPPS* genes and corresponding deduced amino acids were predicted by EditSeq module of DNASTAR software (Lasergene, Madison, WI, USA). Multiple sequence alignment was conducted by MegAlign module of DNASTAR software to determine the sequence identity and divergence. By aligned with genome sequences of *H. pluvialis* (BIG Data Center GSA Database accession no. PRJCA000614) [20], the gene structure was predicted and the schematic diagram was displayed by Gene Structure Display Server 2.0 (http://gsds.cbi.pku.edu.cn/). The domain of deduced amino acid was predicted by SMART online at http://smart.embl-heidelberg.de/. Phylogenetic relationship was analyzed by MEGA7 software with the neighbor-joining method from 1000 bootstrap replicates [41].

4.4. Plasmids Construction and Heterologous Expression

The plasmid used for heterologous expression targeting gene functional analysis was adopted from pFZ153, a plasmid has astaxanthin synthetic gene cluster (*CrtE, CrtI, CrtB, idi, CrtY, CrtZ,* and *CrtW*) and produces astaxanthin in *E. coli* [42]. To investigate the function of *HpGGPPS* genes on astaxanthin synthesis, the pFZ153∆E plasmid was constructed (Figure 6b). Firstly, *CrtE, CrtI,* and *CrtB* genes were removed from pFZ153 (Figure 6a) by *XbaI/EcoRI* digestion. Secondly, the coding sequence of CrtI/CrtB gene was amplified from pFZ153 plasmid using primers CrtIB-F2/CrtIB-R2 containing *XbaI* and *EcoRI* restriction sites, respectively. Finally, the gel-purified fragment of CrtI/CrtB gene was digested with *XbaI/EcoRI* restriction enzyme and then ligated with the pFZ153 fragment without *CrtE*, *CrtI*, and *CrtB* genes to form the new plasmid pFZ153ΔE.

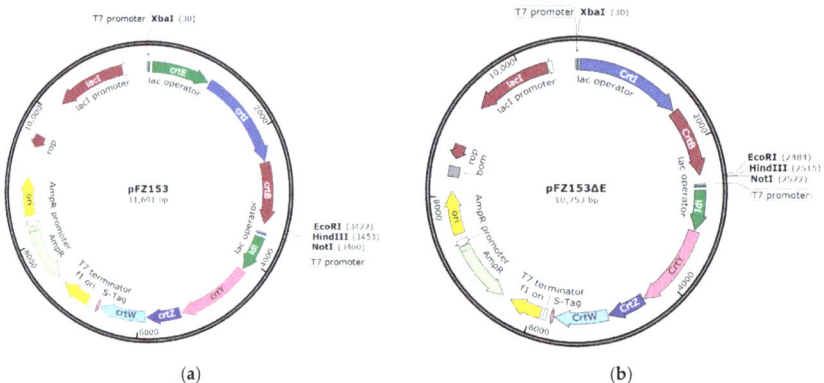

Figure 6. Structure of plasmid pFZ153 and pFZ153ΔE used to confer the function of *HpGGPPS* genes on astaxanthin biosynthesis in *E. coli* (BL21 DE3). The plasmid pFZ153 (**a**) was modified to construct the plasmid pFZ153ΔE (**b**) by removing the *CrtE* gene. In this study, *HpGGPPS* genes were inserted into the plasmid on *EcoRI/HindIII* or *EcoRI/NotI* site to complete the astaxanthin synthetic gene cluster. The *CrtE* gene from pFZ153 was served as the positive control.

To complete the astaxanthin synthetic gene cluster, *HpGGPPS* genes were inserted into pFZ153ΔE to form plasmids pFZ153ΔE/GGPPS. In detail, the coding sequences of *HpGGPPS* genes were amplified from the sequenced plasmids containing *HpGGPPS* genes, using primers listed in Table 1 containing either *EcoRI/HindIII* or *EcoRI/NotI* restriction sites. Similar as described above, the target PCR fragments were gel-purified and ligated into pFZ153ΔE plasmid in either *EcoRI/HindIII* or *EcoRI/NotI* sites. Additionally, the coding sequence of *CrtE* gene amplified from pFZ153 with primers CrtE-F1/CrtE-R1 harboring *EcoRI/HindIII* sites, was also ligated into pFZ153ΔE plasmid to construct the positive control (pFZ153ΔE/CrtE).

The procedures of PCR amplification using Platium SuperFi DNA polymerase and gel-purification using E.Z.N.A. Gel Extraction Kit are the same as described above. The ligation process was performed by T4 ligase (Promega, Madison, WI, USA), as described by the manual. *E. coli* Top10 was used as a host during plasmids construction, as described above. Restriction enzymes used in this study were purchased from Thermo Fisher Scientific Inc. (Waltham, MA, USA).

For the functional analysis of *HpGGPPS* genes, plasmids of pFZ153ΔE/GGPPS and pFZ153ΔE/CrtE were transferred into an expression host, *E. coli* strain BL21 (DE3). The transformed *E. coli* colonies were selected on the LB agar plate with ampicillin (100 μg/mL) and then cultured in 15 mL culture tubes containing 3 mL LB liquid media supplemented with 100 μg/mL ampicillin (LB+Amp100 medium) overnight. The aliquot of 0.5 mL was added into a 250 mL flask containing 100 mL LB+Amp100 medium. The flasks were incubated at 30 °C under dark with shaking (200 rpm) until OD_{600} reached 0.7–0.9, followed by adding IPTG to a final concentration of 0.1 mM. Three hours later, 50 mL of each culture was harvested and pigments were extracted as described below. For each plasmid, at least three independent *E. coli* colonies were selected for pigment extraction as replicates.

4.5. Pigment Extraction from E. coli and HPLC Analysis

The *E. coli* BL21 (DE3) cells expressing plasmids constructed in the study were harvested by centrifugation at 12,000× *g* for 5 min at 4 °C. The pellet was washed by ddH_2O twice and dried using a freeze-dryer. Consequently, the pellet was crashed into powder, weighted, and resuspended in 1 mL acetone for pigment extraction. The suspension was then incubated at a water bath at 55 °C for 15 min with vigorous shaking every 5 min. The supernatant containing pigments was collected by centrifugation at 12,000× g for 10 min at 4 °C. The pigment was subsequently dried using a vacuum evaporator and dissolved in 0.5 mL solution A (methanol/isopropanol, 8:2, V:V) for the following HPLC analysis.

The HPLC assay was performed on a Series 1260 system (Agilent Technologies, Santa Clara, CA, USA). Pigments were separated at a flow rate of 0.6 mL/min on a Phenomenex Gemini-NX C18 column (5 µ, 150 × 3.0 mm, Phenomenex Inc., Aschaffenburg, Germany) using solution A and solution B (ddH$_2$O). The gradient elution was 85% A, 15% B at 0 min, followed by linear gradient to 100% A at 10 min, maintained at 100% A to 12 min, returned to initial condition by 12.1 min, and re-equilibrated at initial condition by 18 min. The injection volume was 5 µL. Column temperature was maintained at 35 °C. The standard astaxanthin (Aladdin Chemistry Co. Ltd., Shanghai, China) was used to identify the target in the pigment. The detection was carried out by UV absorbance at 475 nm. To determine the concentration of astaxanthin in the testing sample, a calibration curve was constructed using a serial of plots with 500, 200, 100, 50, 20, and 10 µg/mL standard astaxanthin. The linearity between concentrations of astaxanthin and their corresponding peak areas was figured out to calculate the concentration of each analyte. The final astaxanthin productivity of each constructed plasmid was calculated by the formula, astaxanthin productivity = cal-con. × 0.5 mL/DW, where cal-con. refers to the calculated astaxanthin concentration in the analyte from the calibration curve, 0.5 mL comes from the final volume for each pigment extraction, DW comes from the amount of dried cells used for a pigment extraction. All organic solvents (acetone, methanol, and isopropanol) used in this study are HPLC grade.

4.6. Statistical Analysis

The data were processed by Pearson t-test to compare two means with replicates. The statistical significance was determined according to the $p < 0.05$.

Supplementary Materials: The following are available online at http://www.mdpi.com/1660-3397/17/12/696/s1, Table S1: Sequence characterization of *HpGGPPS* genes. Figure S1. Sequence similarity and divergence of eight *HpGGPPS* genes in the coding region. The alignment was performed by Clustal W using MegAlign module in the DNASTAR software. Figure S2. The HPLC chromatograms of pigments extracted from transformed *E. coli* cells. (a) the profile of standard astaxanthin purchased from Aladdin Chemistry Co. Ltd (Shanghai, China); (b) an representative profile of the extracted pigment from *E. coli* harboring *HpGGPP* genes and *CrtE* gene.

Author Contributions: D.H. and C.W. conceived and designed the experiments; D.H., W.L., and A.L. performed the experiments; D.H. analyzed the data; D.H. and C.W. wrote the paper; Z.H. reviewed the paper. All authors discussed the results and commented on the manuscript.

Funding: This research was funded by National key research and development plan special project for synthetic biology (2018YFA0902500), National Natural Science Foundation of China (31470389), Postdoctoral Science Foundation of China (2019M653013), and Guangdong Natural Science Foundation (2019A1515011701).

Acknowledgments: We thank Jiang Xia from The Chinese University of Hongkong for kindly providing the pFZ153 plasmid producing astaxanthin and Shuiming Li from Shenzhen University for technique advice on HPLC analysis.

Conflicts of Interest: The authors declare no conflict of interest. The funders had no role in the design of the study; in the collection, analyses, or interpretation of data; in the writing of the manuscript, or in the decision to publish the results.

References

1. Grand View Research. Astaxanthin Market Analysis by Source (Natural [Yeast, Krill/Shrimp, Microalgae] And Synthetic), by Product (Dried Biomass/Powder, Oil, Soft gels, Liquid), by Application, and Segment Forecasts, 2018–2025. Available online: https://www.grandviewresearch.com/industry-analysis/global-astaxanthin-market (accessed on 20 October 2017).
2. Higuera-ciapara, I.; Felix-valenzuela, L.; Goycoolea, F.M. Astaxanthin: A review of its chemistry and applications. *Crit. Rev. Food Sci. Nutr.* **2006**, *46*, 185–196. [CrossRef] [PubMed]
3. Krause, W.; Henrich, K.; Paust, J.; Ernst, H. Preparation of Astaxanthin. Available online: https://www.google.com/patents/US5654488 (accessed on 5 August 1997).
4. Koller, M.; Muhr, A.; Braunegg, G. Microalgae as versatile cellular factories for valued products. *Algal Res.* **2014**, *6*, 52–63. [CrossRef]
5. Lorenz, R.T.; Cysewski, G.R. Commercial potential for *Haematococcus microalgae* as a natural source of astaxanthin. *Trends Biotechnol.* **2000**, *18*, 160–167. [CrossRef]
6. McGarvey, D.J.; Croteau, R. Terpenoid metabolism. *Plant Cell* **1995**, *7*, 1015–1026. [PubMed]
7. Shah, M.M.R.; Yuanmei, L.; Cheng, J.J.; Maurycy, D. Astaxanthin-producing green microalga *Haematococcus pluvialis*: From single cell to high value commercial products. *Front. Plant Sci.* **2016**, *7*, 531. [CrossRef]
8. Rohmer, M.; Knani, M.; Simonin, P.; Sutter, B.; Sahm, H. Isoprenoid biosynthesis in bacteria: A novel pathway for the early steps leading to isopentenyl diphosphate. *Biochem. J.* **1993**, *295*, 517–524. [CrossRef]
9. Liang, C.; Zhang, W.; Zhang, X.; Fan, X.; Xu, D.; Ye, N.; Yang, Q. Isolation and expression analyses of methyl-d-erythritol 4-phosphate (MEP) pathway genes from *Haematococcus pluvialis*. *J. Appl. Phycol.* **2015**, *28*, 1–10. [CrossRef]
10. Sun, Z.; Cunningham, F.X., Jr.; Gantt, E. Differential expression of two isopentenyl pyrophosphate isomerases and enhanced carotenoid accumulation in a unicellular chlorophyte. *Proc. Natl. Acad. Sci. USA* **1998**, *95*, 11482–11488. [CrossRef]
11. Hoeffler, J.F.; Hemmerlin, A.; Grosdemange-Billiard, C.; Bach, T.J.; Rohmer, M. Isoprenoid biosynthesis in higher plants and in *Escherichia coli*: On the branching in the methylerythritol phosphate pathway and the independent biosynthesis of isopentenyl diphosphate and dimethylallyl diphosphate. *Biochem. J.* **2002**, *366*, 573–583. [CrossRef]
12. Gwak, Y.; Hwang, Y.S.; Wang, B.; Kim, M.; Jeong, J.; Lee, C.G.; Jin, E. Comparative analyses of lipidomes and transcriptomes reveal a concerted action of multiple defensive systems against photo oxidative stress in *Haematococcus pluvialis*. *J. Exp. Bot.* **2014**, *65*, 4317–4334. [CrossRef]
13. Britton, G. Biosynthesis of carotenoids. In *Carotenoids in Photosynthesis*; Young, A., Britton, G., Eds.; Springer: London, UK, 1993; pp. 96–126.
14. Mende, K.; Homann, V.; Tudzynski, B. The geranylgeranyl diphosphate synthase gene of *Gibberella fujikuroi*: Isolation and expression. *Mol. Gen. Genet.* **1997**, *255*, 96–105. [CrossRef] [PubMed]
15. Kainou, T.; Kawamura, K.; Tanaka, K.; Matsuda, H.; Kawamukai, M. Identification of the *GGPS1* genes encoding geranylgeranyl diphosphate synthases from mouse and human. *Biochim. Biophys. Acta* **1999**, *1437*, 333–340. [CrossRef]
16. Coman, D.; Altenhoff, A.; Zoller, S.; Gruissem, W.; Vranová, E. Distinct evolutionary strategies in the GGPPS family from plants. *Front. Plant Sci.* **2014**, *5*, 230. [CrossRef] [PubMed]
17. Merchant, S.S.; Prochnik, S.E.; Vallon, O.; Harris, E.H.; Karpowicz, S.J.; Witman, G.B. The *Chlamydomonas* genome reveals the evolution of key animal and plant functions. *Science* **2007**, *318*, 245–250. [CrossRef]
18. Gonzalez-Garay, M.L. Introduction to isoform sequencing using pacific biosciences technology (Iso-Seq). In *Transcriptomics and Gene Regulation*; Wu, J., Ed.; Springer: Dordrecht, The Netherlands, 2016; pp. 141–160.
19. Abdelghany, S.E.; Hamilton, M.; Jacobi, J.L.; Ngam, P.; Devitt, N.; Schilkey, F.; Reddy, A.S. A survey of the sorghum transcriptome using single-molecule long reads. *Nat. Commun.* **2016**, *7*, 11706. [CrossRef]
20. Luo, Q.; Bian, C.; Tao, M.; Huang, Y.; Zheng, Y.; Lv, Y.; Xu, J. Genome and transcriptome sequencing of the astaxanthin-producing green microalga, *Haematococcus pluvialis*. *Genome Biol. Evol.* **2019**, *11*, 166–173. [CrossRef]
21. Wayama, M.; Ota, S.; Matsuura, H.; Nango, N.; Hirata, A.; Kawano, S. Three-dimensional ultra structural study of oil and astaxanthin accumulation during encystment in the green alga *Haematococcus pluvialis*. *PLoS ONE* **2013**, *8*, e53618. [CrossRef]

22. Capelli, B.; Bagchi, D.; Cysewski, G.R. Synthetic astaxanthin is significantly inferior to algal-based astaxanthin as an antioxidant and may not be suitable as a human nutraceutical supplement. *Nutrafoods* **2013**, *12*, 145–152. [CrossRef]
23. Linden, H. Carotenoid hydroxylase from *Haematococcus pluvialis*: cDNA sequence, regulation and functional complementation. *Biochim. Biophys. Acta Gene Struct. Expr.* **1999**, *1446*, 203–212. [CrossRef]
24. Lotan, T.; Hirschberg, J. Cloning and expression in *Escherichia coli* of the gene coding β-C-4-oxygenase, that converts β-carotene to the ketocarotenoid canthaxanthin in *Haematococcus pluvialis*. *FEBS Lett.* **1995**, *364*, 125–128.
25. Kajiwara, S.; Kakizono, T.; Saito, T.; Saito, T.; Kondo, K.; Ohtani, T.; Nishio, N.; Misawa, N. Isolation and functional identification of a novel cDNA for astaxanthin biosynthesis from *Haematococcus pluvialis*, and astaxanthin synthesis in *Escherichia coli*. *Plant Mol. Biol.* **1995**, *29*, 343–352. [CrossRef] [PubMed]
26. Huang, J.C.; Chen, F.; Sandmann, G. Stress-related differential expression of multiple β-carotene ketolase genes in the unicellular green alga *Haematococcus pluvialis*. *J. Biotech.* **2006**, *122*, 176–185. [CrossRef] [PubMed]
27. Ye, L.; Zhu, X.; Wu, T.; Wang, W.; Zhao, D.; Bi, C.; Zhang, X. Optimizing the localization of astaxanthin enzymes for improved productivity. *Biotechnol. Biofuels* **2018**, *11*, 278–287. [CrossRef]
28. Henke, N.A.; Wendisch, V.F. Improved astaxanthin production with *Corynebcterium glutamicum* by application of a membrane fusion protein. *Mar. Drugs* **2019**, *17*, 621. [CrossRef]
29. Wu, Y.; Yan, P.; Liu, X.; Wang, Z.; Tang, Y.J.; Chen, T.; Zhao, X. Combinatorial expression of different β-carotene hydroxylases and ketolases in *Escherichia coli* for increased astaxanthin production. *J. Ind. Microbiol. Biotechnol.* **2019**, *46*, 1505–1516. [CrossRef]
30. Ruiz-Sola, M.A.; Coman, D.; Beck, G.; Barja, M.; Colinas, M.; Graf, A.; Gruissem, W. *Arabidopsis* GERANYLGERANYL DIPHOSPHATE SYNTHASE 11 is a hub isozyme required for the production of most photosynthesis-related isoprenoids. *New Phytol.* **2016**, *209*, 252–264. [CrossRef]
31. Liang, P.H.; Ko, T.P.; Wang, A.H.J. Structure, mechanism and function of prenyltransferases. *Eur. J. Biochem.* **2002**, *269*, 3339–3354. [CrossRef]
32. Tholl, D.; Kish, C.M.; Orlova, I.; Sherman, D.; Gershenzon, J.; Pichersky, E.; Dudareva, N. Formation of monoterpenes in *Antirrhinum majus* and *Clarkia breweri* flowers involves heterodimeric geranyldiphosphate synthases. *Plant Cell* **2004**, *16*, 977–992. [CrossRef]
33. Beck, G.; Coman, D.; Herren, E.; Ruiz-Sola, M.Á.; Rodríguez-Concepción, M.; Gruissem, W.; Vranová, E. Characterization of the GGPP synthase gene family in *Arabidopsis thaliana*. *Plant Mol. Biol.* **2013**, *82*, 393–416. [CrossRef]
34. Hsieh, F.L.; Chang, T.H.; Ko, T.P.; Wang, A.H.J. Structure and mechanism of an *Arabidopsis* medium/long-chain-length prenylpyrophosphate synthase. *Plant Physiol.* **2011**, *155*, 1079–1090. [CrossRef]
35. Lao, Y.M.; Jin, H.; Zhou, J.; Zhang, H.J.; Zhu, X.S.; Cai, Z.H. A novel hydrolytic activity of tri-functional geranylgeranyl pyrophosphate synthase in *Haematococcus pluvialis*. *Plant Cell Physiol.* **2018**, *59*, 2536–2548. [CrossRef] [PubMed]
36. Wang, J.; Lin, H.; Su, P.; Chen, T.; Guo, J.; Gao, W.; Huang, L.Q. Molecular cloning and functional characterization of multiple geranylgeranyl pyrophosphate synthase (ApGGPPS) from *Andrographis paniculata*. *Plant Cell Rep.* **2019**, *38*, 117–128. [CrossRef] [PubMed]
37. Kane, J.F. Effects of rare codon clusters on high-level expression of heterologous proteins in *Escherichia coli*. *Curr. Opin. Biotechnol.* **1995**, *6*, 494–500. [CrossRef]
38. Gustafsson, C.; Govindarajan, S.; Minshull, J. Codon bias and heterologous protein expression. *Trends Biotechnol.* **2004**, *22*, 346–353. [CrossRef] [PubMed]
39. Gao, Z.; Li, Y.; Wu, G.; Li, G.; Sun, H.; Deng, S.; Zhang, X. Transcriptome analysis in *Haematococcus pluvialis*: Astaxanthin induction by salicylic acid (SA) and jasmonic acid (JA). *PLoS ONE* **2015**, *10*, e0140609. [CrossRef]
40. Zheng, Y.; Li, Z.; Tao, M.; Li, J.; Hu, Z. Effects of selenite on green microalga *Haematococcus pluvialis*: Bioaccumulation of selenium and enhancement of astaxanthin production. *Aquat. Toxicol.* **2017**, *183*, 21–27. [CrossRef]

41. Kumar, S.; Stecher, G.; Tamura, K. MEGA7: Molecular Evolutionary Genetics Analysis version 7.0 for bigger datasets. *Mol. Biol. Evol.* **2016**, *33*, 1870–1874. [CrossRef]
42. Ma, T.; Zhou, Y.; Li, X.; Zhu, F.; Cheng, Y.; Liu, Y.; Liu, T. Genome mining of astaxanthin biosynthetic genes from Sphingomonas sp. ATCC 55669 for heterologous overproduction in *Escherichia coli*. *Biotechnol. J.* **2016**, *11*, 228–237. [CrossRef]

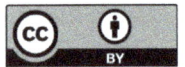

© 2019 by the authors. Licensee MDPI, Basel, Switzerland. This article is an open access article distributed under the terms and conditions of the Creative Commons Attribution (CC BY) license (http://creativecommons.org/licenses/by/4.0/).

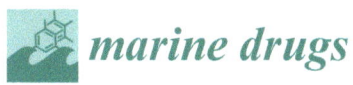

Article

Synthesis of Polysubstituted Tetrahydropyrans by Stereoselective Hydroalkoxylation of Silyl Alkenols: En Route to Tetrahydropyranyl Marine Analogues

Carlos Díez-Poza, Patricia Val, Francisco J. Pulido and Asunción Barbero *

Department of Organic Chemistry, Faculty of Science, Campus Miguel Delibes, 47011 Valladolid, Spain; solracdp@hotmail.com (C.D.-P.); patrivaldo@hotmail.com (P.V.); pulido@qo.uva.es (F.J.P.)
* Correspondence: asuncion.barbero@uva.es; Tel.: +34-983-423-214

Received: 9 September 2018; Accepted: 25 October 2018; Published: 1 November 2018

Abstract: Tetrahydropyrans are abundantly found in marine natural products. The interesting biological properties of these compounds and their analogues make necessary the development of convenient procedures for their synthesis. In this paper, an atom economy access to tetrahydropyrans by intramolecular acid-mediated cyclization of silylated alkenols is described. p-TsOH has shown to be an efficient reagent to yield highly substituted tetrahydropyrans. Moreover, excellent diastereoselectivities are obtained both for unsubstituted and alkylsubstituted vinylsilyl alcohols. The methodology herein developed may potentially be applied to the synthesis of marine drugs derivatives.

Keywords: tetrahydropyrans; acid mediated cyclization; stereoselective; marine drugs analogues

1. Introduction

Tetrahydropyrans are interesting building blocks present in a great number of bioactive marine natural products. Some representative examples include 2,2,5-trisubstituted tetrahydropyrans such as malyngolide [1], antibiotic collected from the lipid extract of cyanobacteria *Lyngbya majuscula* which shows activity against *M. Smegmatis* and *Streptococcus pyogenes*, or 2,5-disubstituted tetrahydropyrans such as rhopaloic acids A and B, which have been isolated from the marine sponge *Rhopaloeides* sp. and show potent inhibitory activity against the embryonic development of the starfish *Asterina pectinifera* [2] (Figure 1). The interesting biological properties of these scaffolds together with their scarce availability has prompted scientists to develop approaches for their synthesis. Moreover, total synthesis has the advantage of enabling the introduction of structural alterations in the molecule for the preparation of analogues with potential biological properties.

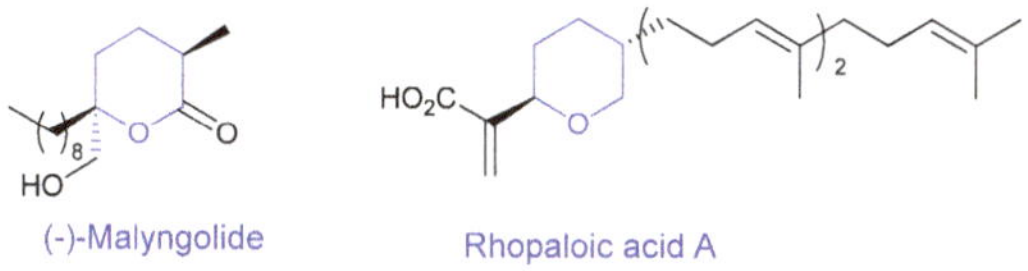

Figure 1. Illustrative examples of THP-containing marine natural products.

The synthesis of these marine products and analogues requires an effective procedure for the stereoselective construction of the tetrahydropyran ring. Different strategies have been devised for the formation of these six membered rings including nucleophilic substitution ring formation, epoxide-mediated annulations or alkene-mediated cyclizations [3,4]. Within the stoichiometric alkene-mediated cyclizations the most common electrophiles used to activate the alkene addition are mercury salts, halogens and seleno reagents. However, few number of approaches have been described on the intramolecular trapping of an alkene by an oxygenated nucleophile in the presence of an appropriate Brønsted [5–7] or Lewis acid [8–10]. Although this protocol could be considered a very efficient atom economy process, the strategy has generally proven to be of limited utility due to frequent side reactions and lack of generality [11,12]. Moreover, as far as we know, most of the described methods are focused on the regioselective formation of tetrahydropyrans with no more than one stereogenic centre. However, very few examples examine the stereoselective aspects of these processes, usually representing specific key transformations in a total synthesis rather than a general established methodology. For instance, Yamamoto has used this protocol in the synthesis of natural caparrapi oxide, where the key step is the stoichiometric acid catalysed cyclization of the corresponding γ-hydroxy alkene [13] (Scheme 1).

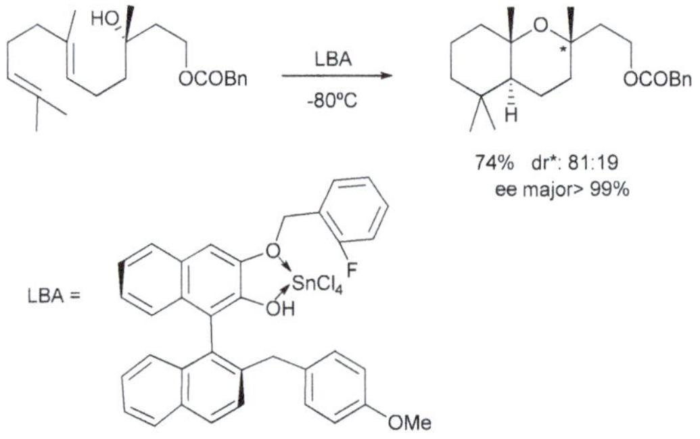

Scheme 1. Towards the synthesis of natural caparrapi oxide.

In another example Nicolaou [14] has reported the formation of the cage-like structure of natural platensimycin by the acid catalysed cyclization of the corresponding alkenol (Scheme 2).

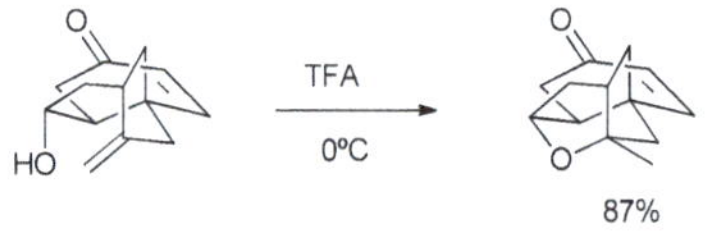

Scheme 2. Towards the synthesis of natural platensimycin.

Therefore, there is a need to develop a general and efficient method for the stereoselective synthesis of tetrahydropyrans through the acid-mediated cyclization of alkenols.

For many years our research group has been devoted to exploring new synthetic approaches to the synthesis of carbo- [15–17] and heterocycles [18,19] using the chemistry of organosilanes. Lately, Hosomi [20,21] and our group [22,23] have reported an efficient synthesis of tetrahydrofurans by intramolecular hydroalkoxylation reaction of vinyl or allylsilanes. In this paper, we report the extension of this work to the stereoselective synthesis of polysubstituted tetrahydropyrans by the acid-mediated cyclization of activated vinylsilyl alcohols.

2. Results

The δ-hydroxy alkenes needed for this study were readily prepared in three steps such as: silylcupration of alkynes and reaction with α,β-unsaturated ketones, formation of the epoxide derivative using sulphur ylides and final S_N1 opening of the epoxide with trialkylaluminum reagents [24] to obtain the corresponding primary alcohol. Unfortunately, primary alcohols **1** showed to be unstable under chromatography conditions, which made necessary to perform the following cyclization without previous purification (Scheme 3).

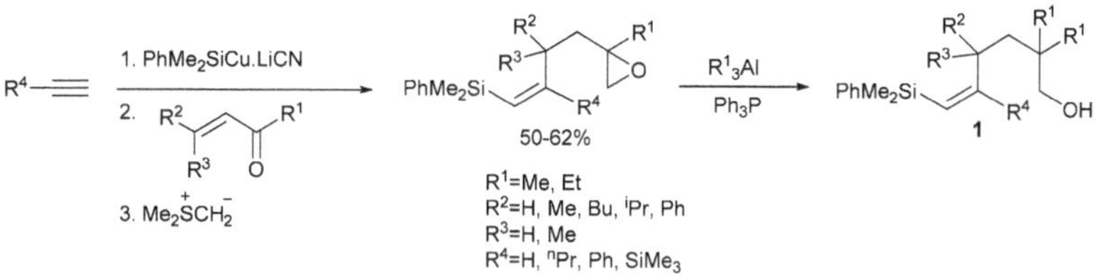

Scheme 3. Preparation of the starting vinylsilyl alcohols.

We used vinylsilyl alcohol **1a** as a model study to get the optimized conditions for this cyclization, using various Lewis and Brønsted acids. The results are shown in Table 1.

Table 1. Optimization of the acid-mediated cyclization.

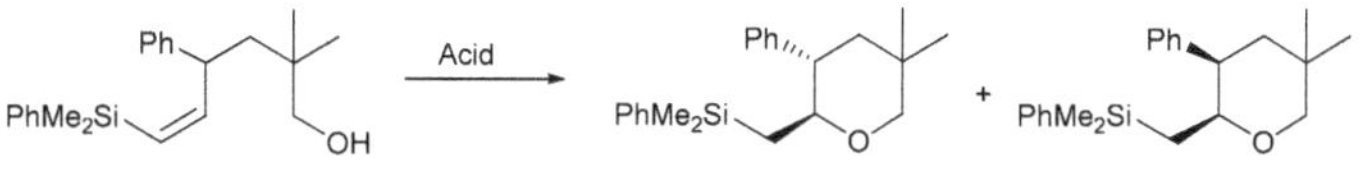

Entry	Acid [1]	Temperature (°C)	Solvent	Ratio 2a/3a [2]	Product, Yield
1	TMSOTf	−78	CH_2Cl_2		Complex mixture
2	TMSOTf	−78	Et_2O		Complex mixture
3	$TiCl_4$	−78	CH_2Cl_2		Complex mixture
4	$ZnCl_2$	−78	CH_2Cl_2		n.r. [3]
5	SiO_2	r. t.	AcOEt		n.r. [3]
6	$BF_3 \cdot OEt_2$	−78	CH_2Cl_2		n.r. [3]
7	$BF_3 \cdot OEt_2$	0	CH_2Cl_2	67:33	2a + 3a (69%)
8	$SnCl_4$	−78	CH_2Cl_2	50:50	2a + 3a (63%)
9	CSA	reflux	CH_2Cl_2		n.r. [3]
10	p-TsOH	reflux	CH_2Cl_2	>95:5	2a (77%)

[1] 1.0 equiv. of acid is used in every example. [2] The ratio of isomers **2a** and **3a** was determined by ^{1}H-NMR analysis.
[3] n.r. stands for no reaction.

p-TsOH showed to be the most efficient reagent for this cyclization (Table 1, entry 10). The reaction in the presence of TMSOTf or $TiCl_4$ gave a complex mixture (Table 1, entries 1–3), while no reaction was observed using $ZnCl_2$ or under a suspension of silica (Table 1, entries 4 and 5). $BF_3 \cdot OEt_2$ was not effective to promote the cyclization at −78 °C, although a 2:1 mixture of both possible stereoisomers was obtained in moderate yield when the reaction temperature was increased to 0 °C (Table 1, entries 6 and 7). Similarly, $SnCl_4$ mediated cyclization provided at −78 °C a 1:1 mixture of isomers in reasonable yield (Table 1, entry 8). Regarding the use of Brønsted acids, the reaction in the presence of CSA resulted to be extremely slow, while the best results were obtained by refluxing the alcohol in the presence of p-TsOH for 1 hour (Table 1, entry 10). Under these conditions tetrahydropyran **2a** was obtained in high yield and excellent diastereoselectivity (a single isomer was observed in the reaction mixture).

With these results in hand and in order to broaden the structural diversity of the tetraydropyrans obtained by this methodology, we decided to apply the optimized conditions (Table 1, entry 10) to different vinylsilyl alcohols. The results are summarized in Table 2.

Table 2. Cyclization of vinylsilyl alcohols **1a–g**.

Entry	R^1	R^2	R^3	R^4	Time (h) [1]	dr [2]	Yield (%) [3]
1	Me	Ph	H	H	1	>95:5	**2a** (77)
2	Me	Ph	H	H	4	>95:5	**2a** (62) [4]
3	Me	Ph	H	H	4	>95:5	**2a** (67) [5]
4	Me	H	H	H	1		**2b** (71)
5	Me	Me	Me	H	1		**2c** (70)
6	Me	Bu	H	H	1	>95:5	**2d** (73)
7	Me	^{i}Pr	H	H	1	>95:5	**2e** (79)
8	Me	Ph	H	^{n}Pr	1	>95:5	**2f** (71)
9	Et	Me	H	^{n}Pr	1	>95:5	**2g** (70)
10	Me	Ph	H	SiMe$_3$	3		n.r. [6]

[1] All the reactions were run at reflux temperature except where indicated. [2] The relative stereochemistry of tetrahydropyrans **2** was assigned based on the 1D-NOE experiments (in every compound 1D-crosspeak was found between CH_2-Si and CH-R^2). [3] Yields over two steps from the corresponding epoxides precursor of **1**. [4] The reaction did not go to completion when 0.5 equiv. of pTsOH were used. [5] The reaction was run at r.t. and partial desilylation of the final THP was observed. [6] n.r. stands for no reaction.

As shown, the process is high yielding and very stereoselective (both for unsubstituted and alkylsubstituted vinylsilyl alcohols) under p-TsOH mediation at reflux temperature. The short reaction time needed to reach completion may indicate the benefit of the gem-dialkyl group (Thorpe-Ingold effect), since the only example of preparation of a THP (a non-substituted one) reported by Hosomi required reflux for 96 hours [21]. The use of stoichiometric amounts of p-TsOH was proven to be the best choice, since under lower loadings of acid the reaction is slower and a certain amount of the starting vinylsilyl alcohol is always recovered (Table 2, entry 2). Moreover, at room temperature the process requires prolonged reaction time which results in lower yields due to partial protodesilylation [25] of the cyclization products (Table 2, entry 3). Furthermore, the reaction seems to be dependent on steric effects, since reaction of alcohol **1h** bearing a vinylic bulky group, such as Me$_3$Si, did not react under the shown conditions (Table 2, entry 10).

We then decided to study the effect of a phenyl group β to silicon in the rate and selectivity of the cyclization. Vinylsilyl alcohol **1i** was chosen as a model substrate for the cyclization process (Table 3).

As expected, the cyclization rate is significantly enhanced by the introduction of the phenyl group in the starting vinylsilyl alcohol. Thus, at reflux temperature the cyclization of **1i** under p-TsOH induction provides only the corresponding desilylated tetrahydropyrans (Table 3, entry 3) while at room temperature a mixture of both silylated and desilylated tetrahydropyrans are obtained. Finally, at 0 °C the reaction is fast enough to produce the cyclization products in 10 min, without side desilylative processes (Table 3, entry 5). Even CSA (either at room temperature or at 0 °C) is reactive enough to provide in good yields the cyclization tetrahydropyrans without any side product (Table 3, entries 6 and 7).

We then studied the scope of the process employing different starting alcohols under the optimized conditions (Table 3, entry 5). The results are shown in Table 4.

Table 3. Optimization of the cyclization of aryl substituted vinylsilyl alcohol **1i**.

Entry	Acid [1]	Temperature (°C)	Solvent	Time (min)	Product (yield)
1	BF$_3$·OEt$_2$	0	CH$_2$Cl$_2$	60	Desilylated THP [2] (52%)
2	SnCl$_4$	−78	CH$_2$Cl$_2$	90	Desilylated THP (48%)
3	p-TsOH	reflux	CH$_2$Cl$_2$	60	Desilylated THP (69%)
4	p-TsOH	r.t.	CH$_2$Cl$_2$	30	2i + 3i + Desilylated THP (55%) [3]
5	p-TsOH	0	CH$_2$Cl$_2$	10	2i + 3i (71%) [4]
6	CSA	r.t.	CH$_2$Cl$_2$	30	2i + 3i (70%) [4]
7	CSA	0	CH$_2$Cl$_2$	60	2i + 3i (69%) [4]

[1] 1.0 equiv. of acid is used in every example. [2] Desilylated THP accounts for 2,3,5,5-tetramethyl-2-phenyl-tetrahydropyran. [3] A 2:1 mixture of the silylated and desilylated tetrahydropyrans was obtained. [4] A 78:22 mixture of **2i**:**3i** was obtained.

Table 4. Cyclization of arylsubstituted vinylsilyl alcohols **1i–l**.

Entry	R^1	R^2	Time (min)	Product (Ratio 2:3)	Yield (%) [1]
1	Me	Me	10	78:22	2i + 3i (71)
2	Me	Ph	10	79:21	2j + 3j (65)
3	Me	^{i}Pr	10	91:9	2k + 3k (72)
4	Et	Me	10	86:14	2l + 3l (73)

[1] Yields over two steps from the epoxide precursor of **1**.

Although the cyclization of alcohols **1i–l** occurs in good yields, the stereoselectivity of the process is decreased, obtaining mixtures of both possible diastereoisomers, in which the stereoisomer with the silylmethyl group *anti* to the R^2 substituent is always predominant. The best stereoselectivity is obtained when a bulky R^2 is present at C-3 (Table 4, entry 3), which indicates that the reaction is influenced by steric effects.

A mechanism that could account for these cyclizations implies an initial protonation of the alcohol, which in turn would deliver the proton to the alkene moiety. The formation of a stabilized β to silicon carbocation will be followed by intramolecular attack of the hydroxyl group to form the tetrahydropyranyl ring.

Regarding the stereoselectivity of the process, one single diastereoisomer is obtained when R^4 is either a hydrogen or an alkyl group. However, a certain loss of stereocontrol is observed when R^4 is a phenyl group (Table 4, entries 1–4). In either case the unique or major isomer is the one in which the silylmethyl group is *anti* to the C-3 substituent.

In accordance with Fleming [26,27] and Hook's [28] models for the reaction of electrophiles with alkenes bearing an allylic stereogenic centre, two different chair-like conformations (**Ia** and **IIa**) could be drawn for vinylsilyl alcohols **1a–e**. In the preferred conformation **Ia** the allylic hydrogen is partially eclipsing the double bond ("inside"), while the largest substituent is antiperiplanar to the alkene moiety (Figure 2). The alternative conformation **IIa** (with R^2 inside) shows a disfavoured 1,3-allylic interaction between R^2 and the silyl group and a 1,3-diaxial interaction between R^2 and the Me group, which would explain the preferred formation of 2,3-*trans*-tetrahydropyranes **2a–e**.

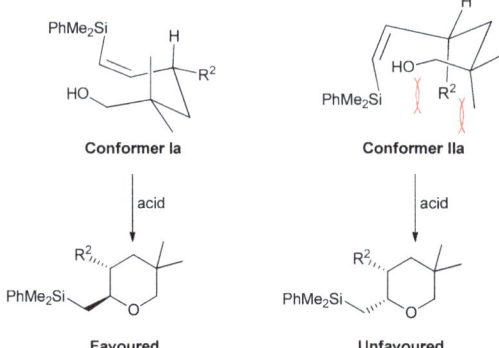

Figure 2. Stereochemical outcome of cyclization of alcohols **1a–e**.

The decrease in stereoselectivity observed for arylsubstituted vinylsilyl alcohols **1i–l** could be explained using the same model, since now, besides a disfavoured 1,3-diaxial interaction in conformer **IIb**, there is a competing 1,2-allylic interaction between R^2 and R^4 in conformer **Ib**. This interaction is especially strong when the phenyl group is coplanar with the double bond, while the possibility of rotating around would cause the loss of the resonance stabilization. For alcohols **1f–g** R^4 is a flexible alkyl chain and this 1,2-allylic interaction seems to be rather small (Figure 3).

Figure 3. Chair-like reactive conformations for arylsubstituted vinylsilyl alcohols **1i–l**.

In addition, the presence of a remaining silyl group in the final tetrahydropyrans offers the attractive possibility of further functionalization. As known, Fleming-Tamao oxidation [29] permits the transformation of the silyl group to a hydroxy group. To demonstrate the potential of these tetrahydropyrans as key intermediates for the synthesis of tetrahydropyranyl marine natural products and their synthetic analogues, we have transformed tetrahydropyran **2d** into the corresponding alcohol **3d** [30] (Scheme 4).

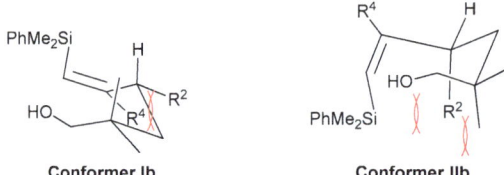

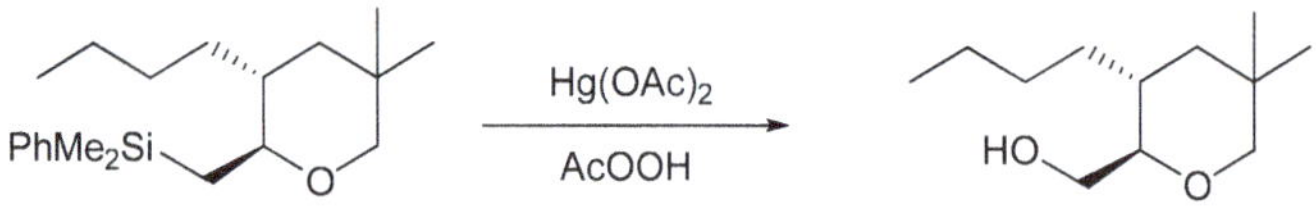

Scheme 4. Synthesis of 2-hydroxymethyltetrahydropyran **3d**.

Finally, we decided to study the effect of the silyl group in the cyclization of silyl alkenols **1**. For this purpose, we synthesized an analogue of alcohol **1e** lacking the silyl moiety (**1m**). Reaction of alcohol **1m** with p-TsOH in DCM did not occur at r.t., nor under reflux conditions, recovering after 5 hours the unreacted starting alcohol. This seems to indicate that the presence of an electron-rich alkene, such as the vinylsilane, is needed for the cyclization to proceed (Scheme 5).

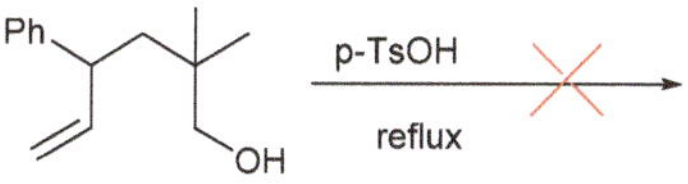

Scheme 5. Influence of the silyl group in the cyclization.

3. Materials and Methods

3.1. General Procedures for the Acid-catalysed Cyclization of Vinylsilyl Alcohols

To a solution of the acid (1 mmol) in dry CH_2Cl_2 (10 mL) is added a solution of the alcohol (1 mmol) in CH_2Cl_2. The mixture is stirred under N_2 in the shown conditions (Tables 1–4) and quenched with saturated solution of $NaHCO_3$ (5 mL). The organic layer was washed 3 times with $NaHCO_3$, dried over $MgSO_4$, evaporated in vacuo and purified by flash chromatography (EtOAc/hexane).

*3.2. Trans-5,5-Dimethyl-2-Dimethylphenylsilylmethyl-3-Phenyl-Tetrahydropyran (**2a**)*

Colourless oil (77%); ^{1}H NMR (400 MHz, $CDCl_3$) δ = 7.49–7.45 (m, 2H), 7.38–7.34 (m, 3H), 7.33–7.24 (m, 3H), 7.14–7.11 (m, 2H), 3.56 (dd, J = 11.4 and 2.4 Hz, 1H), 3.43 (td, J = 9.7 and 3.5 Hz, 1H), 3.23 (d, J = 11.4 Hz, 1H), 2.73–2.64 (m, 1H), 1.67–1.59 (m, 1H), 1.54 (t, J = 13.0 Hz, 1H), 1.19 (s, 3H), 0.92–0.87 (m, 2H, CH_2-Si), 0.88 (s, 3H), 0.33 (s, 3H, CH_3-Si), 0.29 (s, 3H, CH_3-Si); ^{13}C NMR (101 MHz, $CDCl_3$) δ = 143.9 (C), 140.0 (C), 133.7 (CH), 128.6 (CH), 128.0 (CH), 127.6 (CH), 126.3 (CH), 80.4 (CH), 78.2 (CH_2), 48.0 (CH), 46.3 (CH_2), 31.0 (C), 27.2 (CH_3), 24.2 (CH_3), 20.8 (CH_2-Si), −1.5 (CH_3), −2.5 (CH_3); HRMS (ESI+) *m/z* calcd for $C_{22}H_{30}NaOSi$ ([M + Na]$^+$): 361.1958, found 361.1957.

*3.3. 5,5-Dimethyl-2-Dimethylphenylsilylmethyl-Tetrahydropyran (**2b**)*

Colourless oil (71%); ^{1}H NMR (400 MHz, $CDCl_3$) δ = 7.63–7.56 (m, 2H), 7.45–7.38 (m, 3H), 3.46 (dd, J = 11.0 and 2.2 Hz, 1H), 3.35–3.26 (m, 1H), 3.14 (d, J = 11.0 Hz, 1H), 1.51–1.42 (m, 3H), 1.36–1.24 (m, 1H), 1.23–1.18 (m, 1H), 1.09 (dd, J = 14.5 and 7.0 Hz, 1H), 1.04 (s, 3H), 0.81 (s, 3H), 0.37 (s, 3H, CH_3-Si), 0.35 (s, 3H, CH_3-Si); ^{13}C NMR (101 MHz, $CDCl_3$) δ = 139.5 (C), 133.6 (CH), 128.8 (CH), 127.7 (CH), 78.2 (CH_2), 75.9 (CH), 37.1 (CH_2), 31.2 (CH_2), 29.6 (C), 27.2 (CH_3), 24.1 (CH_2), 23.6 (CH_3), −1.8 (CH_3), −2.2 (CH_3); HRMS (ESI+) *m/z* calcd for $C_{16}H_{26}NaOSi$ ([M + Na]$^+$): 285.1645, found 285.1646.

*3.4. 3,3,5,5-Tetramethyl-2-Dimethylphenylsilylmethyl-Tetrahydropyran (**2c**)*

Colourless oil (70%); ^{1}H NMR (400 MHz, $CDCl_3$) δ = 7.59–7.53 (m, 2H), 7.39–7.31 (m, 3H), 3.49 (dd, J = 11.1 and 2.5 Hz, 1H), 2.99–2.94 (m, 2H), 1.35 (dd, J = 13.6 and 2.5 Hz, 1H), 1.17–1.12 (m, 1H), 1.10 (s, 3H), 1.01 (s, 3H), 0.94–0.88 (m, 2H), 0.76 (s, 3H), 0.73 (s, 3H), 0.35 (s, 3H, CH_3-Si), 0.33 (s, 3H, CH_3-Si); ^{13}C NMR (101 MHz, $CDCl_3$) δ = 140.2 (C), 133.8 (CH), 128.6 (CH), 127.6 (CH), 84.0 (CH), 79.1 (CH_2), 52.2 (CH_2), 34.1 (C), 31.3 (C), 29.6 (CH_3), 29.3 (CH_3), 26.5 (CH_3), 21.6 (CH_3), 16.0 (CH_2), −1.2 (CH_3), −2.8 (CH_3); HRMS (ESI+) *m/z* calcd for $C_{18}H_{30}NaOSi$ ([M + Na]$^+$): 313.1958, found 313.1956.

*3.5. Trans-3-Butyl-5,5-Dimethyl-2-Dimethylphenylsilylmethyl-Tetrahydropyran (**2d**)*

Colourless oil (73%); ^{1}H NMR (400 MHz, $CDCl_3$) δ = 7.66–7.60 (m, 2H), 7.45–7.39 (m, 3H), 3.45 (dd, J = 11.0 and 2.6 Hz, 1H), 3.02 (d, J = 11.0 Hz, 1H), 2.94 (td, J = 10.0 and 2.8 Hz, 1H), 1.61–1.56 (m, 1H) 1.50–1.20 (m,8H), 1.06 (s, 3H), 1.00–0.91 (m, 2H), 0.93 (t, J = 7.0, 3H) 0.83 (s, 3H), 0.38 (s, 6H, $(CH_3)_2$-Si); ^{13}C NMR (101 MHz, $CDCl_3$) δ = 140.5 (C), 133.7 (CH), 128.6 (CH), 127.6 (CH), 80.9 (CH), 77.8 (CH_2), 43.2 (CH_2), 39.4 (CH), 31.8 (CH_2), 30.9 (C), 28.4 (CH_2), 27.4 (CH_3), 24.4 (CH_3), 23.0 (CH_2), 20.8 (CH_2), 14.1 (CH_3), −1.4 (CH_3), −2.4 (CH_3); HRMS (ESI+) *m/z* calcd for $C_{20}H_{34}NaOSi$ ([M + Na]$^+$): 341.2271, found 341.2271.

3.6. Trans-3-Isopropy-5,5-Dimethyl-2-Dimethylphenylsilylmethyl-Tetrahydropyran (**2e**)

Colourless oil (75%); ^{1}H NMR (400 MHz, CDCl$_3$) δ = 7.55–7.52 (m, 2H), 7.34–7.32 (m, 3H), 3.35 (dd, *J* = 11.0 and 2.7 Hz, 1H), 3.06 (td, *J* = 10.3 and 3.1 Hz, 1H), 2.92 (d, *J* = 11.0, 1H), 1.89–1.82 (m, 1H), 1.38–1.32 (m, 1H), 1.30–1.25 (m, 1H), 1.17 (dd, *J* = 14.8 and 3.1 Hz, 1H), 0.98 (s, 3H, CH$_3$), 1.00–0.97 (m, 1H), 0.90 (dd, *J* = 14.8 and 10.3 Hz, 1H), 0.81 (d, *J* = 7.0 Hz, 3H, CH$_3$), 0.78 (s, 3H, CH$_3$), 0.63 (d, *J* = 6.9 Hz, 3H, CH$_3$), 0.31 (s, 3H, CH$_3$-Si), 0.30 (s, 3H, CH$_3$-Si);^{13}C NMR (101 MHz, CDCl$_3$) δ = 140.5 (C), 133.6 (CH), 128.5 (CH), 127.6 (CH), 79.1 (CH), 77.9 (CH$_2$), 44.1 (CH), 35.7 (CH$_2$), 30.7 (C), 27.6 (CH), 26.9 (CH$_3$), 24.4 (CH$_3$), 21.0 (CH$_3$), 20.3 (CH$_2$-Si), 15.3 (CH$_3$), −1.4 (CH$_3$), −2.5 (CH$_3$); HRMS (ESI+) *m/z* calcd for C$_{19}$H$_{32}$NaOSi ([M + Na]$^+$): 327.2110, found 327.2115.

3.7. 5,5-Dimethyl-2-Dimethylphenylsilylmethyl-3-Phenyl-2-Propyl-Tetrahydropyran (**2f**)

Colourless oil (71%); ^{1}H NMR (400 MHz, CDCl$_3$) δ = 7.58–7.19 (m, 10H), 3.21 (d, *J* = 11.6, 1H), 3.15 (dd, *J* = 11.6 and 2.4 Hz, 1H), 3.00 (dd, *J* = 13.5 and 3.7 Hz, 1H), 2.17–2.06 (m, 1H), 2.01 (t, *J* = 13.5 Hz, 1H), 1.24–1.17 (m, 2H), 1.34 (dt, *J* = 13.5 and 3.5 Hz,1H), 1.23 (d, *J* = 15.4, 1H, C*H*HSi), 1.13 (d, *J* = 15.4, 1H, CH*H*Si), 1.00 (s, 3H), 0.97–0.92 (m, 1H),0.88 (d, *J* = 7.3 Hz, 3H), 0.85 (s, 3H), 0.50 (s, 3H, CH$_3$-Si), 0.35 (s, 3H, CH$_3$-Si); ^{13}C NMR (101 MHz, CDCl$_3$) δ = 142.9 (C), 141.8 (C), 133.7 (CH), 129.7 (CH), 128.3 (CH), 127.8 (CH), 127.5 (CH), 126.3 (CH), 78.8 (C), 71.1 (CH$_2$), 48.4 (CH), 39.9 (CH$_2$), 32.8 (CH$_2$), 30.8 (C), 27.8 (CH$_3$), 26.6 (CH$_2$-Si), 24.8 (CH$_3$), 15.4 (CH$_2$), 14.7 (CH$_3$), −0.3 (CH$_3$), −0.4 (CH$_3$); HRMS (ESI+) *m/z* calcd for C$_{25}$H$_{36}$NaOSi ([M + Na]$^+$): 406.2428, found 403.2435.

3.8. 5,5-Diethyl-3-Methyl-2-Dimethylphenylsilylmethyl-2-Propyl-Tetrahydropyran (**2g**)

Colourless oil (70%); ^{1}H NMR (400 MHz, CDCl$_3$) δ = 7.54–7.31 (m, 5H), 3.17 (d, *J* = 11.7 Hz, 1H), 3.08 (dd, *J* = 11.7 Hz, 1H), 1.95–1.89 (m, 1H), 1.55–1.41 (m, 7H), 1.31–1.24 (m, 3H), 1.07–0.99 (m, 2H), 0.90–0.82 (m 6H), 0.80 (t, *J* = 7.0 Hz, 3H), 0.73 (t, *J* = 7.5 Hz, 3H), 0.67 (d, *J* = 6.9 Hz, 3H), 0.37 (s, 3H, CH$_3$-Si), 0.31 (s, 3H, CH$_3$-Si); ^{13}C NMR (101 MHz, CDCl$_3$) δ = 141.2 (C), 133.4 (CH), 128.5 (CH), 127.6 (CH), 79.8 (C), 69.0 (CH$_2$), 43.2 (CH$_2$), 37.1 (CH$_2$), 35.5 (C), 30.4 (CH), 28.7 (CH$_2$), 23.6 (CH$_2$), 17.6 (CH$_3$), 17.1 (CH$_2$), 16.1 (CH$_2$), 14.6 (CH$_3$), 7.5 (CH$_3$), 6.9 (CH$_3$), −0.4 (CH$_3$), −1.0 (CH$_3$); HRMS (ESI+) *m/z* calcd for C$_{22}$H$_{38}$NaOSi ([M + Na]$^+$): 369.2584, found 369.2582.

3.9. 3,5,5-Trimethyl-2-Dimethylphenylsilylmethyl-2-Phenyl-Tetrahydropyrans **2i** *and* **3i**

Chromatography gave tetrahydrofurans **2i** and **3i** as a mixture. Colourless oil (71%).

(**2i**): ^{1}H NMR (400 MHz, CDCl$_3$) δ = 7.53–7.51 (m, 2H), 7.49–7.46 (m, 2H), 7.34–7.26 (m, 5H), 7.23–7.19 (m, 1H), 3.26 (d, *J* = 11.8, 1H), 3.19 (dd, *J* = 11.8 and 2.3 Hz, 1H), 1.79–1.73 (m, 1H), 1.74 (d, *J* = 15.4 Hz, 1H, C*H*HSi), 1.44 (d, *J* = 15.4 Hz, 1H, CH*H*Si), 1.35–1.23 (m, 2H), 1.13 (s, 3H), 0.80 (s, 3H), 0.68 (d, *J* = 6.8 Hz, 3H), 0.14 (s, 3H, CH$_3$-Si), −0.13 (s, 3H, CH$_3$-Si); ^{13}C NMR (101 MHz, CDCl$_3$) δ = 147.5 (C), 141.1 (C), 133.4 (CH), 128.5 (CH), 127.6 (CH), 127.4 (CH), 126.3 (CH), 126.1 (CH), 81.6 (C), 71.9 (CH$_2$), 42.7 (CH$_2$), 39.0 (CH), 30.9 (C), 27.4 (CH$_3$), 24.2 (CH$_3$), 17.2 (CH$_3$), 13.7 (CH$_2$-Si), −1.4 (CH$_3$), −1.5 (CH$_3$); HRMS (ESI+) *m/z* calcd for C$_{23}$H$_{32}$OSi ([M + Na]$^+$): 375.2110, found 375.2115.

(**3i**): distinguishable signals: ^{1}H NMR (400 MHz, CDCl$_3$) δ = 3.32 (d, *J* = 11.7, 1H), 2.07–2.00 (m, 1H), 0.96 (s, 3H), 0.89 (s, 3H), 0.78 (d, *J* = 7.2 Hz, 3H), 0.22 (s, 3H), 0.07 (s, 3H); ^{13}C NMR (101 MHz, CDCl$_3$) δ = 28.2 (CH$_3$), 26.4 (CH$_3$), 19.0 (CH$_3$).

3.10. 5,5-Dimethyl-2-Dimethylphenylsilylmethyl-2,3-Diphenyl-Tetrahydropyrans **2j** *and* **3j**

Chromatography gave tetrahydrofurans **2j** and **3j** as a mixture. Colourless oil (65%).

(**2j**): ^{1}H NMR (400 MHz, CDCl$_3$) δ = 7.44–7.13 (m, 13H), 6.74–6.71 (m, 2H), 3.46 (d, *J* = 11.8, 1H), 3.31 (dd, *J* = 11.8 and 2.3 Hz, 1H), 2.98 (dd, *J* = 13.7 and 1.5 Hz, 1H), 2.12–2.05 (m, 2H, C*H*HSi), 1.49 (dt, *J* = 13.6 and 2.8 Hz, 1H), 1.27 (d, *J* = 14.9 Hz, 1H, CH*H*Si), 1.22 (s, 3H), 0.92 (s, 3H), 0.13 (s, 3H, CH$_3$-Si), −0.20 (s, 3H, CH$_3$-Si); ^{13}C NMR (101 MHz, CDCl$_3$) δ = 146.29 (C), 141.56 (C), 140.9 (C), 133.4 (CH), 129.9 (CH), 128.5 (CH), 127.6 (CH), 127.2 (CH), 126.9 (CH), 126.4 (CH), 126.4 (CH), 126.3 (CH), 81.4

(C), 71.7 (CH$_2$), 51.9 (CH), 40.3 (CH$_2$), 31.1 (C), 27.5 (CH$_3$), 24.0 (CH$_3$), 15.4 (CH$_2$-Si), −1.4 (CH$_3$), −1.5 (CH$_3$); HRMS (ESI+) m/z calcd for C$_{28}$H$_{35}$OSi ([M + H]$^+$): 415.2450, found 415.2452.

(**3j**): distinguishable signals: ^{1}H NMR (400 MHz, CDCl$_3$) δ = 3.52 (d, J = 11.9, 1H), 3.38 (dd, J = 11.9 and 1.5 Hz, 1H), 3.16 (dd, J = 13.6 and 2.1 Hz, 1H), 1.89 (d, J = 14.9 Hz, 1H, C*H*HSi), 1.84 (d, J = 14.9 Hz, 1H, CH*H*Si), 1.75 (dd, J = 13.6 and 13.1 Hz, 1H), 1.22 (s, 3H), 0.96 (s, 3H), 0.14 (s, 3H, CH$_3$-Si), −0.26 (s, 3H, CH$_3$-Si); ^{13}C NMR (101 MHz, CDCl$_3$) δ = 129.3 (CH), 128.3 (CH), 127.9 (CH), 127.5 (CH), 127.23 (CH), 126.5 (CH), 126.2 (CH), 126.1 (CH), 82.9 (C), 70.6 (CH$_2$), 51.8 (CH), 38.2 (CH$_2$), 32.8 (C), 29.3 (CH$_3$), 28.1 (CH$_2$), 25.0 (CH$_3$), −2.1 (CH$_3$).

3.11. 3-Isopropyl-5,5-Dimethyl-2-Dimethylphenylsilylmethyl-2-Phenyl-Tetrahydropyrans **2k** and **3k**

Chromatography gave tetrahydrofurans **2k** and **3k** as a mixture. Colourless oil (72%).

(**2k**): ^{1}H NMR (400 MHz, CDCl$_3$) δ = 7.52–7.19 (m, 10H), 3.23 (d, J = 11.6, 1H), 3.15 (dd, J = 11.6 and 2.3 Hz, 1H), 1.85 (d, J = 15.3, 1H, C*H*HSi), 1.60–1.58 (m, 1H), 1.59 (dd, J = 13.1 and 5.4 Hz, 1H), 1.47 (d, J = 15.3, 1H, CH*H*Si), 1.33 (t, J = 13.1 Hz, 1H), 1.25–1.23 (m, 1H), 1.12 (s, 3H), 0.82 (s, 3H), 0.78 (d, J = 6.8 Hz, 3H), 0.48 (d, J = 6.8 Hz, 3H), 0.12 (s, 3H, CH$_3$-Si), −0.10 (s, 3H, CH$_3$-Si); ^{13}C NMR (101 MHz, CDCl$_3$) δ = 147.3 (C), 141.2 (C), 133.5 (CH), 128.4 (CH), 127.6 (CH), 127.3 (CH), 126.5 (CH), 126.3 (CH), 82.3 (C), 72.1 (CH$_2$), 49.4 (CH), 34.0 (CH$_2$), 30.6 (C), 27.8 (CH$_3$), 25.2 (CH), 23.9 (CH$_3$), 23.8 (CH$_3$), 17.9 (CH$_3$), 15.9 (CH$_2$-Si), −1.1 (CH$_3$), −1.3 (CH$_3$); HRMS (ESI+) m/z calcd for C$_{25}$H$_{37}$OSi ([M + H]$^+$): 381.2608, found 381.2610.

(**3k**): distinguishable signals: ^{1}H NMR (400 MHz, CDCl$_3$) δ = 2.00 (d, J = 15.2, 1H, C*H*HSi), 1.79–1.73 (m, 1H), 1.31 (d, J = 15.2, 1H, CH*H*Si), 1.60–1.58 (m, 1H), 1.15 (s, 3H), 1.07–0.92 (m, 2H), 0.82 (d, J = 6.7 Hz, 3H), 0.81 (s, 3H), 0.10 (s, 3H, CH$_3$-Si), −0.18 (s, 3H, CH$_3$-Si), −0.26 (d, J = 6.7 Hz, 3H); ^{13}C NMR (101 MHz, CDCl$_3$) δ = 133.4 (CH), 128.3 (CH), 127.5 (CH), 127.4 (CH), 126.4 (CH), 82.1 (C), 70.2 (CH$_2$), 50.6 (CH), 32.1 (C), 31.9 (CH$_2$), 29.6 (CH$_3$), 26.6 (CH$_2$-Si), 25.9 (CH), 24.9 (CH$_3$), 24.3 (CH$_3$), 16.1 (CH$_3$), −1.5 (CH$_3$), −1.9 (CH$_3$).

3.12. 5,5-Diethyl-3-Methyl-2-Dimethylphenylsilylmethyl-2-Phenyl-Tetrahydropyrans **2l** and **3l**

Chromatography gave tetrahydrofurans **2l** and **3l** as a mixture. Colourless oil (73%).

(**2l**): ^{1}H NMR (400 MHz, CDCl$_3$) δ = 7.51–7.18 (m, 10H), 3.31 (d, J = 11.8, 1H), 3.18 (dd, J = 11.8 and 2.2 Hz, 1H), 1.73 (d, J = 15.5, 1H, C*H*HSi), 1.70–1.60 (m, 3H), 1.42 (d, J = 15.5, 1H, CH*H*Si), 1.41–1.33 (m, 1H), 1.16–1.08 (m, 3H), 0.78 (t, J = 7.4 Hz, 3H,), 0.74 (t, J = 7.3 Hz, 3H), 0.67 (d, J = 6.8 Hz, 3H,), 0.13 (s, 3H, CH$_3$-Si), −0.13 (s, 3H, CH$_3$-Si); ^{13}C NMR (101 MHz, CDCl$_3$) δ = 147.7 (C), 141.1 (C), 133.4 (CH), 128.5 (CH), 127.6 (CH), 127.4 (CH), 126.2 (CH), 126.1 (CH), 81.7 (C), 69.0 (CH$_2$), 38.3 (CH), 38.1 (CH$_2$), 35.4 (C), 28.6 (CH$_2$), 23.8 (CH$_2$), 17.3 (CH$_3$), 13.9 (CH$_2$-Si), 7.5 (CH$_3$), 7.0 (CH$_3$), −1.4 (CH$_3$), −1.5 (CH$_3$); HRMS (ESI+) m/z calcd for C$_{25}$H$_{36}$NaOSi ([M + Na]$^+$): 406.2428, found 403.2436.

(**3l**): distinguishable signals: ^{13}C NMR (101 MHz, CDCl$_3$) δ = 144.2 (C), 128.3 (CH), 127.6 (CH), 127.5 (CH), 127.2 (CH), 68.6 (CH$_2$), 38.5 (CH), 36.7 (CH$_2$), 28.9 (CH$_2$), 28.5 (CH$_2$), 26.4 (CH$_2$), 18.9 (CH$_3$), 14.0 (CH$_3$), 7.6 (CH$_3$), −1.6 (CH$_3$), −1.9 (CH$_3$).

3.13. Procedure for the Fleming-Tamao Oxidation of Silyl Tetrahydropyran **2d**

Mercuric acetate (0.466 mmol, 1.5 eq) was added to a solution of **2d** (0.311 mmol) in peracetic acid (35–40% solution in dilute acetic acid; 2 mL) and the mixture was stirred for 3 h at room temperature. Toluene (6 mL) was added and the mixture of solvents was evaporated under reduced pressure. The residue was taken up in ether, filtered and evaporated under reduced pressure. Purification by flash column chromatography (hexane/EtOAc, 3:1 to pure EtOAc) yielded **3d** (0.186 mmol, 60%) as a white viscous liquid (melting point could not be measured). Rf = 0.4 (silica, hexane/EtOAc, 4:1).

3.14. Trans-2-Hydroxymethyl-3-Butyl-5,5-Dimethyl-Tetrahydropyran (**3d**)

^{1}H NMR (400 MHz, CDCl$_3$) δ = 3.80 (dd, J = 11.4, 2.8 Hz, 1H), 3.56 (dd, J = 11.4, 7.1 Hz, 1H), 3.48 (dd, J = 10.9, 2.5 Hz, 1H), 3.12 (d, J = 10.9 Hz, 1H), 3.04–2.95 (m, 1H), 2.10–1.97 (brs, 1H, OH),

1.65–1.61 (m, 1H), 1.61–1.58 (m, 1H), 1.37–1.13 (m, 5H), 1.01 (s, 3H), 0.98–0.95 (m, 1H), 0.94–0.90 (m, 1H), 0.88 (t, J = 7.1 Hz, 3H), 0.82 (s, 3H); ^{13}C NMR (101 MHz, CDCl$_3$) δ = 82.4 (CH), 77.7 (CH$_2$), 63.9 (CH$_2$OH), 42.7 (CH$_2$), 32.6 (CH, Bu), 31.2 (CH$_2$), 30.9 (C), 28.3 (CH$_2$), 27.2 (CH$_3$), 24.0 (CH$_3$), 22.9 (CH$_2$), 14.0 (CH$_3$, Bu); HRMS (ESI+) m/z calcd for C$_{12}$H$_{24}$NaO$_2$ ([M + Na]$^+$): 223.1669, found 223.1667.

4. Conclusions

In conclusion, a general and efficient methodology for the synthesis of tetrahydropyrans by the acid-mediated cyclizations of vinylsilyl alcohols is described. The reaction leading to polysubstituted tetrahydropyrans is highly stereoselective when R^4 is either H or alkyl group. Worthy of note, quaternary centres adjacent to the oxygen can be formed through the process. The formation of a single diastereoisomer in these cases (THP with the phenyldimethylsilylmethyl group anti to the C-3 substituent) seems to be a consequence of an unfavourable 1,3-diaxial interaction in the alternative reactive conformation. Moreover, the presence of the silyl group bonded to the alkenyl moiety seems to be needed for the cyclization to take place. Further transformation of the silylated tetrahydropyrans thus obtained into the corresponding hydroxymethyl tetrahydropyrans opens an attractive route for the synthesis of marine drugs analogues.

Supplementary Materials: Copies of ^{1}H-NMR and ^{13}C-NMR are available online at http://www.mdpi.com/1660-3397/16/11/421/s1.

Author Contributions: Chemical synthesis and characterization, C.D.-P. and P.V.; supervision, F.J.P.; project conceptualization, supervision, writing—review and editing, A.B.

Funding: We thank the "Junta de Castilla y León" (GR170) for financial support. C.D.-P. acknowledges a predoctoral Grant (Q4718001C), funded by the European Social Fund and the "Junta de Castilla y León".

Conflicts of Interest: The authors declare no conflict of interest.

References

1. Cardllina, J.H.; Moore, R.E. Structure and absolute configuration of malyngolide, an antibiotic from the marine blue-green alga Lyngbya majuscula Gomont. *J. Org. Chem.* **1979**, *44*, 4039–4042. [CrossRef]
2. Yanai, M.; Ohta, S.; Ohta, E.; Ikegami, S. Novel norsesterterpenes, which inhibit gastrulation of the starfish embryo, from the marine sponge Rhopaloeides sp. *Tetrahedron* **1998**, *54*, 15607–15612. [CrossRef]
3. Larrosa, I.; Romea, P.; Urpí, F. Synthesis of six-membered oxygenated heterocycles through carbon–oxygen bond-forming reactions. *Tetrahedron* **2008**, *64*, 2683–2723. [CrossRef]
4. Cossy, J. *Synthesis of Saturated Oxygenated Heterocycles. 5- and 6-Membered Rings I*; Springer: Berlin, Germany, 2014; pp. 43–97, ISBN 13978-3-642-41472-5.
5. Coulombel, L.; Duñach, E. Triflic acid-catalysed cyclisation of unsaturated alcohols. *Green Chem.* **2004**, *6*, 499–501. [CrossRef]
6. Jeong, Y.; Kim, D.Y.; Choi, Y.; Ryu, J.S. Intramolecular hydroalkoxylation in Brønsted acidic ionic liquids and its application to the synthesis of (±)-centrolobine. *Org. Biomol. Chem.* **2011**, *9*, 374–378. [CrossRef] [PubMed]
7. Linares-Palomino, P.J.; Salido, S.; Altarejo, J.; Sánchez, A. Chlorosulfonic acid as a convenient electrophilic olefin cyclization agent. *Tetrahedron Lett.* **2003**, *44*, 6651–6655. [CrossRef]
8. Coulombel, L.; Favier, I.; Duñach, E. Catalytic formation of C–O bonds by alkene activation: Lewis acid-cycloisomerisation of olefinic alcohols. *Chem. Commun.* **2005**, 2286–2288. [CrossRef] [PubMed]
9. Dzudza, A.; Marks, T.J. Efficient Intramolecular Hydroalkoxylation of Unactivated Alkenols Mediated by Recyclable Lanthanide Triflate Ionic Liquids: Scope and Mechanism. *Chem. Eur. J.* **2010**, *16*, 3403–3422. [CrossRef] [PubMed]
10. Zhu, X.; Li, G.; Xu, F.; Zhang, Y.; Xue, M.; Shen, Q. Investigation and mechanistic study into intramolecular hydroalkoxylation of unactivated alkenols catalysed by cationic lanthanide complexes. *Tetrahedron* **2017**, *73*, 1451–1458. [CrossRef]
11. Rosenfeld, D.C.; Shekharm, S.; Takemiya, A.; Utsunomiya, M.; Hartwig, J.F. Hydroamination and Hydroalkoxylation Catalyzed by Triflic Acid. Parallels to Reactions Initiated with Metal Triflates. *Org. Lett.* **2006**, *8*, 4179–4182. [CrossRef] [PubMed]

12. Oe, Y.; Ohta, T.; Ito, Y. Ruthenium catalysed addition reaction of carboxylic acid across olefins without β-hydride elimination. *Chem. Commun.* **2004**, 1620–1621. [CrossRef] [PubMed]
13. Uyanik, M.; Ishihara, K.; Yamamoto, H. Biomimetic synthesis of acid-sensitive (−)- and (+)-caparrapi oxides, (−)- and (+)-8-epicaparrapi oxides and (+)-dysifragin induced by artificial cyclases. *Bioorg. Med. Chem.* **2005**, *13*, 5055–5065. [CrossRef] [PubMed]
14. Nicolaou, K.C.; Li, A.; Edmonds, D.J. Total Synthesis of Platensimycin. *Angew. Chem. Int. Ed.* **2006**, *45*, 7086–7090. [CrossRef] [PubMed]
15. Barbero, A.; Blanco, Y.; Pulido, F.J. Silylcuprates from Allene and Their Reaction with α,β-Unsaturatedd Nitriles and Imines. Synthesis of Silylated Oxo Compounds Leading to Cyclopentane and Cycloheptane Ring Formation. *J. Org. Chem.* **2005**, *70*, 6876–6883. [CrossRef] [PubMed]
16. Barbero, A.; Castreño, P.; Pulido, F.J. Spiro-Cyclopropanation from Oxoallylsilanes. *J. Am. Chem. Soc.* **2005**, *127*, 8022–8023. [CrossRef] [PubMed]
17. Barbero, A.; Castreño, P.; Pulido, F.J. Acid-Catalyzed Cyclization of Epoxyallylsilanes. An Unusual Rearrangement Cyclization Process. *Org. Lett.* **2003**, *5*, 4045–4048. [CrossRef] [PubMed]
18. Diez-Varga, A.; Barbero, H.; Pulido, F.J.; González-Ortega, A.; Barbero, A. Competitive Silyl–Prins Cyclization versus Tandem Sakurai–Prins Cyclization: An Interesting Substitution Effect. *Chem. Eur. J.* **2014**, *20*, 14112–14119. [CrossRef] [PubMed]
19. Barbero, A.; Diez-Varga, A.; Herrero, M.; Pulido, F.J. From Silylated Trishomoallylic Alcohols to Dioxaspiroundecanes or Oxocanes: Catalyst and Substitution Influence. *J. Org. Chem.* **2016**, *81*, 2704–2712. [CrossRef] [PubMed]
20. Miura, K.; Okajima, S.; Hondo, T.; Hosomi, A. Silicon-directed cyclization of vinylsilanes bearing hydroxy group catalysed by an acid. *Tetrahedron Lett.* **1995**, *36*, 1483–1486. [CrossRef]
21. Miura, K.; Okajima, S.; Hondo, T.; Nakagawa, T.; Takahashi, T.; Hosomi, A. Acid-Catalyzed Cyclization of Vinylsilanes Bearing a Hydroxy Group: A New Method for Stereoselective Synthesis of Disubstituted Tetrahydrofurans. *J. Am. Chem. Soc.* **2000**, *122*, 11348–11357. [CrossRef]
22. Pulido, F.J.; Barbero, A.; Val, P.; Diez, A.; González-Ortega, A. Efficiency of Acid- and Mercury-Catalyzed Cyclization Reactions in the Synthesis of Tetrahydrofurans from Allylsilyl Alcohols. *Eur. J. Org. Chem.* **2012**, 5350–5356. [CrossRef]
23. Barbero, A.; Barbero, H.; González-Ortega, A.; Pulido, F.J.; Val, P.; Diez-Varga, A.; Morán, J.R. Efficient access to polysubstituted tetrahydrofurans by electrophilic cyclization of vinylsilyl alcohols. *RSC Adv.* **2015**, *5*, 49541–49551. [CrossRef]
24. Schneider, C.; Brauner, J. Lewis Base-Catalyzed Addition of Trialkylaluminum Compounds to Epoxides. *Eur. J. Org. Chem.* **2001**, 4445–4450. [CrossRef]
25. Hatakeyama, S.; Sugawara, K.; Takano, S. Stereocontrolled construction of substituted pyrrolidines based on intramolecular protodesilylation reaction. Enantiospecific synthesis of (−)-kainic acid and (+)-allokainic acid from L-serine. *J. Chem. Soc. Chem. Commun.* **1993**, *2*, 125–127. [CrossRef]
26. Fleming, I. Stereocontrol in Organic Synthesis using silicon compounds. In *Frontiers in Natural Product Chemistry*; Atta-ur-Rahman, Choudhary, M.I., Kahn, K.M., Eds.; Bentham Scientific Publishers: Karachi, Pakistan, 2005; pp. 55–64, ISBN 978-1-60805-676-7.
27. Fleming, I.; Barbero, A.; Walter, D. Stereochemical Control in Organic Synthesis Using Silicon-Containing Compounds. *Chem. Rev.* **1997**, *97*, 2063–2192. [CrossRef] [PubMed]
28. Paddon-Row, M.N.; Rondan, N.G.; Houk, K.N. Staggered models for asymmetric induction: Attack trajectories and conformations of allylic bonds from ab initio transition structures of addition reactions. *J. Am. Chem. Soc.* **1982**, *104*, 7162–7166. [CrossRef]
29. Fleming, I.; Henning, R.; Parker, D.C.; Plaut, H.E.; Sanderson, P.E.J. The phenyldimethylsilyl group as a masked hydroxy group. *J. Chem. Soc. Perkin Trans. 1* **1995**, *4*, 317–337. [CrossRef]
30. Maezaki, N.; Matsumori, Y.; Shogaki, T.; Soejima, M.; Ohishi, H.; Tanaka, T.; Iwata, C. Stereoselective Synthesis of a 2,2,5-Trisubstituted Tetrahydropyran Chiron via 1,3- and 1,6-Asymmetric Induction: A Total Synthesis of (−)-Malyngolide. *Tetrahedron* **1998**, *54*, 13087–13104. [CrossRef]

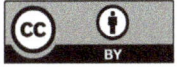

© 2018 by the authors. Licensee MDPI, Basel, Switzerland. This article is an open access article distributed under the terms and conditions of the Creative Commons Attribution (CC BY) license (http://creativecommons.org/licenses/by/4.0/).

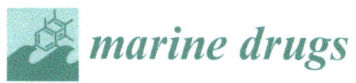

Article

Asymmetric Synthesis of the C15–C32 Fragment of Alotamide and Determination of the Relative Stereochemistry

Hao-yun Shi [1,2], Yang Xie [1], Pei Hu [1], Zi-qiong Guo [1,2], Yi-hong Lu [1,2], Yu Gao [1,*] and Cheng-gang Huang [1,2,*]

1. Shanghai Institute of Materia Medica, Chinese Academy of Sciences, 501 Haike Road, Shanghai 201203, China; baiyinyun@hotmail.com (H.-y.S.), sunshine_xie@163.com (Y.X.); hupeishtcm@126.com (P.H.); 18673675362@163.com (Z.-q.G.); xiong1743771101@163.com (Y.-h.L.)
2. School of Pharmacy, University of Chinese Academy of Sciences, No. 19A Yuquan Road, Beijing 100049, China
* Corresponding: gaoyucpu@126.com (Y.G.); cghsimm@126.com (C.-g.H.); Tel.: +86-21-2023-1963 (Y.G.)

Received: 15 October 2018; Accepted: 24 October 2018; Published: 30 October 2018

Abstract: Alotamide is a cyclic depsipetide isolated from a marine cyanobacterium and possesses a unique activation of calcium influx in murine cerebrocortical neurons (EC$_{50}$ 4.18 µM). Due to its limited source, the three stereocenters (C19, C28, and C30) in its polyketide fragment remain undetermined. In this study, the first asymmetric synthesis of its polyketide fragment was achieved. Four relative possible diastereomers were constructed with a boron-mediated enantioselective aldol reaction and Julia–Kocienski olefination as the key steps. Comparison of ^{13}C NMR spectra revealed the relative structure of fragment C15–C32 of alotamide.

Keywords: alotamide; asymmetric synthesis; relative structural determination

1. Introduction

Recently, several active secondary metabolites have been isolated from marine cyanobacterium and some of these metabolites demonstrate excellent bioactivities such as cytotoxic, antimicrobial, and antiprotozoal properties [1,2]. For example, apratoxins display potent cytotoxicity against several cancer cells at the nanoscale level and have become the new lead compounds in anticancer drug discovery [3–6].

Alotamide was also isolated from the marine cyanobacterium *Lyngbya bouillonii* in 2009 [7]. It is a cyclic depsipetide and structurally has two parts. The northern part is a tripetide that consists of N-Me-Val, Cys-derived thiazolene ring, and Pro and the southern part is a special unsaturated polyketide with three undetermined stereocenters (C19, C28, and C30). Functionally, alotamide is a unique calcium influx activator in murine cerebrocortical neurons (EC$_{50}$ 4.18 µM). Given that calcium overload is involved in physiological processes and may lead to several nervous diseases such as AD and epilepsy, this compound has gained increasing attention as a new neurotoxin from the marine resource [8]. In view of the limited natural source, a concise synthetic strategy of alotamide should be developed. In this study, we described the first asymmetric synthesis of its polyketide fragment C15–C32 and obtained four possible diastereomers. The relative stereochemistry was assigned after the NMR comparison.

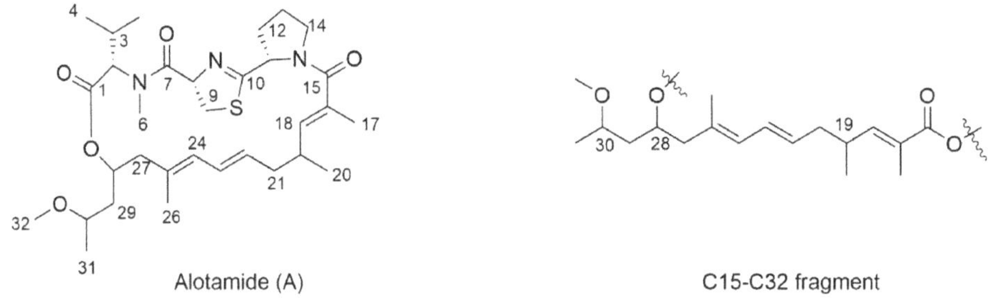

Figure 1. Structure of alotamide.

2. Results

The chemical structure of alotamide is shown in Figure 1. The southern polyketide with three undetermined stereocenters established eight possible isomers and only four needed to be evaluated for relative stereochemical determination. In this regard, we set C19 as R and listed four diastereomers, which are shown in Figure 2 (**1a–1d**).

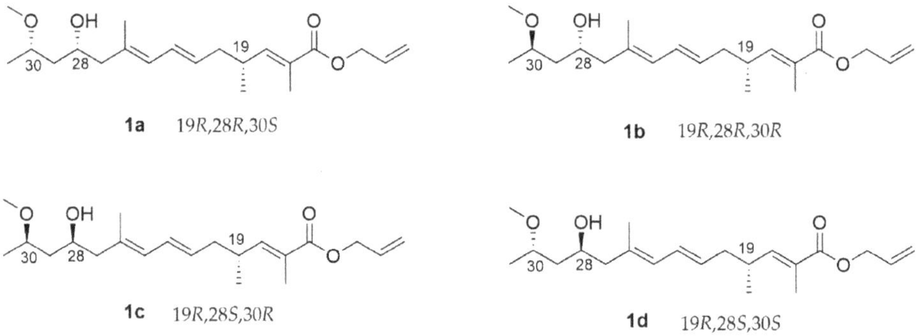

Figure 2. Structures of four diastereomers **1a–1d**.

According to the retrosynthetic analysis (Scheme 1), the dihydroxy unit would arise from an asymmetric aldol reaction and the Julia–Kocienski olefination would be applied to form the diene part. The polyketide fragment would be separated into two subunits, **2** and **3**, which both could be prepared from commercial compounds.

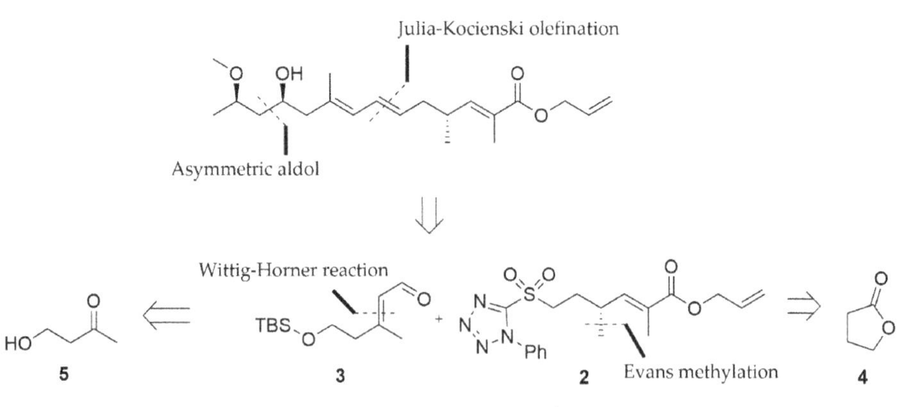

Scheme 1. Retrosynthetic analysis.

Compound **2** was prepared from commercial lactone **4** and treated with LiOH to open the lactone ring (Scheme 2) [9]. The resulting compound was subjected to TBS protection and condensation with Evan's protocol **6** [10] in sequence to obtain **7** in 71% yield over three steps. Compound **7** was treated with NaHMDS/MeI at −78 °C to obtain the desired R-methyl **8** in 89% yield (dr = 12:1). After the reduction of **8** by LiBH$_4$ [11], alcohol **9** was oxidized into the corresponding aldehyde, which was immediately refluxed with the Wittig reagent **10** to generate olefin **11**. In this reaction, the E/Z selectivity reached 30:1 and the little Z isomer was separated in the following DIBAL-H reduction. The sequential oxidation with IBX and Pinnick reaction generated a free acid and the allyl protection was conducted to acquire **12** in 64% yield for the above four steps. After the deprotection of the TBS group, the Mitsunobu reaction was applied to convert the compound **13** into tetrazole **15** in 94% yield. Then the SPT part was oxidized by H$_2$O$_2$ (20 eq) in the presence of (NH$_4$)$_6$Mo$_7$O$_{24}$ (0.2 eq) to obtain the desired **2** without the Z isomer [12].

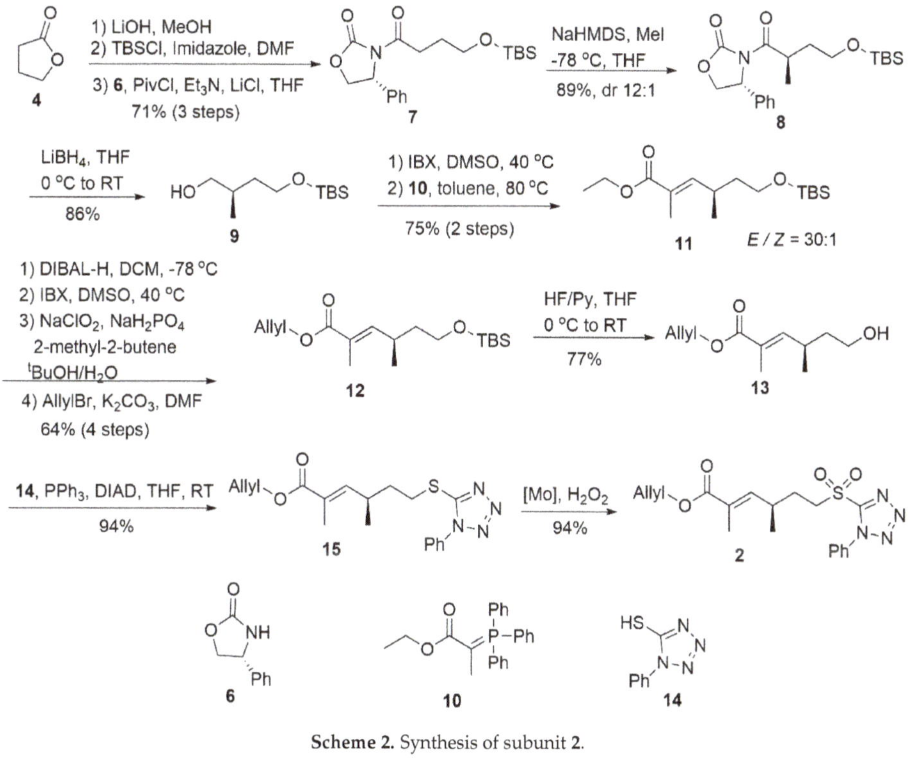

Scheme 2. Synthesis of subunit 2.

The preparation of subunit **3** was initiated with 4-hydroxy-2-butanone (Scheme 3). The Wittig–Horner reaction was conducted after PMB protection to smoothly obtain the desired product **17** (70% yield, E/Z = 3:1) while a complex mixture appeared when TBS protected alcohol was applied in this HWE reaction [13,14]. After the removal of the PMB group followed by the TBS protection, compound **19** was obtained and then converted into the corresponding aldehyde **3** by sequential steps of DIBAL-H reduction and IBX oxidation prior to the Julia–Kocienski olefination.

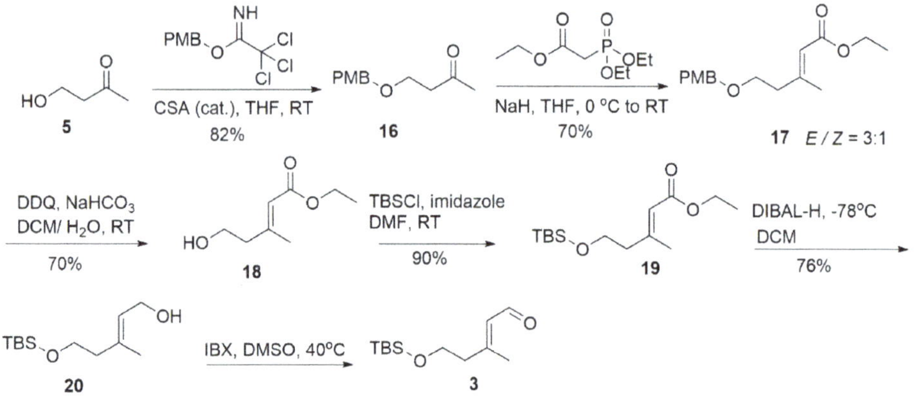

Scheme 3. Synthesis of subunit 3.

The different bases were tested through olefination (Table 1). When 1 eq KHMDS (entry 1) was applied, the yield was 50% and numerous reactants **2** and **3** remained. The product diene was an E/Z mixture with E/Z selectivity of up to 15:1. When the amount of KHMDS was increased to 1.5 eq, the yield improved and the two reactants remained in small quantities. When 2 eq KHMDS was used, the two reactants were completely consumed and the yield reached 86% while the high selectivity (15:1) was maintained. Other bases such as LiHMDS were also tried, but the resulting E/Z selectivity was low. We also exchanged the aldehyde and SO_2PT functional groups and subjected them to olefination (entry 5). The yield of the Z isomer greatly increased and the selectivity was 1.5:1 [15,16].

Table 1. Optimization of the Julia–Kocienski olefination.

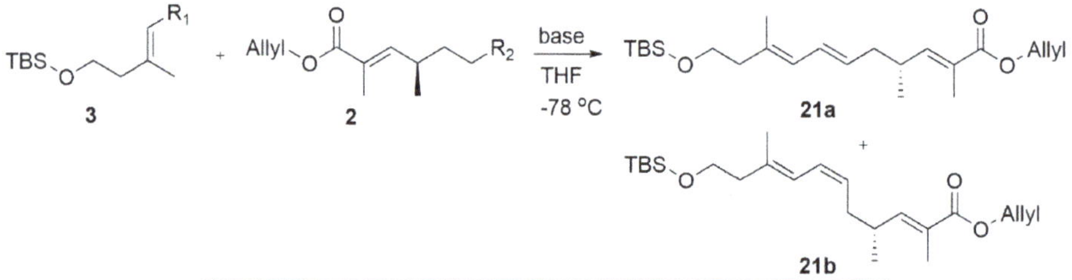

Entry	R 1	R 2	Base (equiv)	Yield [1]	21a:21b [2]
1	CHO	SO_2PT	KHMDS (1eq)	50%	15:1
2	CHO	SO_2PT	KHMDS (1.5eq)	72%	15:1
3	CHO	SO_2PT	KHMDS (2eq)	86%	15:1
4	CHO	SO_2PT	LiHMDS (2eq)	83%	3.5:1
5	SO_2PT	CHO	KHMDS (2eq)	94%	1.5:1

[1] Combined yield of **21a** and **21b**. [2] Determined by LC-MS.

Having completed the construction of diene **21a**, we started to prepare the dihydroxy unit (Scheme 4). To our delight, under the condition of the HF/Py complex, we fairly achieved the alcohol **22** and oxidized it to corresponding aldehyde **23** by DMP prior to the aldol reaction (deprotection of PMB group in this step led to a complex mixture).

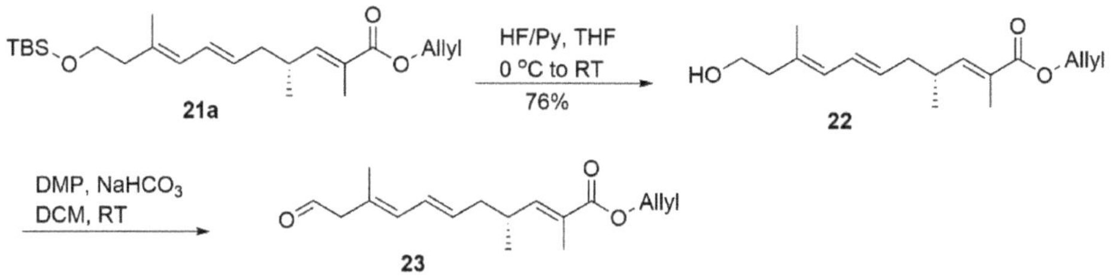

Scheme 4. Synthesis of compound **23**.

IPCBCl-controlled aldol reaction [17,18] was selected to install the C28 stereo-center (Table 2). The application of (−)-IPCBCl at −20 °C successfully generated **24b** with the C28 (*S*) configuration in 59% yield (dr = 99:1). The chiral reactant was changed into (+)-IPCBCl, which afforded the C28 (*R*) product as expected and maintained the high diastereoselectivity (dr = 98:2). LiHMDS also proceeded and a 1:1 mixture was obtained in this aldol reaction.

Table 2. Boron-mediated aldol reaction.

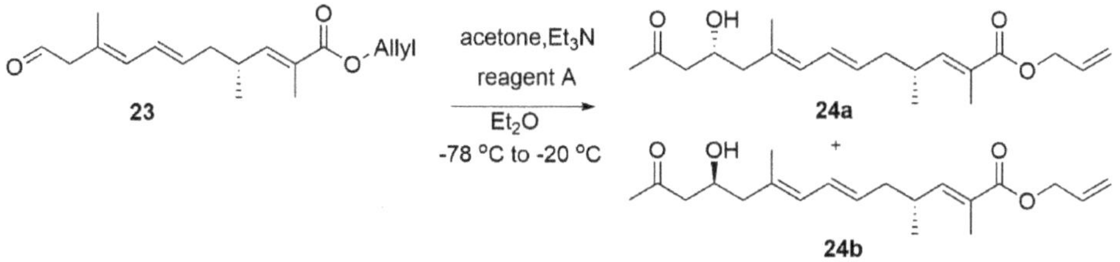

Entry	Reagent A	Yield [1]	24a:24b [2]
1	(−)-IPCBCl	59%	1:99
2	(+)-IPCBCl	55%	98:2
3	LiHMDS	47%	1:1

[1] Combined yield of **24a** and **24b**. [2] Determined by LC-MS.

After TBS protection followed by the reduction of the combination of BH_3-DMS and CBS catalysts, we obtained **26a** (dr = 4:1, determined by ^1H NMR) and **26b** (dr = 17:1, determined by ^1H NMR), respectively. Compounds **26c** (dr = 3.6:1, determined by ^1H NMR) and **26d** (dr = 14:1, determined by ^1H NMR) were achieved from **25b** with the similar dr value (Scheme 5).

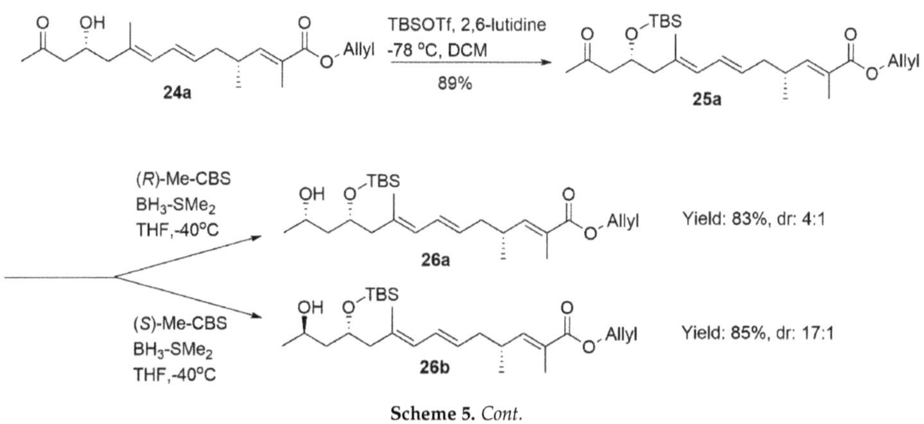

Scheme 5. *Cont.*

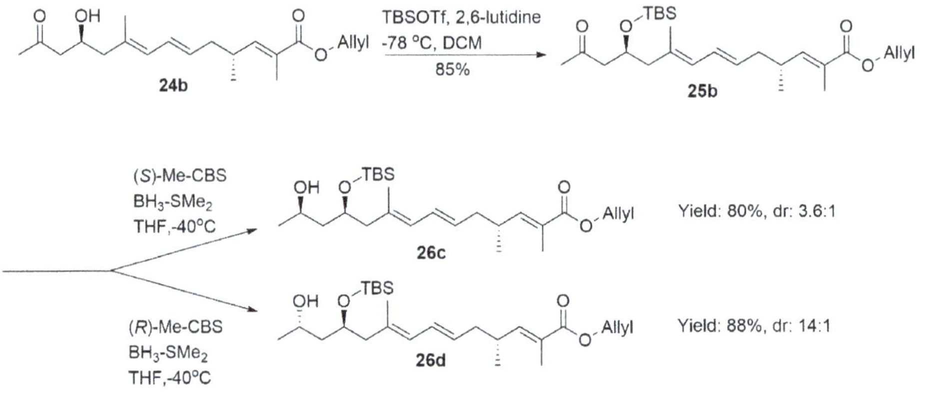

Scheme 5. Synthesis of 26a–26d.

The stereochemistries of the 1,3-diol part in **26a–26d** were confirmed by their ^{13}C NMR chemical shifts of the corresponding acetonides **28a–28d** (Scheme 6). *Syn*-diol acetonide preferred a chair conformation and two ketal methyl groups were significantly different (e.g., 19.94 and 30.46 ppm for **28a**). Meanwhile *anti*-diol acetonide preferred a twist-boat conformation and two similar methyl groups existed (e.g., 25.24 and 25.13 ppm for **28b**) [19–21].

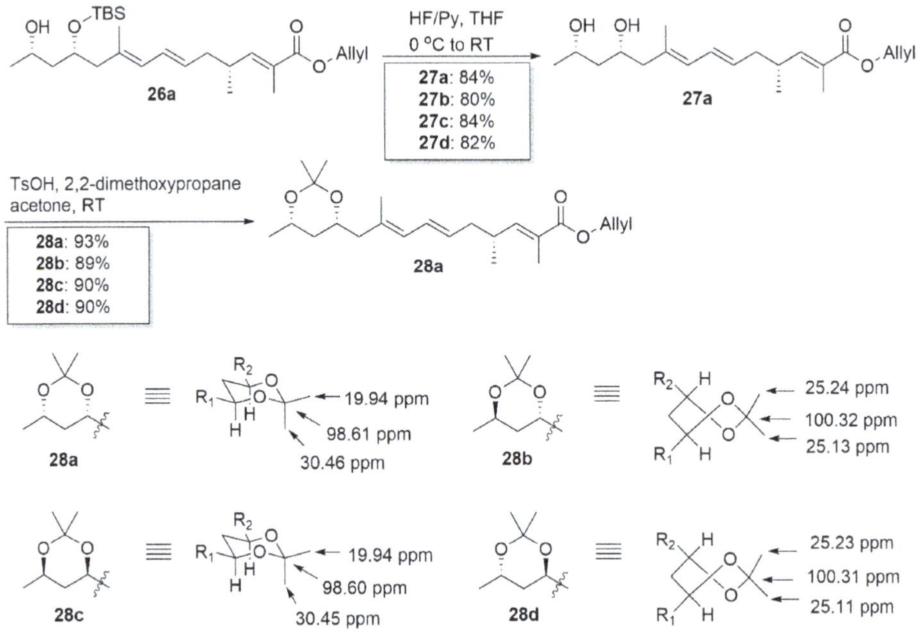

Scheme 6. Stereo-chemical assignments of 28a–28d.

After the sequential methylation and removal of the TBS group from **26a–26d**, we successfully furnished the four desired analogues **1a–1d** (Scheme 7). The total yield was 2.5% for **1a** from the lactone and 2.7% for **1b**, 2.5% for **1c**, and 2.6% for **1d**.

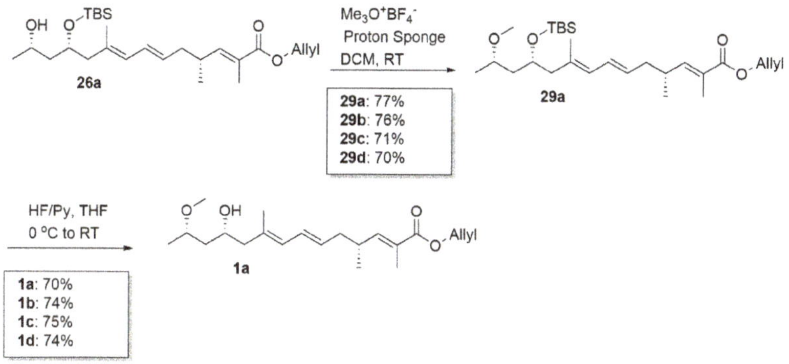

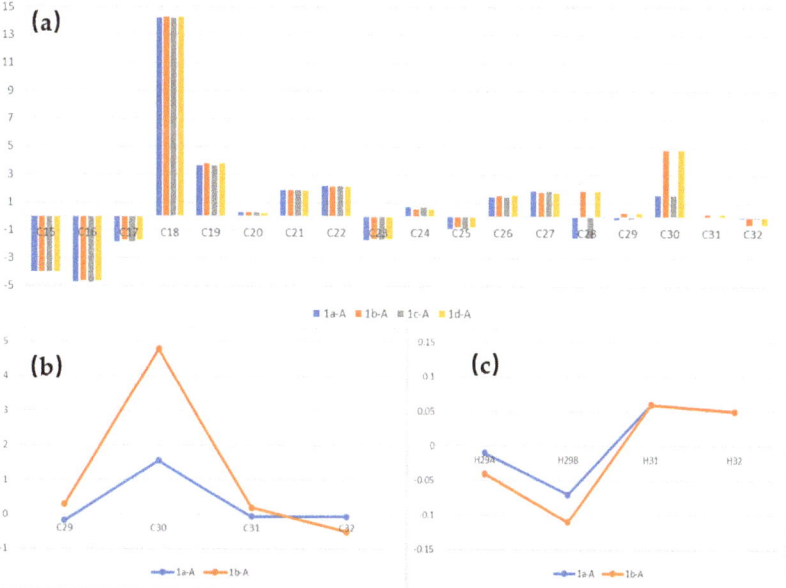

Scheme 7. Synthesis of 1a–1d.

3. Discussion

A careful comparison between four isomers and alotamide was conducted. The differences in ^{13}C NMR chemical shifts are shown in Figure 3a. From C15 to C28, several significant variations ($\Delta\delta > 1$ ppm) existed between all four isomers and alotamide possibly because of the difference between the "straight-chain" mode in our analogues and the "ring" mode in the original structure. From C28 to C32, the dihydroxy unit is a linear chain both in our analogues and natural compound. Thus, comparing the data in this portion is suitable for relative stereochemistry determination.

At the same time, several obvious variations in ^{13}C spectra were observed between 1,3-*syn* isomers (**1a** and **1c**) and 1,3-*anti* isomers (**1b** and **1d**) from C29 to C32 (Figure 3a). Therefore, we chose **1a** and **1b** to represent the *syn*-analogues and *anti*-analogues to distinguish *syn*-configurations and *anti*-configurations (Figure 3b,c).

Figure 3. (a) $\Delta\delta$ ^{13}C (ppm) between alotamide and **1a–1d**, (b) $\Delta\delta$ ^{13}C (ppm) between alotamide and **1a** and **1b** from C29–C32, (c) $\Delta\delta$ ^{1}H (ppm) between alotamide and **1a** and **1b** in dihydroxy unit.

A significant variation at C30 position of **1b** (Δδ > 4 ppm) and a closer correlation of **1a** at C29, C31 and C32 in the ^{13}C spectra revealed the *syn* configuration in the C28–C30 unit. In addition, smaller variations with alotamide in ^{1}H spectra were noticed for analogue **1a** at protons H29A and H29B (differences between alotamide and **1a** and **1b** at proton H30 were not plotted in Figure 3c because the differences were all greater than 0.4 ppm and insignificant). This finding confirmed the 1,3-*syn* structure in the dihydroxy unit.

Two 1,3-*syn* isomers **1a** and **1c** were also compared. Their ^{1}H spectra were the same and the differences in ^{13}C NMR chemical shifts are listed in Table 3. A closer correlation of **1c** was observed especially at the sites C20, C29, and C31. Thus, it appeared that **1c** (19*R*, 28*S*, 30*R*) most closely fit the original natural alotamide. The total synthesis of alotamide with fragment **1c** and another (19*S*, 28*R*, 30*S*) enantiomer is in progress.

Table 3. Δδ ^{13}C (ppm) between alotamide and **1a** and **1c**.

Isomer	C20	C21	C23	C26	C29	C31
1a	0.30	1.90	−1.67	1.40	−0.18	−0.06
1c	0.28	1.88	−1.65	1.41	−0.13	−0.04

4. Materials and Methods

All anaerobic and moisture-sensitive manipulations were carried out with standard Schlenk techniques under argon. Solvents were dried and distilled by standard procedures. ^{1}H- NMR and ^{13}C-NMR spectra were recorded in CDCl$_3$ on a Bruker Ascend-400 400 MHz or Bruker Ascend-500 500 MHz at room temperature. Chemical shifts (δ) are reported in ppm and are referenced to chloroform (δ 7.26 ppm for 1H, δ 77.16 ppm for ^{13}C). Data for NMR spectra are reported as follows: s = singlet, d = doublet, t = triplet, q = quartet, quint. = quintet, sext. = sextet, m = multiplet, br = broad signal, J = coupling constant in Hz. HRMS were recorded on an Agilent 6530-Q-TOF mass spectrometer equipped with an Agilent 1260- HPLC. Optical rotations were measured on a PerkinElmer 241 MC polarimeter.

4.1. (R)-3-(4-((Tert-Butyldimethylsilyl)Oxy)Butanoyl)-4-Phenyloxazolidin-2-One (7)

To a solution of the lactone (5 g, 58 mmol) in MeOH (50 mL) at room temperature was added LiOH (2.44 g, 58 mmol) and stirred overnight. The solvent was removed from the reaction and the residue was dissolved in dimethylformamide (50 mL) at 0 °C. Imidazole (8 g, 116 mmol) was added to this solution, which was followed by TBSCl (8.7 g, 58 mmol) in two portions over 15 min. The reaction mixture was warmed to room temperature overnight with stirring and then diluted with 1 M HCl and extracted with EtOAc (3 × 100 mL). The combined organic layers were washed with brine and dried over Na$_2$SO$_4$. The organic layer was removed under vacuum and the crude acid was used without further purification.

To a stirred solution of the acid in dry THF (200 mL) at 0 °C under argon, Et$_3$N (20 mL, 145 mmol) and PivCl (7.1 mL, 58 mmol) were added sequentially. After 1 h stirring at 0 °C, LiCl (0.62 g, 14.5 mmol), followed by oxazolidinone **6** (9.4 g, 58 mmol), were added. The reaction was continued for 1 h at 0 °C and another 2 h at room temperature prior to quenching with a saturated NH$_4$Cl solution (50 mL) and extracted with DCM (2 × 200 mL). The combined organic layers were washed with brine, dried over Na$_2$SO$_4$, and concentrated in vacuum. Purification by column chromatography (PE/EA = 9:1) afforded compound **7** (15 g, 71% for three steps) as a colorless oil.

^{1}**H NMR** (400 MHz, CDCl$_3$) δ 7.47–7.21 (m, 5H), 5.43 (dd, J = 8.7, 3.6 Hz, 1H), 4.69 (td, J = 8.8, 1.0 Hz, 1H), 4.28 (ddd, J = 8.9, 3.6, 1.3 Hz, 1H), 3.64 (t, J = 6.3 Hz, 2H), 3.03 (qt, J = 17.7, 7.4 Hz, 2H), 1.92–1.77 (m, 2H), 0.90 (s, 9H), 0.04 (d, J = 1.3 Hz, 6H). ^{13}**C NMR** (101 MHz, CDCl$_3$) δ 172.62, 153.76, 139.27, 129.18, 128.68, 125.93, 70.00, 62.25, 61.91, 57.56, 32.08, 27.09, 25.96, 18.32, −5.34, −5.62. $[\alpha]_D^{20}$ = −42.63, (c 3.38, CHCl$_3$). HRMS (ESI+): calcd. for C$_{19}$H$_{29}$NO$_4$Si [M + H]$^+$, 364.1939; found 364.1940.

4.2. (R)-3-((R)-4-((Tert-Butyldimethylsilyl)oxy)-2-Methylbutanoyl)-4-Phenyloxazolidin-2-one (8)

To a stirred solution of compound **7** (15 g, 41.2 mmol) in dry THF (100 mL) at −78 °C under argon, NaHMDS (2.0 M solution in THF, 24.7 mL, 49.4 mmol) was added dropwise. After 1 h, MeI (7.7 mL, 123.5 mmol) was added and the mixture was stirred overnight at the same temperature. The reaction mixture was quenched with a saturated NH_4Cl solution (100 mL) and warmed up to room temperature before being extracted with DCM (2 × 100 mL). The combined organic extracts were washed with water and brine, dried over Na_2SO_4, and concentrated in vacuum. Purification by column chromatography (PE/EA = 13:1) gave pure **8** (13.8 g, 89%) as a white solid.

^{1}H NMR (400 MHz, $CDCl_3$) δ 7.45–7.23 (m, 5H), 5.44 (dd, J = 8.7, 3.7 Hz, 1H), 4.67 (t, J = 8.8 Hz, 1H), 4.25 (dd, J = 8.9, 3.7 Hz, 1H), 4.02–3.85 (m, 1H), 3.73–3.55 (m, 2H), 2.00 (td, J = 13.9, 6.4 Hz, 1H), 1.59 (dq, J = 12.2, 6.1 Hz, 1H), 1.15 (d, J = 7.0 Hz, 3H), 0.91 (s, 9H), 0.06 (s, 6H). **^{13}C NMR** (101 MHz, $CDCl_3$) δ 176.36, 153.35, 139.47, 129.28, 128.70, 125.75, 69.80, 61.02, 57.74, 35.72, 34.71, 26.00, 18.39, 17.83, −5.33. $[\alpha]_D^{20}$ = −79.14, (c 2.34, $CHCl_3$). HRMS (ESI+): calcd. for $C_{20}H_{31}NO_4Si$ $[M + H]^+$, 378.2095, found 378.2095.

4.3. (R)-4-((Tert-Butyldimethylsilyl)Oxy)-2-Methylbutan-1-Ol (9)

To an ice-cold solution of compound **8** (13.8 g, 36.6 mmol) in THF (100 mL) moist with a catalytic amount of water, $LiBH_4$ (1.2 g, 54.9 mmol) was added portion wise under argon. After 12 h of stirring at room temperature, the reaction was quenched cautiously with a saturated NH_4Cl solution (50 mL) and then distilled under a reduced pressure followed by extraction with DCM. The combined organic solution was dried over Na_2SO_4 and concentrated in vacuum. Purification by column chromatography (PE/EA = 9:1) provided pure compound **9** (6.86 g, 86%) as a colorless oil [11].

^{1}H NMR (400 MHz, $CDCl_3$) δ 3.81–3.69 (m, 1H), 3.68–3.60 (m, 1H), 3.46 (s, 1H), 3.43–3.33 (m, 1H), 3.19 (s, 1H), 1.86–1.70 (m, 1H), 1.59–1.46 (m, 2H), 0.89 (m, 12H), 0.05 (s, 6H). **^{13}C NMR** (101 MHz, $CDCl_3$) δ 68.21, 61.82, 37.53, 34.46, 25.98, 18.34, 17.46, −5.33, −5.36. $[\alpha]_D^{20}$ = −10.98, (c 1.82, $CHCl_3$). HRMS (ESI+): calcd. for $C_{11}H_{26}O_2Si$ $[M + H]^+$, 219.1775, found 219.1771.

4.4. Ethyl (R,E)-6-((Tert-Butyldimethylsilyl)Oxy)-2,4-Dimethylhex-2-Enoate (11)

To a stirred solution of **9** (6.86 g, 31.5 mmol) in DMSO (50 mL) IBX (10.6 g, 37.8 mmol) was added. After 1 h stirring at 40 °C, the reaction was quenched with water (50 mL) and extracted with ether (2 × 100 mL). The combined organic layers were washed with brine, dried over Na_2SO_4, and removed under vacuum. The residue was refluxed with **10** (22 g, 63 mmol) in toluene (100 mL) at 80 °C for 3 h and the solvent was removed under vacuum. Purification by column chromatography (PE/EA = 40:1) provided pure compound **11** (7 g, 75%) as a colorless oil [22].

^{1}H NMR (400 MHz, $CDCl_3$) δ 6.53 (dd, J = 10.1, 1.4 Hz, 1H), 4.17 (q, J = 7.1 Hz, 2H), 3.70–3.41 (m, 2H), 2.80–2.45 (m, 1H), 1.83 (d, J = 1.4 Hz, 3H), 1.66–1.44 (m, 2H), 1.28 (t, J = 7.1 Hz, 3H), 1.00 (d, J = 6.7 Hz, 3H), 0.87 (s, 9H), 0.01 (d, J = 2.1 Hz, 6H). **^{13}C NMR** (101 MHz, $CDCl_3$) δ 168.57, 147.56, 126.83, 61.02, 60.52, 39.83, 29.78, 26.04, 20.06, 18.37, 14.42, 12.59, −5.23, −5.25. $[\alpha]_D^{20}$ = −2.167, (c 0.1, $CHCl_3$). HRMS (ESI+): calcd. for $C_{16}H_{32}O_3Si$ $[M + H]^+$, 301.2193, found 301.2194.

4.5. Allyl (R,E)-6-((Tert-Butyldimethylsilyl)oxy)-2,4-Dimethylhex-2-Enoate (12)

To a stirred solution of compound **11** (7 g, 23.6 mmol) in dry DCM (60 mL) at −78 °C under argon, DIBAL-H (1.5 M solution in toluene, 18.0 mL, 27.0 mmol) was added dropwise. After 1 h, the reaction mixture was quenched with aqueous sodium-potassium tartrate solution (20 mL) and warmed up to room temperature before being extracted with DCM (2 × 100 mL). The combined organic extracts were washed with water and brine, dried over Na_2SO_4, and concentrated in vacuum. Purification by column chromatography (PE/EA = 8:1) gave alcohol (4.8 g, 79%) as a colorless oil.

To a stirred solution of above alcohol in DMSO (50 mL), IBX (6.2 g, 22 mmol) was added. After 1 h stirring at 40 °C, the reaction was quenched with water (50 mL) and extracted with ether (2 × 100 mL). The combined organic layers were washed with brine, dried over Na_2SO_4, and removed under vacuum. The crude anhydride was used without further purification.

To the solution of above crude aldehyde in ^tBuOH (40 mL), NaH_2PO_4 (11 g, 93 mmol) in H_2O (40 mL), 2-methyl-2-butene (19 mL, 186 mmol), and $NaClO_2$ (3.1 g, 28 mmol, >79.0% purity) were added. After stirring for 2 h at room temperature, the mixture was extracted with EA (50 mL × 3) and the combined organic layers were washed with brine, dried over Na_2SO_4, filtrated, and concentrated. The crude acid was taken into the next step without future purification.

To a stirred solution of above acid in dry DMF (50 mL) allylBr (3.2 g, 37.2 mmol) and K_2CO_3 (5.1 g, 37.2 mmol) were added separately. After being stirred for 12 h, the mixture was quenched with a saturated aqueous solution of NH_4Cl and extracted with EA (100 mL × 3). The combined organic layers were washed with brine, dried over Na_2SO_4, filtrated, and concentrated. The residue was purified by column chromatography on silica gel (PE/EA = 40:1) to give **12** (4.7 g, 81%) for three steps as a colorless oil.

^{1}H NMR (400 MHz, $CDCl_3$) δ 6.58 (dd, *J* = 10.1, 1.4 Hz, 1H), 5.96 (ddt, *J* = 17.1, 10.5, 5.6 Hz, 1H), 5.32 (ddd, *J* = 17.2, 3.0, 1.5 Hz, 1H), 5.23 (dd, *J* = 10.4, 1.3 Hz, 1H), 4.64 (dt, *J* = 5.6, 1.4 Hz, 2H), 3.66–3.42 (m, 2H), 2.82–2.58 (m, 1H), 1.86 (d, *J* = 1.4 Hz, 3H), 1.68–1.55 (m, 2H), 1.01 (d, *J* = 6.7 Hz, 3H), 0.88 (s, 10H), 0.02 (d, *J* = 2.2 Hz, 6H). **^{13}C NMR** (101 MHz, $CDCl_3$) δ 168.16, 148.14, 132.76, 126.60, 117.84, 65.27, 61.00, 39.80, 29.82, 26.04, 20.02, 18.38, 12.62, −5.22. $[\alpha]_D^{20}$ = −53.365, (*c* 0.52, $CHCl_3$). HRMS (ESI+): calcd. for $C_{17}H_{32}O_3Si$ [M + H]$^+$, 313.2193, found 313.2186.

4.6. Allyl (R,E)-6-Hydroxy-2,4-Dimethylhex-2-Enoate (13)

To a stirred solution of **12** (4.7 g, 15 mmol) in dry THF (10 mL), the HF/Py complex (2 mL) was added at 0 °C. After being stirred for 1 h, the mixture was quenched with a saturated aqueous solution of $NaHCO_3$ and extracted with DCM (20 mL × 3). The combined organic layers were washed with 1 M HCl brine, dried over Na_2SO_4, filtrated, and concentrated. The residue was purified by column chromatography on silica gel (PE/EA = 6:1) to give **13** (2.3 g, 77%) as a colorless oil.

^{1}H NMR (400 MHz, $CDCl_3$) δ 6.59 (dd, *J* = 10.1, 1.4 Hz, 1H), 5.97 (ddt, *J* = 17.1, 10.6, 5.6 Hz, 1H), 5.34 (dq, *J* = 17.2, 1.5 Hz, 1H), 5.24 (ddd, *J* = 10.5, 2.6, 1.3 Hz, 1H), 4.65 (dt, *J* = 5.6, 1.4 Hz, 2H), 3.75–3.44 (m, 2H), 2.78–2.63 (m, 1H), 1.88 (d, *J* = 1.4 Hz, 3H), 1.75–1.62 (m, 1H), 1.62–1.50 (m, 2H), 1.05 (d, *J* = 6.7 Hz, 3H). **^{13}C NMR** (101 MHz, $CDCl_3$) δ 168.07, 147.61, 132.63, 126.88, 117.97, 65.34, 60.94, 39.55, 29.97, 20.09, 12.62. $[\alpha]_D^{20}$ = −55.72, (*c* 0.79, $CHCl_3$). HRMS (ESI+): calcd. for $C_{11}H_{18}O_3$ [M + H]$^+$, 199.1329, found 199.1328.

4.7. Allyl (R,E)-2,4-Dimethyl-6-((1-Phenyl-1H-Tetrazol-5-yl)Thio)Hex-2-Enoate (15)

To a stirred solution of **13** (2.3 g, 11.6 mmol) in anhydrous dry THF (50 mL) at 0 °C under argon, PPh_3 (6.1 g, 23.2 mmol), **14** (2 g, 11.6 mmol), and DIAD (4.6 mL, 23.2 mmol) were added sequentially. The reaction was continued further for 1 h at room temperature prior to quenching with the saturated NH_4Cl solution (50 mL) and extracted with DCM (2 × 100 mL). The combined organic layers were washed with brine, dried over Na_2SO_4, and concentrated in vacuum. Purification by column chromatography (PE/EA = 15:1) afforded compound **15** (3.9 g, 94%) as a colorless oil.

^{1}H NMR (400 MHz, $CDCl_3$) δ 7.67–7.46 (m, 5H), 6.55 (dd, *J* = 10.1, 1.4 Hz, 1H), 5.94 (ddt, *J* = 17.1, 10.5, 5.6 Hz, 1H), 5.42–5.29 (m, 1H), 5.22 (dd, *J* = 10.4, 1.3 Hz, 1H), 4.62 (dt, *J* = 5.6, 1.4 Hz, 2H), 3.41–3.13 (m, 2H), 2.77–2.60 (m, 1H), 2.06–1.90 (m, 1H), 1.89–1.74 (m, 4H), 1.05 (d, *J* = 6.7 Hz, 3H). **^{13}C NMR** (101 MHz, $CDCl_3$) δ 167.69, 154.18, 146.10, 133.74, 132.49, 130.22, 129.89, 127.82, 123.90, 118.07, 65.40, 35.95, 32.63, 31.37, 19.89, 12.76. $[\alpha]_D^{20}$ = −58.87, (*c* 1.47, $CHCl_3$). HRMS (ESI+): calcd. for $C_{18}H_{22}N_4O_2S$ [M + H]$^+$, 359.1536, found 359.1532.

4.8. Allyl (R,E)-2,4-Dimethyl-6-((1-Phenyl-1H-Tetrazol-5-yl)sulfonyl)Hex-2-Enoate (2)

To a stirred solution of **15** (3.9 g, 10.1 mmol) in ethanol (100 mL) at 0 °C, $(NH_4)_6Mo_7O_{24}$ (2.9 g, 2.2 mmol) and H_2O_2 (20 mL) were added sequentially. The reaction was continued further for 12 h at room temperature prior to quenching with saturated NH_4Cl solution (50 mL) and extracted with DCM (2 × 100 mL). The combined organic layers were washed with brine, dried over Na_2SO_4, and concentrated in vacuum. Purification by column chromatography (PE/EA = 8:1) afforded compound **2** (3.6 g, 94%) as a white solid.

^{1}H NMR (400 MHz, CDCl$_3$) δ 7.76–7.51 (m, 5H), 6.53 (dd, J = 10.1, 1.4 Hz, 1H), 5.97 (ddt, J = 17.1, 10.5, 5.6 Hz, 1H), 5.48–5.32 (m, 1H), 5.25 (dd, J = 10.4, 1.3 Hz, 1H), 4.65 (dt, J = 5.6, 1.3 Hz, 2H), 3.77–3.58 (m, 2H), 2.95–2.62 (m, 1H), 2.24–2.04 (m, 1H), 2.01–1.92 (m, 1H), 1.88 (d, J = 1.4 Hz, 3H), 1.11 (d, J = 6.7 Hz, 3H). **^{13}C NMR** (101 MHz, CDCl$_3$) δ 167.47, 153.49, 144.44, 133.12, 132.42, 131.64, 129.88, 128.93, 125.17, 118.32, 65.61, 54.40, 32.31, 28.74, 19.98, 12.86. $[\alpha]_D^{20}$ = −13.87, (c 0.79, CHCl$_3$). HRMS (ESI+): calcd. for $C_{18}H_{22}N_4O_2S_2$ [M + H]$^+$, 391.1435, found 391.1435.

4.9. 4-((4-Methoxybenzyl)Oxy)Butan-2-One (16)

To a stirred solution of 4-hydroxy-2-butanone (1.1 mL, 12.8 mmol) in dry THF (20 mL) at 0 °C, 4-methoxybenzyl 2,2,2-trichloroacetimidate (2 mL, 10.7 mmol) and triphenylcarbenium tetrafluoroborate (cat.) were added sequentially. The reaction was continued further for 1 h at room temperature prior to quenching with the saturated NH_4Cl solution (50 mL) and extracted with DCM (2 × 100 mL). The combined organic layers were washed with brine, dried over Na_2SO_4, and concentrated in vacuum. Purification by column chromatography (PE/EA = 6:1) afforded compound **16** (1.8 g, 82%) as a colorless oil [14].

^{1}H NMR (400 MHz, CDCl$_3$) δ 7.33–7.18 (m, 2H), 6.94–6.81 (m, 2H), 4.45 (s, 2H), 3.81 (s, 3H), 3.72 (t, J = 6.3 Hz, 2H), 2.71 (t, J = 6.3 Hz, 2H), 2.18 (s, 3H). **^{13}C NMR** (101 MHz, CDCl$_3$) δ 207.51, 159.27, 130.16, 129.42, 113.84, 72.91, 64.96, 55.31, 43.81, 30.48. HRMS (ESI+): calcd. for $C_{12}H_{16}O_3$ [M + H]$^+$, 209.1172, found 209.1170.

4.10. Ethyl (E)-5-((4-Methoxybenzyl)Oxy)-3-Methylpent-2-Enoate (17)

To a stirred solution of triethyl phosphonoacetate (3.5 mL, 17.5 mmol) in dry THF (50 mL) at 0 °C, NaH (0.7 g, 17.5 mmol) was added. After stirring at room temperature for 1 h, **16** (1.8 g, 8.8 mmol) in THF (5 mL) was added at 0 °C. The reaction was continued further for 12 h at room temperature prior to quenching with a saturated NH_4Cl solution (50 mL) and extracted with DCM (2 × 100 mL). The combined organic layers were washed with brine, dried over Na_2SO_4, and concentrated in vacuum. Purification by column chromatography (PE/EA = 20:1) afforded compound **17** in the E/Z mixture (1.7 g, 70%) as a colorless oil.

^{1}H NMR (400 MHz, CDCl$_3$) δ 7.27 (d, J = 8.6 Hz, 2H), 6.99–6.72 (m, 2H), 5.82–5.63 (m, 1H), 4.47 (d, J = 2.8 Hz, 2H), 4.23–4.08 (m, 2H), 3.82 (d, J = 2.1 Hz, 3H), 3.70–3.51 (m, 2H), 2.98 (t, J = 6.6 Hz, 1H), 2.45 (t, J = 6.4 Hz, 2H), 2.19 (d, J = 1.2 Hz, 2H), 1.96 (d, J = 1.3 Hz, 1H), 1.29 (td, J = 7.1, 5.4 Hz, 3H). **^{13}C NMR** (101 MHz, CDCl$_3$) δ 166.73, 166.34, 159.33, 159.19, 157.81, 156.72, 130.70, 130.30, 129.38, 129.27, 117.46, 117.10, 113.90, 113.81, 72.76, 72.46, 68.74, 67.59, 59.60, 55.35, 40.89, 33.73, 26.16, 19.00, 14.42. HRMS (ESI+): calcd. for $C_{16}H_{22}O_4$ [M + H]$^+$, 279.1591; found 279.1589.

4.11. Ethyl (E)-5-Hydroxy-3-Methylpent-2-Enoate (18)

To a stirring solution of **17** (1.7 g, 6.1 mmol) in DCM (20 mL) and water (4 mL) DDQ (1.67 g, 7.3 mmol) was added at room temperature. After 1 h, the reaction mixture was quenched with saturated aqueous $NaHCO_3$ (10 mL) and 1 M aqueous $NaHSO_3$ (10 mL) and extracted with DCM (30 mL × 3). The combined organic layers were washed with brine, dried over Na_2SO_4, and concentrated. The crude product was purified by column chromatography (PE/EA = 3:1) to give the desired compound **18** as a colorless oil (672 mg, 70% yield) [13].

¹H NMR (400 MHz, CDCl$_3$) δ 5.71 (d, *J* = 1.2 Hz, 1H), 4.12 (q, *J* = 7.1 Hz, 2H), 3.76 (t, *J* = 6.4 Hz, 2H), 2.47–2.30 (m, 2H), 2.16 (d, *J* = 1.2 Hz, 3H), 1.92 (s, 1H), 1.25 (t, *J* = 7.1 Hz, 3H). **¹³C NMR** (101 MHz, CDCl$_3$) δ 166.67, 156.12, 117.73, 60.22, 59.78, 43.82, 18.82, 14.37. HRMS (ESI+): calcd. for C$_8$H$_{14}$O$_3$ [M + H]$^+$, 159.1016, found 159.1014.

4.12. Ethyl (E)-5-((Tert-Butyldimethylsilyl)Oxy)-3-Methylpent-2-Enoate (19)

To a stirred solution of **18** (672 mg, 4.3 mmol) in anhydrous DMF (10 mL) at 0 °C, imidazole (7.7 g, 11.4 mmol) and TBSCl (1.1 g, 6.84 mmol) were added sequentially. The reaction was continued further for 12 h at room temperature prior to quenching with saturated NH$_4$Cl solution (20 mL) and extracted with EA (2 × 20 mL). The combined organic layers were washed with brine, dried over Na$_2$SO$_4$, and concentrated in vacuum. Purification by column chromatography (PE/EA = 40:1) created compound **19** (1.05 g, 90%) as a colorless oil [13].

¹H NMR (400 MHz, CDCl$_3$) δ 5.66 (d, *J* = 1.1 Hz, 1H), 4.12 (q, *J* = 7.1 Hz, 2H), 2.32 (t, *J* = 6.6 Hz, 2H), 2.15 (d, *J* = 1.2 Hz, 3H), 1.24 (t, *J* = 7.1 Hz, 3H), 0.86 (s, 9H), 0.02 (s, 6H). **¹³C NMR** (101 MHz, CDCl$_3$) δ 166.74, 156.92, 117.34, 61.41, 59.53, 44.12, 25.97, 19.21, 18.36, 14.42, −5.29. HRMS (ESI+): calcd. for C$_{14}$H$_{28}$O$_3$Si [M + H]$^+$, 273.1880, found 273.1880.

4.13. (E)-5-((Tert-Butyldimethylsilyl)Oxy)-3-Methylpent-2-En-1-Ol (20)

To a stirred solution of compound **19** (1.05 g, 3.87 mmol) in dry DCM (15 mL) at −78 °C under argon, DIBAL-H (1.5 M solution in toluene, 3.9 mL, 5.8 mmol) was added dropwise. After 1 h, the reaction mixture was quenched with the aqueous sodium-potassium tartrate solution (20 mL) and warmed up to room temperature before being extracted with DCM (2 × 20 mL). The combined organic extracts were washed with water and brine, dried over Na$_2$SO$_4$, and concentrated in vacuum. Purification by column chromatography (PE/EA = 7:1) gave **20** (680 mg, 76%) as a colorless oil [23].

¹H NMR (400 MHz, CDCl$_3$) δ 5.45 (td, *J* = 6.9, 1.2 Hz, 1H), 4.16 (d, *J* = 6.9 Hz, 2H), 3.71 (t, *J* = 7.0 Hz, 2H), 2.25 (t, *J* = 7.0 Hz, 2H), 1.71 (s, 3H), 1.53 (s, 1H), 0.90 (s, 9H), 0.06 (s, 6H). **¹³C NMR** (101 MHz, CDCl$_3$) δ 136.95, 125.38, 62.20, 59.42, 42.91, 26.05, 18.45, 16.80, −5.17. HRMS (ESI+): calcd. for C$_{12}$H$_{26}$O$_2$Si ([M + H]$^+$, 231.1775, found 231.1775.

4.14. Allyl (R,2E,6E,8E)-11-((Tert-butyldimethylsilyl)Oxy)-2,4,9-Trimethylundeca-2,6,8-Trienoate (21a)

To a stirred solution of **20** (680 mg, 3.0 mmol) in DMSO (10 mL) IBX (990 mg, 3.5 mmol) was added. After 1 h of stirring at 40 °C, the reaction was quenched with water (10 mL) and extracted with ether (2 × 20 mL). The combined organic layers were washed with brine, dried over Na$_2$SO$_4$, and removed under vacuum. The crude aldehyde **3** was used without further purification.

To a stirred solution of crude **3** and compound **2** (1.3 g, 3.3 mmol) in dry THF (30 mL) at −78 °C under argon, KHMDS (1.0 M solution in THF, 27.0 mL, 27.0 mmol) was added dropwise. After 1 h, the reaction mixture was quenched with the saturated NH$_4$Cl solution (20 mL) and warmed up to room temperature before being extracted with DCM (2 × 100 mL). The combined organic extracts were washed with water and brine, dried over Na$_2$SO$_4$, and concentrated in vacuum. Purification by column chromatography (PE/EA = 40:1) gave **21a** (1.0 g, 86%, 2 steps) as a colorless oil.

¹H NMR (400 MHz, CDCl$_3$) δ 6.61 (dd, *J* = 10.0, 1.4 Hz, 1H), 6.23 (dd, *J* = 15.0, 10.8 Hz, 1H), 5.97 (ddt, *J* = 17.1, 10.5, 5.6 Hz, 1H), 5.79 (d, *J* = 10.8 Hz, 1H), 5.48 (dt, *J* = 14.8, 7.3 Hz, 1H), 5.33 (ddd, *J* = 17.2, 3.1, 1.5 Hz, 1H), 5.23 (dd, *J* = 10.4, 1.3 Hz, 1H), 4.64 (d, *J* = 5.5 Hz, 2H), 3.68 (t, *J* = 7.0 Hz, 2H), 2.64–2.47 (m, 1H), 2.24 (t, *J* = 7.0 Hz, 2H), 2.14 (t, *J* = 7.1 Hz, 2H), 1.85 (d, *J* = 1.3 Hz, 3H), 1.74 (s, 3H), 1.02 (d, *J* = 6.7 Hz, 3H), 0.88 (s, 9H), 0.04 (s, 6H). **¹³C NMR** (101 MHz, CDCl$_3$) δ 168.13, 147.84, 134.13, 132.75, 129.61, 128.53, 126.49, 126.40, 117.83, 65.27, 62.39, 43.29, 40.02, 33.96, 26.09, 19.68, 18.47, 17.20, 12.73, −5.14. $[\alpha]_D^{20}$ = −32.72, (*c* 0.38, CHCl$_3$). HRMS (ESI+): calcd. for C$_{23}$H$_{40}$O$_3$Si [M + H]$^+$, 293.2819, found 293.2819.

4.15. Allyl (R,2E,6E,8E)-11-Hydroxy-2,4,9-Trimethylundeca-2,6,8-Trienoate (22)

To a stirred solution of **21a** (1.0 g, 2.6 mmol) in dry THF (5 mL), HF/Py complex (1 mL) was added at 0 °C. After being stirred for 1 h, the mixture was quenched with a saturated aqueous solution of NaHCO$_3$ and extracted with DCM (20 mL × 3). The combined organic layers were washed with 1 M HCl, brine, dried over Na$_2$SO$_4$, filtrated, and concentrated. The residue was purified by column chromatography on silica gel (PE/EA = 6:1) to give **22** (550 mg, 76%) as a colorless oil.

^{1}H NMR (400 MHz, CDCl$_3$) δ 6.60 (dd, *J* = 10.0, 1.4 Hz, 1H), 6.24 (dd, *J* = 15.0, 10.8 Hz, 1H), 5.96 (ddt, *J* = 17.1, 10.5, 5.6 Hz, 1H), 5.85 (d, *J* = 10.8 Hz, 1H), 5.52 (dt, *J* = 14.8, 7.3 Hz, 1H), 5.32 (ddd, *J* = 17.2, 3.0, 1.5 Hz, 1H), 5.22 (dd, *J* = 10.4, 1.3 Hz, 1H), 4.63 (d, *J* = 5.6 Hz, 2H), 3.69 (t, *J* = 6.3 Hz, 2H), 2.65–2.51 (m, 1H), 2.29 (t, *J* = 6.3 Hz, 2H), 2.15 (t, *J* = 7.0 Hz, 2H), 1.84 (d, *J* = 1.4 Hz, 3H), 1.75 (s, 3H), 1.54 (s, 1H), 1.01 (d, *J* = 6.7 Hz, 3H). **^{13}C NMR** (101 MHz, CDCl$_3$) δ 168.09, 147.69, 132.93, 132.70, 130.49, 128.14, 127.38, 126.53, 117.82, 65.26, 60.49, 42.95, 39.97, 33.84, 19.67, 16.50, 12.72. $[\alpha]_D^{20}$ = −38.23, (*c* 0.96, CHCl$_3$). HRMS (ESI+): calcd. for C$_{17}$H$_{26}$O$_3$ [M + H]$^+$, 279.1955, found 279.1954.

4.16. Allyl (2E,4R,6E,8E,11R)-11-Hydroxy-2,4,9-Trimethyl-13-Oxotetradeca-2,6,8-Trienoate (24a)

To the above alcohol **22** (200 mg, 0.72 mmol) in dry DCM (5 mL, 0 °C), DMP (610 mg, 1.44 mmol) and NaHCO$_3$ (240 mg, 2.9 mmol) was added sequentially. After being stirred for 30 min, the mixture was carefully quenched with a solution of saturated aqueous NaHCO$_3$ and Na$_2$S$_2$O$_3$. The resulting mixture was extracted with DCM (20 mL × 3) and the combined organic layers were washed with brine, dried over Na$_2$SO$_4$, and concentrated. The crude aldehyde **23** was used without future purification.

To a stirred solution of (+)-IPCBCl (1.8 M in heptane, 1.08 mmol, 0.6 mL) in dry ether (3 mL) at −0 °C under argon, Et$_3$N (0.2 mL, 1.44 mmol) and acetone (80 uL, 1.08 mmol) were added sequentially. After 1 h stirring at −0 °C, aldehyde **23** in ether (2 mL) was added at −78 °C. The reaction was continued further for 1 h at −78 °C and another 12 h at −20 °C prior to quenching with a mixture of PH 7 buffer (1 mL), methanol (1 mL), and H$_2$O$_2$ (1 mL). The mixture was warmed up to room temperature before being extracted with ether (2 × 10 mL). The combined organic extracts were washed with water and brine, dried over Na$_2$SO$_4$, and concentrated in vacuum. Purification by column chromatography (PE/EA = 4:1) created **24a** (132 mg, 55%) as a colorless oil.

^{1}H NMR (400 MHz, CDCl$_3$) δ 6.60 (dd, *J* = 10.0, 1.2 Hz, 1H), 6.22 (dd, *J* = 15.0, 10.8 Hz, 1H), 5.96 (ddt, *J* = 17.1, 10.5, 5.6 Hz, 1H), 5.83 (d, *J* = 10.8 Hz, 1H), 5.52 (dt, *J* = 14.8, 7.3 Hz, 1H), 5.32 (dd, *J* = 17.2, 1.4 Hz, 1H), 5.23 (dd, *J* = 10.4, 1.1 Hz, 1H), 4.64 (d, *J* = 5.5 Hz, 2H), 4.20 (tt, *J* = 11.6, 5.9 Hz, 1H), 2.79 (s, 1H), 2.66–2.47 (m, 3H), 2.24 (dd, *J* = 13.4, 7.5 Hz, 1H), 2.19–2.07 (m, 6H), 1.84 (d, *J* = 1.2 Hz, 3H), 1.75 (s, 3H), 1.02 (d, *J* = 6.7 Hz, 3H). **^{13}C NMR** (101 MHz, CDCl$_3$) δ 209.56, 168.10, 147.68, 132.82, 132.72, 130.79, 128.10, 127.99, 126.58, 117.85, 65.91, 65.29, 49.62, 47.13, 40.02, 33.86, 30.98, 19.72, 16.89, 12.75. $[\alpha]_D^{20}$ = −33.92, (*c* 0.34, CHCl$_3$). HRMS (ESI+): calcd. for C$_{20}$H$_{30}$O$_4$ [M + H]$^+$, 335.2217, found 335.2217.

4.17. Allyl (2E,4R,6E,8E,11S)-11-Hydroxy-2,4,9-Trimethyl-13-Oxotetradeca-2,6,8-Trienoate (24b)

To a stirred solution of (−)-IPCBCl (1.7 M in heptane, 1.08 mmol, 0.64 mL) in dry ether (3 mL) at 0 °C under argon, Et$_3$N (0.2 mL, 1.44 mmol) and acetone (80 uL, 1.08 mmol) were added sequentially. After 1 h stirring at 0 °C, aldehyde **23** in ether (2 mL) was added at −78 °C. The reaction was continued further for 1 h at −78 °C and another 12 h at −20 °C prior to quenching with a mixture of PH 7 buffer (1 mL), methanol (1 mL), and H$_2$O$_2$ (1 mL). The mixture was warmed up to room temperature before being extracted with ether (2 × 10 mL). The combined organic extracts were washed with water and brine, dried over Na$_2$SO$_4$, and concentrated in vacuum. Purification by column chromatography (PE/EA = 4:1) provided **24b** (142 mg, 59%) as a colorless oil.

^{1}H NMR (400 MHz, CDCl$_3$) δ 6.60 (dd, *J* = 10.0, 1.2 Hz, 1H), 6.23 (dd, *J* = 15.0, 10.8 Hz, 1H), 5.96 (ddt, *J* = 17.1, 10.5, 5.6 Hz, 1H), 5.83 (d, *J* = 10.8 Hz, 1H), 5.53 (dt, *J* = 14.8, 7.3 Hz, 1H), 5.32 (dd, *J* = 17.2, 1.4 Hz, 1H), 5.23 (dd, *J* = 10.4, 1.1 Hz, 1H), 4.64 (d, *J* = 5.5 Hz, 2H), 4.29–4.12 (m, 1H), 2.66–2.51 (m, 3H), 2.23 (dd, *J* = 13.5, 7.6 Hz, 1H), 2.19–2.08 (m, 6H), 1.84 (d, *J* = 1.2 Hz, 3H),

1.75 (s, 3H), 1.02 (d, J = 6.7 Hz, 3H). ^{13}C NMR (101 MHz, CDCl$_3$) δ 209.53, 168.10, 147.67, 132.83, 132.72, 130.76, 128.12, 127.98, 126.57, 117.86, 65.92, 65.29, 49.66, 47.11, 39.97, 33.86, 30.98, 19.69, 16.91, 12.74. $[α]_D^{20}$ = −26.04, (c 0.37, CHCl$_3$). HRMS (ESI+): calcd. for C$_{20}$H$_{30}$O$_4$ [M + H]$^+$, 335.2217, found 335.2216.

4.18. Allyl (2E,4R,6E,8E,11R)-11-((Tert-Butyldimethylsilyl)oxy)-2,4,9-Trimethyl-13-Oxotetradeca-2,6,8-Trienoate (25a)

To a stirred solution of compound **24a** (132 mg, 0.4 mmol) in dry DCM (3 mL) at −78 °C under argon, 2,6-lutidine (0.23 mL, 2 mmol) and TBSOTf (0.35 mL, 1.5 mmol) were added sequentially. After 1 h, the reaction mixture was quenched with aqueous NaHCO$_3$ (5 mL) and warmed up to room temperature before being extracted with DCM (2 × 10 mL). The combined organic extracts were washed with 1 M HCl and brine, dried over Na$_2$SO$_4$, and concentrated in vacuum. Purification by column chromatography (PE/EA = 40:1) created **25a** (160 mg, 89%) as a colorless oil.

^{1}**H NMR** (400 MHz, CDCl$_3$) δ 6.60 (dd, J = 10.0, 1.3 Hz, 1H), 6.19 (dd, J = 15.0, 10.8 Hz, 1H), 5.96 (ddt, J = 17.1, 10.5, 5.6 Hz, 1H), 5.75 (d, J = 10.8 Hz, 1H), 5.48 (dt, J = 14.8, 7.3 Hz, 1H), 5.33 (dd, J = 17.2, 1.5 Hz, 1H), 5.23 (dd, J = 10.4, 1.2 Hz, 1H), 4.64 (d, J = 5.6 Hz, 2H), 4.38–4.20 (m, 1H), 2.67–2.41 (m, 3H), 2.29–2.20 (m, 1H), 2.19–2.00 (m, 6H), 1.84 (d, J = 1.1 Hz, 3H), 1.73 (s, 3H), 1.01 (d, J = 6.7 Hz, 3H), 0.85 (s, 9H), 0.03 (d, J = 8.1 Hz, 6H). ^{13}C NMR (101 MHz, CDCl$_3$) δ 208.04, 168.10, 147.75, 133.24, 132.74, 130.28, 128.31, 128.07, 126.53, 117.86, 68.06, 65.29, 50.86, 48.64, 40.00, 33.93, 31.85, 25.96, 19.67, 18.12, 17.30, 12.74, −4.41, −4.71. $[α]_D^{20}$ = −40.90, (c 0.26, CHCl$_3$). HRMS (ESI+): calcd. for C$_{26}$H$_{44}$O$_4$Si [M + H]$^+$, 449.3082, found 449.3078.

4.19. Allyl (2E,4R,6E,8E,11S)-11-((Tert-Butyldimethylsilyl)oxy)-2,4,9-Trimethyl-13-Oxotetradeca-2,6,8-Trienoate (25b)

The procedure was identical to **25a**. Compound **25b** (160 mg, 85%) was obtained as a colorless oil.

^{1}**H NMR** (400 MHz, CDCl$_3$) δ 6.60 (dd, J = 10.0, 1.3 Hz, 1H), 6.19 (dd, J = 15.0, 10.8 Hz, 1H), 5.96 (ddt, J = 17.1, 10.5, 5.6 Hz, 1H), 5.74 (d, J = 10.8 Hz, 1H), 5.48 (dt, J = 14.8, 7.3 Hz, 1H), 5.32 (dd, J = 17.2, 1.5 Hz, 1H), 5.23 (dd, J = 10.4, 1.3 Hz, 1H), 4.64 (d, J = 5.5 Hz, 2H), 4.35–4.23 (m, 1H), 2.66–2.42 (m, 3H), 2.23 (dd, J = 13.2, 5.7 Hz, 1H), 2.19–2.05 (m, 6H), 1.84 (d, J = 1.2 Hz, 3H), 1.73 (s, 3H), 1.01 (d, J = 6.7 Hz, 3H), 0.84 (s, 9H), 0.02 (d, J = 7.1 Hz, 6H). ^{13}C NMR (101 MHz, CDCl$_3$) δ 208.07, 168.09, 147.76, 133.25, 132.74, 130.27, 128.31, 128.04, 126.52, 117.85, 68.09, 65.28, 50.84, 48.60, 40.04, 33.92, 31.84, 25.95, 19.71, 18.11, 17.33, 12.73, −4.42, −4.74. $[α]_D^{20}$ = −17.13, (c 0.51, CHCl$_3$). HRMS (ESI+): calcd. for C$_{26}$H$_{44}$O$_4$Si [M + H]$^+$, 449.3082, found 449.3079.

4.20. Allyl (2E,4R,6E,8E,11R,13S)-11-((Tert-Butyldimethylsilyl)Oxy)-13-Hydroxy-2,4,9-Trimethyltetradeca-2,6,8-Trienoate (26a)

To a solution of (R)-Me-CBS (1 M in toluene, 0.05 mL, 0.05 mmol) in dry THF (5 mL) was slowly added BH$_3$·DMS (12 uL, 0.13 mmol) at −40 °C. After being stirred for 30 min at the same temperature, a solution of **25a** (57 mg, 0.13 mmol) in THF (2 mL) was slowly added. After being stirred for 2 h at −40 °C, the mixture was diluted with MeOH. The resulting mixture was concentrated and extracted with DCM (30 mL × 3). The combined organic layers were washed with brine, dried, filtrated, and concentrated. The residue was purified by column chromatography on silica gel (PE/EA = 15:1) to give a mixture of **26a** and **26b** (4:1, 48 mg, 83%) as a colorless oil (pure major isomer **26a** can be obtained by repeating the purification on silica gel).

^{1}**H NMR** (400 MHz, CDCl$_3$) δ 6.60 (d, J = 9.9 Hz, 1H), 6.18 (dd, J = 14.7, 11.0 Hz, 1H), 5.96 (ddt, J = 17.1, 10.5, 5.6 Hz, 1H), 5.77 (d, J = 10.8 Hz, 1H), 5.49 (dt, J = 14.8, 7.3 Hz, 1H), 5.32 (dd, J = 17.2, 1.4 Hz, 1H), 5.23 (dd, J = 10.5, 1.0 Hz, 1H), 4.63 (d, J = 5.5 Hz, 2H), 4.27–4.06 (m, 2H), 2.66–2.47 (m, 1H), 2.35 (dd, J = 13.4, 6.3 Hz, 1H), 2.23 (dd, J = 13.3, 7.6 Hz, 1H), 2.16 (dd, J = 20.8, 13.7 Hz, 2H), 1.84 (s, 3H), 1.71 (s, 3H), 1.61 (ddd, J = 14.0, 10.0, 3.7 Hz, 1H), 1.48 (ddd, J = 14.5, 9.4, 3.7 Hz, 1H), 1.14 (d, J = 6.2 Hz, 3H), 0.99 (d, J = 11.9 Hz, 3H), 0.88 (s, 9H), 0.07 (d, J = 18.8 Hz, 6H). ^{13}C NMR (101 MHz, CDCl$_3$) δ 168.12, 147.74, 133.01, 132.72, 130.26, 128.29, 127.95, 126.52, 117.86, 70.36, 65.29, 64.58, 46.98, 43.26, 40.03, 33.91, 25.95, 23.98, 19.68, 18.06, 17.15, 12.76, −4.51, −4.70. $[α]_D^{20}$ = −17.67, (c 0.1, CHCl$_3$). HRMS (ESI+): calcd. for C$_{26}$H$_{46}$O$_4$Si [M + H]$^+$, 451.3238, found 451.3241.

4.21. Allyl (2E,4R,6E,8E,11R,13R)-11-((Tert-Butyldimethylsilyl)Oxy)-13-Hydroxy-2,4,9-Trimethyltetradeca-2,6,8-Trienoate (26b)

To a solution of (S)-Me-CBS (1 M in toluene, 0.1 mL, 0.1 mmol) in dry THF (5 mL), BH$_3$·DMS (24 uL, 0.25 mmol) was slowly added at −40 °C. After being stirred for 30 min at the same temperature, a solution of **25a** (110 mg, 0.24 mmol) in THF (2 mL) was slowly added. After being stirred for 2 h at −40 °C, the mixture was diluted with MeOH. The resulting mixture was concentrated and extracted with DCM (30 mL × 3). The combined organic layers were washed with brine, dried, filtrated, and concentrated. The residue was purified by column chromatography on silica gel (PE/EA = 15:1) to create **26b** (92 mg, 85%) as a colorless oil.

^{1}**H NMR** (400 MHz, CDCl$_3$) δ 6.60 (dd, *J* = 10.0, 1.3 Hz, 1H), 6.19 (dd, *J* = 15.0, 10.8 Hz, 1H), 6.04–5.92 (m, 1H), 5.77 (d, *J* = 10.8 Hz, 1H), 5.51 (dd, *J* = 14.9, 7.4 Hz, 1H), 5.33 (dd, *J* = 17.2, 1.5 Hz, 1H), 5.23 (dd, *J* = 10.4, 1.3 Hz, 1H), 4.64 (d, *J* = 5.5 Hz, 2H), 4.01 (dq, *J* = 13.0, 4.3 Hz, 1H), 3.96–3.83 (m, 1H), 3.18 (s, 1H), 2.66–2.50 (m, 1H), 2.32 (dd, *J* = 13.1, 4.6 Hz, 1H), 2.12 (dt, *J* = 13.2, 7.9 Hz, 3H), 1.84 (d, *J* = 1.1 Hz, 3H), 1.72 (s, 3H), 1.59–1.52 (m, 1H), 1.47–1.37 (m, 1H), 1.14 (d, *J* = 6.2 Hz, 3H), 1.02 (d, *J* = 6.7 Hz, 3H), 0.89 (s, 9H), 0.12 (d, *J* = 8.4 Hz, 6H). ^{13}**C NMR** (101 MHz, CDCl$_3$) δ 168.12, 147.73, 132.79, 132.72, 130.34, 128.23, 127.93, 126.54, 117.86, 72.22, 67.43, 65.29, 49.26, 44.82, 40.01, 33.91, 25.95, 23.70, 19.70, 18.03, 17.28, 12.75, −3.77, −4.55. $[\alpha]_D^{20}$ = −40.33, (*c* 0.35, CHCl$_3$). HRMS (ESI+): calcd. for C$_{26}$H$_{46}$O$_4$Si [M + H]$^+$, 451.3238, found 451.3241.

4.22. Allyl (2E,4R,6E,8E,11S,13R)-11-((Tert-Butyldimethylsilyl)Oxy)-13-Hydroxy-2,4,9-Trimethyltetradeca-2,6,8-Trienoate (26c)

To a solution of (S)-Me-CBS (1 M in toluene, 0.05 mL, 0.05 mmol) in dry THF (5 mL), BH$_3$·DMS (12 uL, 0.13 mmol) was slowly added at −40 °C. After being stirred for 30 min at the same temperature, a solution of **25b** (55 mg, 0.12 mmol) in THF (2 mL) was slowly added. After being stirred for 2 h at −40 °C, the mixture was diluted with MeOH. The resulting mixture was concentrated and extracted with DCM (30 mL × 3). The combined organic layers were washed with brine, dried, filtrated, and concentrated. The residue was purified by column chromatography on silica gel (PE/EA = 15:1) to give a mixture of **26c** and **26d** (3.6:1, 44 mg, 80%) as a colorless oil (pure major isomer **26c** can be obtained by repeating the purification on silica gel).

^{1}**H NMR** (400 MHz, CDCl$_3$) δ 6.60 (dd, *J* = 10.0, 1.3 Hz, 1H), 6.19 (dd, *J* = 15.0, 10.9 Hz, 1H), 5.96 (ddt, *J* = 17.1, 10.5, 5.6 Hz, 1H), 5.77 (d, *J* = 10.8 Hz, 1H), 5.49 (dt, *J* = 14.8, 7.3 Hz, 1H), 5.32 (dd, *J* = 17.2, 1.5 Hz, 1H), 5.23 (dd, *J* = 10.4, 1.2 Hz, 1H), 4.64 (d, *J* = 5.5 Hz, 2H), 4.23–4.07 (m, 2H), 3.36 (s, 1H), 2.67–2.49 (m, 1H), 2.35 (dd, *J* = 13.3, 6.2 Hz, 1H), 2.29–2.21 (m, 1H), 2.14 (t, *J* = 7.0 Hz, 2H), 1.84 (d, *J* = 1.1 Hz, 3H), 1.71 (s, 3H), 1.64–1.56 (m, 1H), 1.49 (ddd, *J* = 14.5, 9.5, 3.7 Hz, 1H), 1.14 (d, *J* = 6.2 Hz, 3H), 1.01 (d, *J* = 6.6 Hz, 3H), 0.88 (s, 9H), 0.06 (d, *J* = 20.4 Hz, 6H). ^{13}**C NMR** (101 MHz, CDCl$_3$) δ 168.09, 147.74, 133.01, 132.71, 130.27, 128.27, 127.94, 126.52, 117.86, 70.43, 65.29, 64.58, 46.92, 43.25, 40.04, 33.93, 25.95, 23.98, 19.73, 18.06, 17.21, 12.73, −4.52, −4.71. $[\alpha]_D^{20}$ = −14.83, (*c* 0.1, CHCl$_3$). HRMS (ESI+): calcd. for C$_{26}$H$_{46}$O$_4$Si [M + H]$^+$, 451.3238, found 451.3240.

4.23. Allyl (2E,4R,6E,8E,11S,13S)-11-((Tert-Butyldimethylsilyl)Oxy)-13-Hydroxy-2,4,9-Trimethyltetradeca-2,6,8-Trienoate (26d)

To a solution of (R)-Me-CBS (1 M in toluene, 0.1 mL, 0.1 mmol) in dry THF (5 mL), BH$_3$·DMS (24 uL, 0.25 mmol) was slowly added at −40 °C. After being stirred for 30 min at the same temperature, a solution of **25b** (113 mg, 0.25 mmol) in THF (2 mL) was slowly added. After being stirred for 2 h at −40 °C, the mixture was diluted with MeOH. The resulting mixture was concentrated and extracted with DCM (30 mL × 3). The combined organic layers were washed with brine, dried, filtrated, and concentrated. The residue was purified by column chromatography on silica gel (PE/EA = 15:1) to provide **26d** (100 mg, 88%) as a colorless oil.

^{1}**H NMR** (400 MHz, CDCl$_3$) δ 6.60 (dd, *J* = 10.0, 1.3 Hz, 1H), 6.19 (dd, *J* = 15.0, 10.8 Hz, 1H), 5.96 (ddt, *J* = 17.1, 10.5, 5.6 Hz, 1H), 5.76 (d, *J* = 10.8 Hz, 1H), 5.50 (dt, *J* = 14.8, 7.3 Hz, 1H), 5.32 (dd, *J* = 17.2, 1.5 Hz, 1H), 5.23 (dd, *J* = 10.4, 1.3 Hz, 1H), 4.64 (d, *J* = 5.5 Hz, 2H), 4.11–3.98 (m, 1H), 3.95–3.82 (m, 1H), 3.12 (s, 1H), 2.67–2.51 (m, 1H), 2.32 (dd, *J* = 13.2, 4.7 Hz, 1H), 2.19–2.06 (m, 3H), 1.84 (d, *J* = 1.2 Hz, 3H),

1.71 (s, 3H), 1.56 (dt, J = 14.4, 3.2 Hz, 1H), 1.46–1.38 (m, 1H), 1.14 (d, J = 6.2 Hz, 3H), 1.02 (d, J = 6.7 Hz, 3H), 0.89 (s, 9H), 0.11 (d, J = 8.9 Hz, 6H). ^{13}C NMR (101 MHz, CDCl$_3$) δ 168.10, 147.74, 132.78, 132.71, 130.32, 128.22, 127.91, 126.53, 117.84, 72.26, 67.41, 65.28, 49.21, 44.81, 40.03, 33.90, 25.95, 23.70, 19.72, 18.02, 17.33, 12.74, −3.78, −4.56. $[\alpha]_D^{20}$ = −15.29, (c 0.63, CHCl$_3$). HRMS (ESI+): calcd. for C$_{26}$H$_{46}$O$_4$Si [M + H]$^+$, 451.3238, found 451.3228.

4.24. Synthetic Procedure of 27a–27d

To a stirred solution of **26a** (35 mg) in dry THF (2 mL), the HF/Py complex (0.7 mL) was added at 0 °C. After being stirred for 1 h, the mixture was quenched with a saturated aqueous solution of NaHCO$_3$ and extracted with DCM (10 mL × 3). The combined organic layers were washed with 1 M HCl, brine, dried over Na$_2$SO$_4$, filtrated, and concentrated. The residue was purified by a column chromatography on silica gel (PE/EA = 2:1) to create **27a** (22 mg, 84%) as a colorless oil.

^{1}H NMR (400 MHz, CDCl$_3$) δ 6.64–6.56 (m, 1H), 6.23 (dd, J = 15.0, 10.8 Hz, 1H), 5.96 (ddt, J = 17.1, 10.5, 5.6 Hz, 1H), 5.84 (d, J = 10.8 Hz, 1H), 5.54 (dt, J = 14.8, 7.3 Hz, 1H), 5.32 (dd, J = 17.2, 1.4 Hz, 1H), 5.23 (dd, J = 10.5, 0.9 Hz, 1H), 4.64 (d, J = 5.5 Hz, 2H), 4.13–4.02 (m, 1H), 4.02–3.92 (m, 1H), 2.65–2.51 (m, 1H), 2.24–2.10 (m, 4H), 1.84 (d, J = 1.3 Hz, 3H), 1.75 (s, 3H), 1.61–1.55 (m, 1H), 1.55–1.47 (m, 1H), 1.20 (d, J = 6.2 Hz, 3H), 1.02 (d, J = 6.7 Hz, 3H). ^{13}C NMR (101 MHz, CDCl$_3$) δ 168.11, 147.65, 132.71, 132.58, 130.99, 128.31, 128.00, 126.60, 117.87, 70.45, 68.91, 65.30, 48.84, 44.80, 40.00, 33.83, 24.07, 19.72, 16.88, 12.75. $[\alpha]_D^{20}$ = −29.76, (c 0.34, CHCl$_3$). HRMS (ESI+): calcd. for C$_{20}$H$_{32}$O$_4$ [M + Na]$^+$, 337.2373, found 337.2375.

Compound **27b** (20.9 mg, 80%) was obtained as a colorless oil. ^{1}H NMR (400 MHz, CDCl$_3$) δ 6.60 (dd, J = 10.0, 1.3 Hz, 1H), 6.23 (dd, J = 15.0, 10.8 Hz, 1H), 5.96 (ddt, J = 17.1, 10.5, 5.6 Hz, 1H), 5.85 (d, J = 10.7 Hz, 1H), 5.54 (dt, J = 14.8, 7.3 Hz, 1H), 5.32 (dd, J = 17.2, 1.5 Hz, 1H), 5.23 (dd, J = 10.4, 1.2 Hz, 1H), 4.64 (d, J = 5.5 Hz, 2H), 4.21–4.12 (m, 1H), 4.08 (ddd, J = 12.4, 7.8, 5.3 Hz, 1H), 2.65–2.51 (m, 1H), 2.22–2.18 (m, 2H), 2.16 (d, J = 7.2 Hz, 2H), 1.84 (d, J = 1.3 Hz, 3H), 1.76 (s, 3H), 1.67–1.54 (m, 2H), 1.23 (d, J = 6.3 Hz, 3H), 1.02 (d, J = 6.7 Hz, 3H). ^{13}C NMR (101 MHz, CDCl$_3$) δ 168.11, 147.65, 133.00, 132.71, 130.92, 128.15, 128.03, 126.59, 117.86, 66.73, 65.47, 65.30, 48.14, 44.09, 40.01, 33.84, 23.69, 19.72, 16.81, 12.75. $[\alpha]_D^{20}$ = −14.00, (c 0.05, CHCl$_3$). HRMS (ESI+): calcd. for C$_{20}$H$_{32}$O$_4$ [M + Na]$^+$, 337.2373, found 337.2377.

Compound **27c** (22 mg, 84%) was obtained as a colorless oil. ^{1}H NMR (400 MHz, CDCl$_3$) δ 6.60 (dd, J = 10.0, 1.3 Hz, 1H), 6.23 (dd, J = 14.9, 10.8 Hz, 1H), 5.96 (ddt, J = 17.1, 10.5, 5.6 Hz, 1H), 5.84 (d, J = 10.8 Hz, 1H), 5.54 (dt, J = 14.9, 7.3 Hz, 1H), 5.33 (dd, J = 17.2, 1.5 Hz, 1H), 5.23 (dd, J = 10.4, 1.2 Hz, 1H), 4.64 (d, J = 5.5 Hz, 2H), 4.10–4.02 (m, 1H), 4.01–3.94 (m, 1H), 2.62–2.52 (m, 1H), 2.20–2.11 (m, 4H), 1.84 (d, J = 1.3 Hz, 3H), 1.75 (s, 3H), 1.61–1.55 (m, 1H), 1.54–1.46 (m, 1H), 1.20 (d, J = 6.2 Hz, 3H), 1.02 (d, J = 6.7 Hz, 3H). ^{13}C NMR (101 MHz, CDCl$_3$) δ 168.12, 147.64, 132.71, 132.57, 130.99, 128.32, 128.01, 126.60, 117.87, 70.45, 68.91, 65.31, 48.84, 44.81, 39.99, 33.85, 24.07, 19.70, 16.88, 12.75. $[\alpha]_D^{20}$ = −29.37, (c 0.32, CHCl$_3$). HRMS (ESI+): calcd. for C$_{20}$H$_{32}$O$_4$ [M + Na]$^+$, 337.2373, found 337.2374.

Compound **27d** (21.4 mg, 82%) was obtained as a colorless oil. ^{1}H NMR (400 MHz, CDCl$_3$) δ 6.23 (dd, J = 15.0, 10.8 Hz, 1H), 5.96 (ddt, J = 17.1, 10.5, 5.6 Hz, 1H), 5.86 (d, J = 10.8 Hz, 1H), 5.54 (dt, J = 14.8, 7.3 Hz, 1H), 5.33 (dd, J = 17.2, 1.5 Hz, 1H), 5.23 (dd, J = 10.4, 1.3 Hz, 1H), 4.64 (d, J = 5.5 Hz, 2H), 4.21–4.11 (m, 1H), 4.12–4.02 (m, 1H), 2.65–2.51 (m, 1H), 2.23–2.18 (m, 2H), 2.15 (t, J = 7.2 Hz, 2H), 1.84 (d, J = 1.3 Hz, 3H), 1.76 (s, 3H), 1.65–1.56 (m, 2H), 1.23 (d, J = 6.3 Hz, 3H), 1.02 (d, J = 6.6 Hz, 3H). ^{13}C NMR (101 MHz, CDCl$_3$) δ 168.12, 147.64, 132.99, 132.72, 130.95, 128.18, 128.04, 126.60, 117.87, 66.72, 65.48, 65.31, 48.14, 44.10, 39.99, 33.86, 23.69, 19.70, 16.82, 12.76. $[\alpha]_D^{20}$ = −17.62, (c 0.32, CHCl$_3$). HRMS (ESI+): calcd. for C$_{20}$H$_{32}$O$_4$ [M + Na]$^+$, 337.2373, found 337.2374.

4.25. Synthetic Procedure of 28a–28d

To a stirred solution of compound **27a** (22 mg, 0.065 mmol) in dry acetone (2 mL) under argon, PTSA·H$_2$O (1.14 mg, 0.006 mmol) and 2,2-dimethylpropane (0.08 mL, 0.65 mmol) were added sequentially. After 1 h, the reaction mixture was quenched with a saturated aqueous solution of

NaHCO$_3$ and extracted with DCM (2 × 10 mL). The combined organic extracts were washed with water and brine, dried over Na$_2$SO$_4$, and concentrated in vacuum. Purification by column chromatography (PE/EA = 20:1) provided **28a** (23 mg, 93%) as a colorless oil.

^{1}H NMR (400 MHz, CDCl$_3$) δ 6.61 (dd, J = 9.9, 1.3 Hz, 1H), 6.23 (dd, J = 15.0, 10.8 Hz, 1H), 5.96 (ddt, J = 17.1, 10.5, 5.6 Hz, 1H), 5.80 (d, J = 10.8 Hz, 1H), 5.50 (dt, J = 14.8, 7.3 Hz, 1H), 5.32 (dd, J = 17.2, 1.5 Hz, 1H), 5.23 (dd, J = 10.4, 1.3 Hz, 1H), 4.64 (d, J = 5.5 Hz, 2H), 4.04–3.88 (m, 2H), 2.65–2.50 (m, 1H), 2.30 (dd, J = 13.6, 5.9 Hz, 1H), 2.15 (t, J = 7.1 Hz, 2H), 2.06 (dd, J = 13.6, 7.0 Hz, 1H), 1.84 (d, J = 1.1 Hz, 3H), 1.74 (s, 3H), 1.49–1.42 (m, 4H), 1.41–1.34 (m, 4H), 1.15 (d, J = 6.1 Hz, 3H), 1.02 (d, J = 6.7 Hz, 3H). ^{13}C NMR (101 MHz, CDCl$_3$) δ 168.11, 147.77, 133.12, 132.72, 129.98, 128.39, 127.15, 126.52, 117.83, 98.61, 67.97, 65.34, 65.27, 46.85, 40.00, 38.60, 33.90, 30.46, 22.38, 19.94, 19.69, 17.34, 12.74. $[α]_D^{20}$ = −30.22, (c 0.26, CHCl$_3$). HRMS (ESI+): calcd. for C$_{23}$H$_{36}$O$_4$ [M + Na]$^+$, 377.2686, found 377.2689.

Compound **28b** (20.8 mg, 89%) was obtained as a colorless oil. ^{1}H NMR (400 MHz, CDCl$_3$) δ 6.61 (dd, J = 10.0, 1.3 Hz, 1H), 6.23 (dd, J = 15.0, 10.8 Hz, 1H), 5.96 (ddt, J = 17.1, 10.5, 5.6 Hz, 1H), 5.81 (d, J = 10.7 Hz, 1H), 5.49 (dt, J = 14.8, 7.3 Hz, 1H), 5.33 (dd, J = 17.2, 1.5 Hz, 1H), 5.23 (dd, J = 10.4, 1.3 Hz, 1H), 4.64 (d, J = 5.5 Hz, 2H), 4.04–3.88 (m, 2H), 2.64–2.51 (m, 1H), 2.31 (dd, J = 14.1, 6.9 Hz, 1H), 2.22–2.07 (m, 3H), 1.84 (d, J = 1.3 Hz, 3H), 1.74 (s, 3H), 1.63–1.57 (m, 2H), 1.35 (s, 6H), 1.18 (d, J = 6.3 Hz, 3H), 1.02 (d, J = 6.7 Hz, 3H). ^{13}C NMR (101 MHz, CDCl$_3$) δ 168.13, 147.79, 133.39, 132.74, 129.93, 128.43, 126.83, 126.52, 117.84, 100.32, 65.40, 65.28, 62.94, 46.16, 40.00, 39.83, 33.93, 25.24, 25.13, 21.86, 19.70, 17.07, 12.75. $[α]_D^{20}$ = −47.32, (c 0.11, CHCl$_3$). HRMS (ESI+): calcd. for C$_{23}$H$_{36}$O$_4$ [M + Na]$^+$, 377.2686, found 377.2684.

Compound **28c** (22 mg, 90%) was obtained as a colorless oil. ^{1}H NMR (400 MHz, CDCl$_3$) δ 6.61 (dd, J = 9.9, 1.3 Hz, 1H), 6.23 (dd, J = 15.0, 10.8 Hz, 1H), 5.96 (ddt, J = 17.1, 10.5, 5.6 Hz, 1H), 5.80 (d, J = 10.8 Hz, 1H), 5.50 (dt, J = 14.8, 7.3 Hz, 1H), 5.32 (dd, J = 17.2, 1.5 Hz, 1H), 5.23 (dd, J = 10.4, 1.2 Hz, 1H), 4.64 (d, J = 5.5 Hz, 2H), 4.02–3.88 (m, 2H), 2.66–2.50 (m, 1H), 2.30 (dd, J = 13.6, 5.9 Hz, 1H), 2.15 (t, J = 7.1 Hz, 2H), 2.06 (dd, J = 13.7, 7.0 Hz, 1H), 1.84 (d, J = 1.2 Hz, 3H), 1.74 (s, 3H), 1.49–1.42 (m, 4H), 1.41–1.34 (m, 4H), 1.15 (d, J = 6.1 Hz, 3H), 1.02 (d, J = 6.7 Hz, 3H). ^{13}C NMR (101 MHz, CDCl$_3$) δ 168.10, 147.76, 133.12, 132.72, 129.96, 128.39, 127.11, 126.51, 117.83, 98.60, 67.97, 65.34, 65.27, 46.81, 40.00, 38.60, 33.89, 30.45, 22.38, 19.94, 19.70, 17.35, 12.73. $[α]_D^{20}$ = −25.76, (c 0.69, CHCl$_3$). HRMS (ESI+): calcd. for C$_{23}$H$_{36}$O$_4$ [M + Na]$^+$, 377.2686, found 377.2685.

Compound **28d** (21.5 mg, 90%) was obtained as a colorless oil. ^{1}H NMR (400 MHz, CDCl$_3$) δ 6.61 (dd, J = 10.0, 1.3 Hz, 1H), 6.23 (dd, J = 15.0, 10.8 Hz, 1H), 5.96 (ddt, J = 17.1, 10.5, 5.6 Hz, 1H), 5.49 (dt, J = 14.8, 7.3 Hz, 1H), 5.32 (dd, J = 17.2, 1.5 Hz, 1H), 5.23 (dd, J = 10.4, 1.3 Hz, 1H), 4.64 (d, J = 5.5 Hz, 2H), 4.04–3.86 (m, 2H), 2.65–2.48 (m, 1H), 2.31 (dd, J = 14.1, 7.0 Hz, 1H), 2.20–2.06 (m, 3H), 1.84 (d, J = 1.3 Hz, 3H), 1.74 (s, 3H), 1.68–1.57 (m, 2H), 1.35 (s, 6H), 1.18 (d, J = 6.3 Hz, 3H), 1.02 (d, J = 6.7 Hz, 3H). ^{13}C NMR (101 MHz, CDCl$_3$) δ 168.11, 147.78, 133.38, 132.73, 129.90, 128.42, 126.79, 126.51, 117.83, 100.31, 65.38, 65.27, 62.93, 46.13, 40.00, 39.84, 33.92, 25.23, 25.11, 21.85, 19.70, 17.07, 12.74. $[α]_D^{20}$ = −17.71, (c 0.23, CHCl$_3$). HRMS (ESI+): calcd. for C$_{23}$H$_{36}$O$_4$ [M + Na]$^+$, 377.2686, found 377.2692.

4.26. Synthetic Procedure of 29a–29d

To a stirred solution of compound **26a** (48 mg, 0.11 mmol) in dry DCM (3 mL) and 4A molecular sieve under argon, the Proton Sponge (107 mg, 0.5 mmol) and trimethyloxonium tetrafluoroborate (60 mg, 0.4 mmol) were added sequentially. After 1 h, the reaction mixture was quenched with 1 M HCl (10 mL) and extracted with DCM (2 × 10 mL). The combined organic extracts were washed with water and brine, dried over Na$_2$SO$_4$, and concentrated in vacuum. Purification by column chromatography (PE/EA = 40:1) created **29a** (38 mg, 77%) as a colorless oil.

^{1}H NMR (400 MHz, CDCl$_3$) δ 6.60 (d, J = 9.9 Hz, 1H), 6.20 (dd, J = 15.0, 10.8 Hz, 1H), 5.96 (ddt, J = 17.1, 10.5, 5.6 Hz, 1H), 5.75 (d, J = 10.8 Hz, 1H), 5.47 (dt, J = 14.8, 7.3 Hz, 1H), 5.28 (ddd, J = 13.8, 11.6, 1.3 Hz, 2H), 4.64 (d, J = 5.6 Hz, 2H), 4.00 (tdd, J = 8.7, 5.4, 3.2 Hz, 1H), 3.54–3.37 (m, 1H), 3.28 (d, J = 2.2 Hz, 3H), 2.71–2.44 (m, 1H), 2.36–2.21 (m, 1H), 2.21–2.01 (m, 3H), 1.84 (d, J = 1.2 Hz, 3H), 1.72 (s, 3H), 1.62–1.54 (m, 1H), 1.37–1.28 (m, 1H), 1.11 (d, J = 6.1 Hz, 3H), 1.01 (d, J = 6.6 Hz, 3H), 0.88 (s, 9H),

0.05 (d, J = 6.1 Hz, 6H). ^{13}**C NMR** (101 MHz, CDCl$_3$) δ 168.12, 147.85, 133.80, 132.75, 129.65, 128.52, 127.56, 126.47, 117.85, 73.13, 67.86, 65.27, 55.62, 49.18, 44.92, 39.99, 33.96, 26.08, 19.64, 19.38, 18.20, 17.36, 12.72, −3.96, −4.53. $[α]_D^{20}$ = −38.67, (c 0.05, CHCl$_3$). HRMS (ESI+): calcd. for C$_{27}$H$_{48}$O$_4$Si [M + H]$^+$, 465.3395, found 465.3388.

Compound **29b** (72 mg, 76%) was obtained as a colorless oil. ^{1}**H NMR** (500 MHz, CDCl$_3$) δ 6.61 (dd, J = 9.9, 1.1 Hz, 1H), 6.20 (dd, J = 14.9, 10.9 Hz, 1H), 5.96 (ddt, J = 17.1, 10.5, 5.6 Hz, 1H), 5.77 (d, J = 10.8 Hz, 1H), 5.46 (dt, J = 14.8, 7.3 Hz, 1H), 5.33 (dd, J = 17.2, 1.5 Hz, 1H), 5.23 (dd, J = 10.4, 1.2 Hz, 1H), 4.64 (dd, J = 5.5, 1.1 Hz, 2H), 3.93–3.83 (m, 1H), 3.41 (dd, J = 12.5, 6.3 Hz, 1H), 3.29 (s, 3H), 2.64–2.47 (m, 1H), 2.28–2.05 (m, 4H), 1.84 (d, J = 1.3 Hz, 3H), 1.72 (s, 4H), 1.48–1.39 (m, 1H), 1.11 (d, J = 6.1 Hz, 3H), 1.01 (d, J = 6.7 Hz, 3H), 0.86 (s, 9H), 0.02 (d, J = 9.8 Hz, 6H). ^{13}**C NMR** (126 MHz, CDCl$_3$) δ 168.14, 147.87, 133.66, 132.73, 129.73, 128.47, 127.73, 126.45, 117.85, 74.24, 68.48, 65.28, 55.97, 48.38, 44.21, 40.01, 33.97, 26.01, 19.64, 19.43, 18.16, 17.33, 12.74, −4.15, −4.47. $[α]_D^{20}$ = −34.83, (c 0.38, CHCl$_3$). HRMS (ESI+): calcd. for C$_{27}$H$_{48}$O$_4$Si [M + H]$^+$, 465.3395, found 465.3391.

Compound **29c** (32 mg, 71%) was obtained as a colorless oil. ^{1}**H NMR** (400 MHz, CDCl$_3$) δ 6.59 (d, J = 9.7 Hz, 1H), 6.18 (dd, J = 15.0, 10.9 Hz, 1H), 5.94 (ddt, J = 17.1, 10.5, 5.6 Hz, 1H), 5.73 (d, J = 10.7 Hz, 1H), 5.45 (dt, J = 14.7, 7.2 Hz, 1H), 5.31 (dd, J = 17.2, 1.1 Hz, 1H), 5.21 (d, J = 10.5 Hz, 1H), 4.62 (d, J = 5.5 Hz, 2H), 3.98 (dt, J = 16.1, 6.0 Hz, 1H), 3.51–3.35 (m, 1H), 3.26 (s, 3H), 2.62–2.44 (m, 1H), 2.27 (ddd, J = 19.7, 13.8, 9.4 Hz, 1H), 2.18–2.01 (m, 3H), 1.82 (s, 3H), 1.70 (s, 3H), 1.60–1.52 (m, 1H), 1.37–1.25 (m, 1H), 1.09 (d, J = 6.1 Hz, 3H), 0.99 (d, J = 6.6 Hz, 3H), 0.86 (s, 9H), 0.03 (d, J = 6.8 Hz, 6H). ^{13}**C NMR** (101 MHz, CDCl$_3$) δ 168.11, 147.86, 133.79, 132.74, 129.66, 128.51, 127.55, 126.46, 117.84, 73.13, 67.86, 65.27, 55.63, 49.18, 44.91, 40.05, 33.97, 26.08, 19.71, 19.38, 18.20, 17.39, 12.72, −3.96, −4.54. $[α]_D^{20}$ = −26.17, (c 0.1, CHCl$_3$). HRMS (ESI+): calcd. for C$_{27}$H$_{48}$O$_4$Si [M + H]$^+$, 465.3395, found 465.3389.

Compound **29d** (72 mg, 70%) was obtained as a colorless oil. ^{1}**H NMR** (400 MHz, CDCl$_3$) δ 6.61 (dd, J = 10.0, 1.2 Hz, 1H), 6.20 (dd, J = 15.0, 10.9 Hz, 1H), 5.96 (ddt, J = 17.1, 10.5, 5.6 Hz, 1H), 5.77 (d, J = 10.8 Hz, 1H), 5.46 (dt, J = 14.7, 7.2 Hz, 1H), 5.33 (dd, J = 17.2, 1.5 Hz, 1H), 5.23 (dd, J = 10.4, 1.2 Hz, 1H), 4.64 (d, J = 5.5 Hz, 2H), 3.94–3.79 (m, 1H), 3.51–3.36 (m, 1H), 3.29 (s, 3H), 2.70–2.50 (m, 1H), 2.25–2.07 (m, 4H), 1.85 (d, J = 1.3 Hz, 3H), 1.79–1.67 (m, 4H), 1.45 (m, 1H), 1.12 (d, J = 6.1 Hz, 3H), 1.01 (d, J = 6.6 Hz, 3H), 0.86 (s, 9H), 0.01 (d, J = 9.0 Hz, 6H). ^{13}**C NMR** (101 MHz, CDCl$_3$) δ 168.12, 147.87, 133.67, 132.75, 129.73, 128.47, 127.72, 126.47, 117.84, 74.25, 68.54, 65.28, 55.97, 48.39, 44.20, 40.07, 33.96, 26.02, 19.70, 19.44, 18.17, 17.37, 12.74, −4.15, −4.47. $[α]_D^{20}$ = −16.46, (c 0.41, CHCl$_3$). HRMS (ESI+): calcd. for C$_{27}$H$_{48}$O$_4$Si [M + H]$^+$, 465.3395, found 465.3389.

*4.27. Synthetic Procedure of **1a**–**1d***

To a stirred solution of **29a** in dry THF (2 mL), the HF/Py complex (0.4 mL) was added at 0 °C. After being stirred for 1 h, the mixture was quenched with a saturated aqueous solution of NaHCO$_3$ and extracted with DCM (10 mL × 3). The combined organic layers were washed with 1 M HCl, brine, dried over Na$_2$SO$_4$, filtrated, and concentrated. The residue was purified by column chromatography on silica gel (PE/EA = 4:1) to create **1a** (20 mg, 70%) as a colorless oil.

^{1}**H NMR** (400 MHz, CDCl$_3$) δ 6.60 (dd, J = 9.9, 1.3 Hz, 1H), 6.23 (dd, J = 15.0, 10.8 Hz, 1H), 5.96 (ddt, J = 17.1, 10.5, 5.6 Hz, 1H), 5.83 (d, J = 10.8 Hz, 1H), 5.59–5.42 (m, 1H), 5.32 (dd, J = 17.2, 1.5 Hz, 1H), 5.22 (dd, J = 10.4, 1.2 Hz, 1H), 4.63 (d, J = 5.5 Hz, 2H), 4.10–3.98 (m, 1H), 3.69–3.61 (m, 1H), 3.34 (s, 3H), 2.57 (m, 1H), 2.17 (m, 4H), 1.84 (d, J = 1.3 Hz, 3H), 1.75 (s, 3H), 1.59–1.55 (m, 2H), 1.17 (d, J = 6.2 Hz, 3H), 1.01 (d, J = 6.6 Hz, 3H). ^{13}**C NMR** (101 MHz, CDCl$_3$) δ 168.11, 147.75, 133.68, 132.71, 130.36, 128.23, 127.58, 126.52, 117.85, 74.75, 66.38, 65.28, 56.34, 48.36, 42.82, 40.00, 33.89, 19.70, 18.94, 16.91, 12.73. $[α]_D^{20}$ = −25.83, (c 0.46, CHCl$_3$). HRMS (ESI+): calcd. for C$_{21}$H$_{34}$O$_4$ [M + Na]$^+$, 373.2349, found 373.2346.

Compound **1b** (40 mg, 74%) was obtained as a colorless oil. ^{1}**H NMR** (400 MHz, CDCl$_3$) δ 6.60 (dd, J = 9.9, 1.1 Hz, 1H), 6.23 (dd, J = 15.0, 10.8 Hz, 1H), 5.95 (ddt, J = 17.1, 10.5, 5.6 Hz, 1H), 5.82 (d, J = 10.8 Hz, 1H), 5.50 (dt, J = 14.8, 7.3 Hz, 1H), 5.32 (dd, J = 17.2, 1.5 Hz, 1H), 5.22 (dd, J = 10.4, 1.2 Hz, 1H), 4.63 (d, J = 5.5 Hz, 2H), 3.98–3.87 (m, 1H), 3.61–3.49 (m, 1H), 3.33 (s, 3H), 2.65–2.47 (m, 1H),

2.26–2.05 (m, 4H), 1.83 (s, 3H), 1.75 (s, 3H), 1.59–1.50 (m, 2H), 1.17 (d, J = 6.0 Hz, 3H), 1.01 (d, J = 6.7 Hz, 3H). ^{13}C NMR (101 MHz, CDCl$_3$) δ 168.10, 147.78, 133.68, 132.70, 130.13, 128.30, 127.42, 126.48, 117.82, 77.98, 69.74, 65.25, 55.89, 48.24, 43.29, 40.00, 33.88, 19.68, 19.20, 17.00, 12.71. $[α]_D^{20}$ = −29.17, (c 0.80, CHCl$_3$). HRMS (ESI+): calcd. for C$_{21}$H$_{34}$O$_4$ [M + Na]$^+$, 373.2349, found 373.2348.

Compound **1c** (18 mg, 75%) was obtained as a colorless oil. ^{1}H NMR (400 MHz, CDCl$_3$) δ 6.60 (dd, J = 9.9, 1.3 Hz, 1H), 6.23 (dd, J = 15.0, 10.8 Hz, 1H), 5.96 (ddt, J = 17.1, 10.5, 5.6 Hz, 1H), 5.83 (d, J = 10.8 Hz, 1H), 5.59–5.42 (m, 1H), 5.32 (dd, J = 17.2, 1.5 Hz, 1H), 5.22 (dd, J = 10.4, 1.2 Hz, 1H), 4.63 (d, J = 5.5 Hz, 2H), 4.10–3.98 (m, 1H), 3.69–3.61 (m, 1H), 3.34 (s, 3H), 2.57 (m, 1H), 2.17 (m, 4H), 1.84 (d, J = 1.3 Hz, 3H), 1.75 (s, 3H), 1.59–1.55 (m, 2H), 1.17 (d, J = 6.2 Hz, 3H), 1.01 (d, J = 6.6 Hz, 3H). ^{13}C NMR (101 MHz, CDCl$_3$) δ 168.11, 147.74, 133.68, 132.71, 130.34, 128.24, 127.58, 126.52, 117.85, 74.74, 66.38, 65.28, 56.34, 48.36, 42.87, 39.98, 33.89, 19.68, 18.96, 16.91, 12.73. $[α]_D^{20}$ = −21.89, (c 0.52, CHCl$_3$). HRMS (ESI+): calcd. for C$_{21}$H$_{34}$O$_4$ [M + Na]$^+$, 373.2349, found 373.2349.

Compound **1d** (40 mg, 74%) was obtained as a colorless oil. ^{1}H NMR (400 MHz, CDCl$_3$) δ 6.60 (dd, J = 9.9, 1.1 Hz, 1H), 6.23 (dd, J = 15.0, 10.8 Hz, 1H), 5.95 (ddt, J = 17.1, 10.5, 5.6 Hz, 1H), 5.82 (d, J = 10.8 Hz, 1H), 5.50 (dt, J = 14.8, 7.3 Hz, 1H), 5.32 (dd, J = 17.2, 1.5 Hz, 1H), 5.22 (dd, J = 10.4, 1.2 Hz, 1H), 4.63 (d, J = 5.5 Hz, 2H), 3.98–3.87 (m, 1H), 3.61–3.49 (m, 1H), 3.33 (s, 3H), 2.65–2.47 (m, 1H), 2.26–2.05 (m, 4H), 1.83 (s, 3H), 1.75 (s, 3H), 1.59–1.50 (m, 2H), 1.17 (d, J = 6.0 Hz, 3H), 1.01 (d, J = 6.7 Hz, 3H). ^{13}C NMR (101 MHz, CDCl$_3$) δ 168.10, 147.78, 133.69, 132.70, 130.11, 128.31, 127.41, 126.48, 117.83, 77.96, 69.75, 65.26, 55.89, 48.22, 43.30, 39.96, 33.88, 19.66, 19.20, 17.04, 12.71. $[α]_D^{20}$ = −38.68, (c 0.76, CHCl$_3$). HRMS (ESI+): calcd. for C$_{21}$H$_{34}$O$_4$ [M + Na]$^+$, 373.2349, found 373.2350. Detailed NMR data tables of **1a–1d** are in the Supplementary Material.

5. Conclusions

Asymmetric synthesis of the alotamdie fragment C15–C32 was established and four diastereomers were achieved concisely. Boron-mediated enantioselective aldol reaction led to a good diastereoselectivity and Julia-Kocienski olefination constructed the diene part in excellent E/Z selectivity and yield. A careful NMR comparison between four isomers and natural alotamide suggested the relative structure.

Supplementary Materials: A supplementary file is available online at http://www.mdpi.com/1660-3397/16/11/414/s1. Supplementary Information shows the NMR spectra of the synthetic compounds and the NMR data tables of **1a–1d**.

Author Contributions: Y.G. and C.-g.H. designed the experiments. H.-y.S., Y.X., P.H., Z.-Q.G., and Y.-h.L. performed the experiments. H.-y.S. and C.-g.H. wrote the paper.

Funding: We acknowledge financial support from the National Natural Science Foundation of China for Young Scientists [no. 81602998] and the National Science and Technology Major Project of the Ministry of Science and Technology of China (No. 2018ZX09731016-003 and No. 2018ZX09201001-001-008).

Conflicts of Interest: The authors declare no conflict of interest.

References

1. Nagarajan, M.; Maruthanayagam, V.; Sundararaman, M. A review of pharmacological and toxicological potentials of marine cyanobacterial metabolites. *J. Appl. Toxicol.* **2012**, *32*, 153–185. [CrossRef] [PubMed]
2. Mayer, A.M.; Rodriguez, A.D.; Taglialatela-Scafati, O.; Fusetani, N. Marine pharmacology in 2009–2011: Marine compounds with antibacterial, antidiabetic, antifungal, anti-inflammatory, antiprotozoal, antituberculosis, and antiviral activities; affecting the immune and nervous systems, and other miscellaneous mechanisms of action. *Mar. Drugs* **2013**, *11*, 2510–2573. [CrossRef] [PubMed]
3. Luesch, H.; Yoshida, W.Y.; Moore, R.E.; Paul, V.J.; Corbett, T.H. Total Structure Determination of Apratoxin A, a Potent Novel Cytotoxin from the Marine CyanobacteriumLyngbyamajuscula. *J. Am. Chem Soc.* **2001**, *123*, 5418–5423. [CrossRef] [PubMed]

4. Gutierrez, M.; Suyama, T.L.; Engene, N.; Wingerd, J.S.; Matainaho, T.; Gerwick, W.H. Apratoxin D, a potent cytotoxic cyclodepsipeptide from papua new guinea collections of the marine cyanobacteria Lyngbya majuscula and Lyngbya sordida. *J. Nat. Prod.* **2008**, *71*, 1099–1103. [CrossRef] [PubMed]
5. Matthew, S.; Schupp, P.J.; Luesch, H. Apratoxin E, a cytotoxic peptolide from a guamanian collection of the marine cyanobacterium Lyngbya bouillonii. *J. Nat. Prod.* **2008**, *71*, 1113–1116. [CrossRef] [PubMed]
6. Masuda, Y.; Suzuki, J.; Onda, Y.; Fujino, Y.; Yoshida, M.; Doi, T. Total synthesis and conformational analysis of apratoxin C. *J. Org. Chem.* **2014**, *79*, 8000–8009. [CrossRef] [PubMed]
7. Soria-Mercado, I.E.; Pereira, A.; Cao, Z.; Murray, T.F.; Gerwick, W.H. Alotamide A, a novel neuropharmacological agent from the marine cyanobacterium Lyngbya bouillonii. *Org. Lett.* **2009**, *11*, 4704–4707. [CrossRef] [PubMed]
8. Liu, L.; Rein, K.S. New Peptides Isolated from Lyngbya Species: A Review. *Mar. Drugs* **2010**, *8*, 1817–1837. [CrossRef] [PubMed]
9. Matinkhoo, K.; Pryyma, A.; Todorovic, M.; Patrick, B.O.; Perrin, D.M. Synthesis of the Death-Cap Mushroom Toxin alpha-Amanitin. *J. Am. Chem. Soc.* **2018**, *140*, 6513–6517. [CrossRef] [PubMed]
10. Hu, W.; Zhang, F.; Xu, Z.; Liu, Q.; Cui, Y.; Jia, Y. Stereocontrolled and efficient total synthesis of (−)-stephanotic acid methyl ester and (−)-celogentin C. *Org. Lett.* **2010**, *12*, 956–959. [CrossRef] [PubMed]
11. Ren, R.-G.; Li, M.; Si, C.-M.; Mao, Z.-Y.; Wei, B.-G. Studies toward asymmetric synthesis of leiodelide A. *Tetrahedron Lett.* **2014**, *55*, 6903–6906. [CrossRef]
12. Bosch, L.; Mola, L.; Petit, E.; Saladrigas, M.; Esteban, J.; Costa, A.M.; Vilarrasa, J. Formal Total Synthesis of Amphidinolide E. *J. Org. Chem.* **2017**, *82*, 11021–11034. [CrossRef] [PubMed]
13. Lin, L.; Romano, C.; Mazet, C. Palladium-Catalyzed Long-Range Deconjugative Isomerization of Highly Substituted alpha,beta-Unsaturated Carbonyl Compounds. *J. Am. Chem Soc.* **2016**, *138*, 10344–10350. [CrossRef] [PubMed]
14. Menche, D.; Hassfeld, J.; Li, J.; Mayer, K.; Rudolph, S. Modular total synthesis of archazolid A and B. *J. Org. Chem.* **2009**, *74*, 7220–7229. [CrossRef] [PubMed]
15. Takano, D.; Nagamitsu, T.; Ui, H.; Shiomi, K.; Yamaguchi, Y.; Masuma, R.; Kuwajima, I.; Ōmura, S. Total Synthesis of Nafuredin, a Selective NADH-fumarate Reductase Inhibitor. *Org. Lett.* **2001**, *3*, 2289–2291. [CrossRef] [PubMed]
16. Chen, K.; Xu, Z.; Ye, T. Total synthesis of amphidinins E, F and epi-amphidinin F. *Org. Chem. Front.* **2018**, *5*, 629–632. [CrossRef]
17. ElMarrouni, A.; Joolakanti, S.R.; Colon, A.; Heras, M.; Arseniyadis, S.; Cossy, J. Two concise total syntheses of (−)-bitungolide F. *Org. Lett.* **2010**, *12*, 4074–4077. [CrossRef] [PubMed]
18. Brun, E.; Bellosta, V.; Cossy, J. Synthesis of the Acyclic Carbon Skeleton of Filipin III. *J. Org. Chem.* **2016**, *81*, 8206–8221. [CrossRef] [PubMed]
19. Rychnovsky, S.D.; Rogers, B.N.; Richardson, T.I. Configurational Assignment of Polyene Macrolide Antibiotics Using the [^{13}C]Acetonide Analysis. *Acc. Chem. Res.* **1998**, *31*, 9–17. [CrossRef]
20. Huang, W.; Ren, R.G.; Dong, H.Q.; Wei, B.G.; Lin, G.Q. Diverse synthesis of marine cyclic depsipeptide lagunamide A and its analogues. *J. Org. Chem.* **2013**, *78*, 10747–10762. [CrossRef] [PubMed]
21. Kaneda, M.; Sueyoshi, K.; Teruya, T.; Ohno, H.; Fujii, N.; Oishi, S. Total synthesis of odoamide, a novel cyclic depsipeptide, from an Okinawan marine cyanobacterium. *Org. Biomol. Chem.* **2016**, *14*, 9093–9104. [CrossRef] [PubMed]
22. Babu, V.S.; Zhou, Y.; Kishi, Y. Design, synthesis, and cytotoxicity of stabilized mycolactone analogs. *Bioorg. Med. Chem. Lett.* **2017**, *27*, 1274–1277. [CrossRef] [PubMed]
23. O'Neil, G.; Black, M. A Synthesis of the C3-C15 Fragment of the Archazolids. *Synlett* **2009**, *2010*, 107–110. [CrossRef]

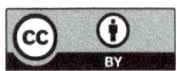

© 2018 by the authors. Licensee MDPI, Basel, Switzerland. This article is an open access article distributed under the terms and conditions of the Creative Commons Attribution (CC BY) license (http://creativecommons.org/licenses/by/4.0/).

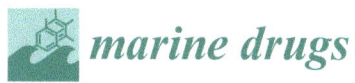

Article

Smenamide A Analogues. Synthesis and Biological Activity on Multiple Myeloma Cells

Alessia Caso [1,†], Ilaria Laurenzana [2,†], Daniela Lamorte [2], Stefania Trino [2], Germana Esposito [1], Vincenzo Piccialli [3,*] and Valeria Costantino [1,*]

1. Department of Pharmacy, University of Naples Federico II, 80131 Napoli, Italy; alessia.caso@unina.it (A.C.); germana.esposito@unina.it (G.E.)
2. Laboratory of Pre-Clinical and Translational Research, IRCCS—Referral Cancer Center of Basilicata (CROB), 85028 Rionero in Vulture, Italy; ilaria.laurenzana@crob.it (I.L.); daniela.lamorte@crob.it (D.L.); stefania.trino@crob.it (S.T.)
3. Department of Chemical Sciences, University of Naples Federico II, via Cintia 4, 80126 Naples, Italy
* Correspondence: vinpicci@unina.it (V.P.); valeria.costantino@unina.it (V.C.); Tel.: +39-081-674-111 (V.P.); +39-081-678-504 (V.C.)
† These authors contribute equally to this work.

Received: 29 May 2018; Accepted: 10 June 2018; Published: 13 June 2018

Abstract: Smenamides are an intriguing class of peptide/polyketide molecules of marine origin showing antiproliferative activity against lung cancer Calu-1 cells at nanomolar concentrations through a clear pro-apoptotic mechanism. To probe the role of the activity-determining structural features, the 16-*epi*-analogue of smenamide A and eight simplified analogues in the 16-*epi* series were prepared using a flexible synthetic route. The synthetic analogues were tested on multiple myeloma (MM) cell lines showing that the configuration at C-16 slightly affects the activity, since the 16-*epi*-derivative is still active at nanomolar concentrations. Interestingly, it was found that the truncated compound **8**, mainly composed of the pyrrolinone terminus, was not active, while compound **13**, essentially lacking the pyrrolinone moiety, was 1000-fold less active than the intact substance and was the most active among all the synthesized compounds.

Keywords: smenamides; marine natural products; peptide/polyketide molecules; synthetic analogues; functional-analogues; antiproliferative activity; MM cell line

1. Introduction

Marine sponges, together with their symbiotic microorganisms, have proven to be a rich source of skeletally new substances [1–3], which have often inspired novel strategies in anticancer drug discovery. Targeted cancer therapies consist of "drugs" which interfere with specific molecules necessary for tumor growth and progression. A primary goal of these therapies is to fight cancer cells with more precision without hitting normal cells. These drugs are classified into monoclonal antibodies, directed against antigens expressed on the neoplastic cell surface, and small molecules, usually designed to interfere with protein targets [4].

Smenamides A (**1**) and B (**2**) (Figure 1) are highly functionalized peptide/polyketide substances isolated by our group in 2013 from the Caribbean sponge *Smenospongia aurea* [5]. They have proven to be interesting for their structural features, such as the unusual *N*-methylacetamide western terminus, the dolapyrrolidone eastern terminus, typical of dolastatin-15 (**3**), a potent antimitotic agent derived from *Dolabella auricularia* [6], and the chlorovinyl functional group, common to some cyanobacterial metabolites, such as jamaicamides (**4–6**, Figure 1), isolated from *Lyngbiamajuscula* [7]. The only difference between the two smenamides resides in the configuration of the C-13/C-15 double bond positioned close to the middle part of the polyketide portion of the molecule. It has been speculated that this could determine a different overall shape and, as a consequence, the different biological behavior observed for smenamides [5].

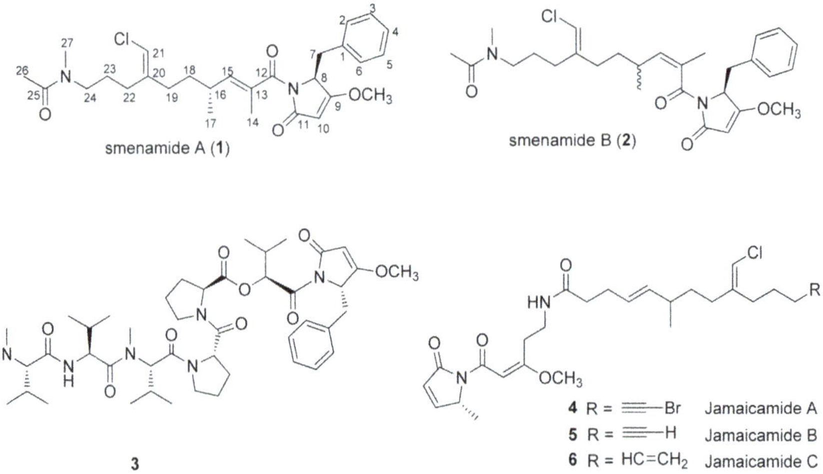

Figure 1. Smenamide A (**1**) and B (**2**), dolastatin-15 (**3**), and jamaicamides (**4–6**). Configuration at C-16 in smenamide A as determined by synthesis [8].

Smenamides have proven to be active in blocking the proliferation of the Calu-1 cancer cell line at nanomolar concentrations, working, however, with a different mechanism of action. Smenamide A, more interestingly, acts with a clear pre-apoptotic mechanism proving to be the more promising as a lead compound. It is worth stating that the configuration at C-16 in both smenamides remained unassigned in the original study due to the limited amount of the natural substances available. In a recent study, a chiral protocol strategy aimed at the total synthesis of the smenamide family was designed, starting from commercially available S-citronellene, a cheap starting material [8]. Two stereoisomers of smenamide A, namely *ent*-smenamide A and 16-*epi*-smenamide A (**7**, Figure 2), were synthesized. This synthetic effort allowed us to determine the C-16 configuration of smenamide A as *R* (Figure 1), as well as to develop a flexible synthetic route towards this class of substances.

In the present study, the antiproliferative activity of 16-*epi*-smenamide A has been evaluated on multiple myeloma (MM) cell lines. MM is a clonal plasma cell malignancy accounting for approximately 13% of all hematological cancers [9]. It originates from post-germinal centre B cells that accumulate somatic hypermutation and immunoglobulin heavy-chain class switching [8]. Several novel agents have been introduced into clinical practice but, after an initial response, most patients relapse or progress with a treatment-refractory disease [10]. For this reason, MM still proves to be incurable for most patients. In this scenario, it is necessary to develop new agents targeting novel pathways relevant for the MM cells, thereby increasing the range of available therapies.

In addition to 16-*epi*-smenamide A, the eight simplified synthetic analogues **8–15** (Figure 2) have also been synthesized. They were conceived as "functional-analogues" of smenamide A, incorporating some of the potential activity-determining structural features of the natural product. They were easily prepared thanks to the flexible nature of the previously developed synthetic route, with the aim of probing the importance of the main structural features of the smenamides, that is, the pyrrolinone, chlorovinyl and *N*-methylacetamido functional groups. In this paper, we illustrate a case-example of the application of this strategy to the design and study of functional-analogues of complex natural lead compounds.

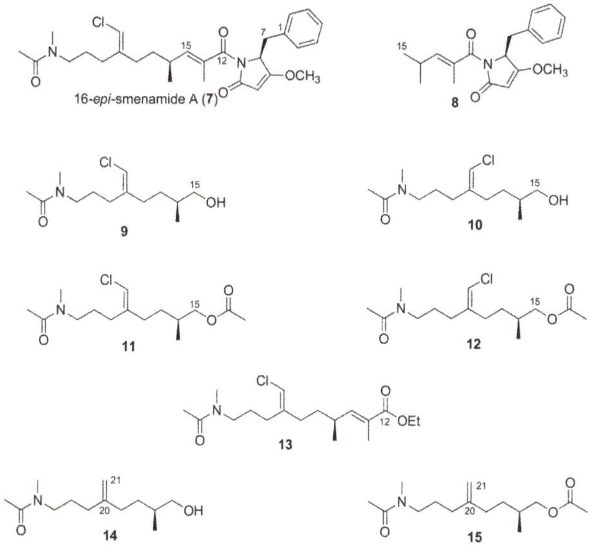

Figure 2. 16-*epi*-smenamide A (**7**) and its analogues **8–15**. For structural comparison, numeration of analogues is in agreement with that of 16-*epi*-smenamide A.

2. Results and Discussion

2.1. Compounds 7–15

16-*epi*-smenamide A (**7**, Figure 2) is the C-16 epimer of the natural smenamide A (**1**, Figure 1). It was synthesized starting from *S*-citronellene using the chiral protocol previously reported. 16-*epi*-smenamide A was tested on SKM-M1 and RPMI-8226 cells, two MM cell lines, showing it to be able to reduce cell viability in a dose-dependent way at nanomolar concentrations (see Section 2.2). We demonstrated that 16-*epi*-smenamide A, despite possessing the opposite configuration at C-16, retains the potent antiproliferative activity shown by the natural compound, smenamide-A, thus suggesting that this configuration does not affect the nature of its activity. Therefore, as a working hypothesis for the design of simplified analogues of 16-*epi*-smenamide A (**7**), this compound was hypothetically disconnected into two main building blocks, corresponding to the polyketide and the peptide moieties. To probe the importance of the main structural features of smenamides, eight "functional-analogues" of 16-*epi*-smenamide-A were prepared. In particular, the truncated compound **8**, retaining the C1–C18 portion of smenamide A, was synthesized to investigate the role of the pyrrolinone moiety. Compounds **9–12**, in turn, represent the simplified C15–C27 polyketide portion and retain only the chlorovinyl and *N*-methylacetamide functional groups. They also served to investigate the role of the geometric isomerism around the C20/C21 double bond. The modulation of the polarity within the 9/11 and 10/12 pairs was achieved by acetylation. Ester **13**, only lacking the pyrrolinone moiety, was prepared to simulate the entire polyketide portion, while compound **14** and its acetyl-derivative **15** allowed us to investigate the role of the chlorine atom. In fact, it is well known that the presence of halogens in natural products is important for the modulation of the biological activity [11,12], as previously reported.

Thus, the activation of 2,4-dimethyl-2-pentenoic acid as the pentafluorophenylester (**16**) (Figure 3) and its subsequent coupling with the previously synthesized pyrrolinone subunit **17** [8], afforded compound **8** in an 85% yield.

Ketone **18** (Figure 4) is a versatile intermediate to access 16-*epi*-smenamide analogues. It was easily prepared from commercially available *S*-citronellene, as depicted in Figure 4, and used as the starting material to obtain the seven analogues **9–15** by the introduction of the chlorovinyl, methylene and α,β-unsaturated ethyl ester functionalities (Figure 5). Thus, the Wittig olefination of **18** gave the two isomeric chlorovinyl derivatives **19** and **20** in a 3:2 ratio in favor of **19**, which could be separated by column chromatography.

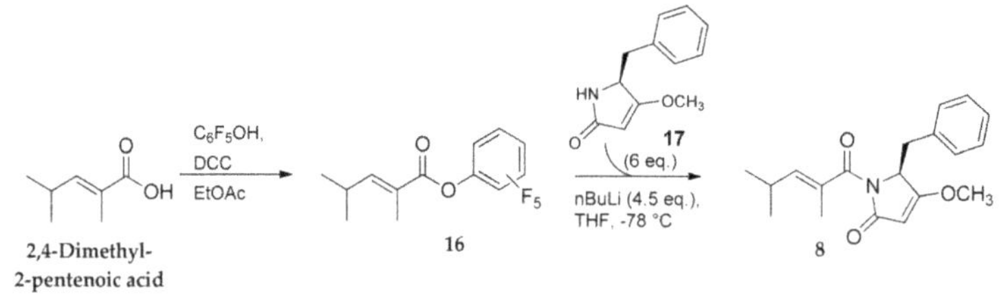

Figure 3. Preparation of pyrrolinone derivative **8**.

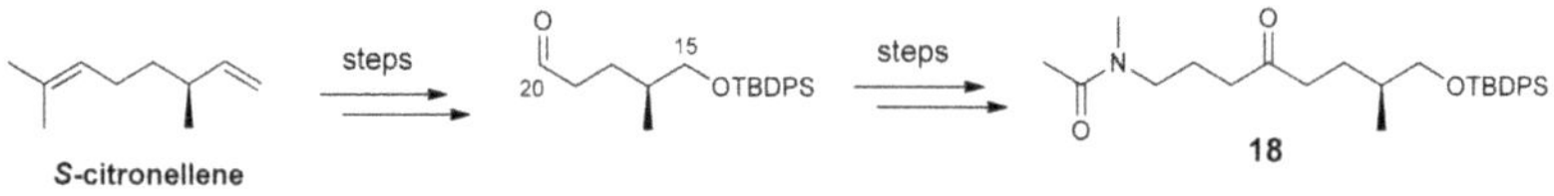

Figure 4. Synthesis of the ketone intermediate **18**.

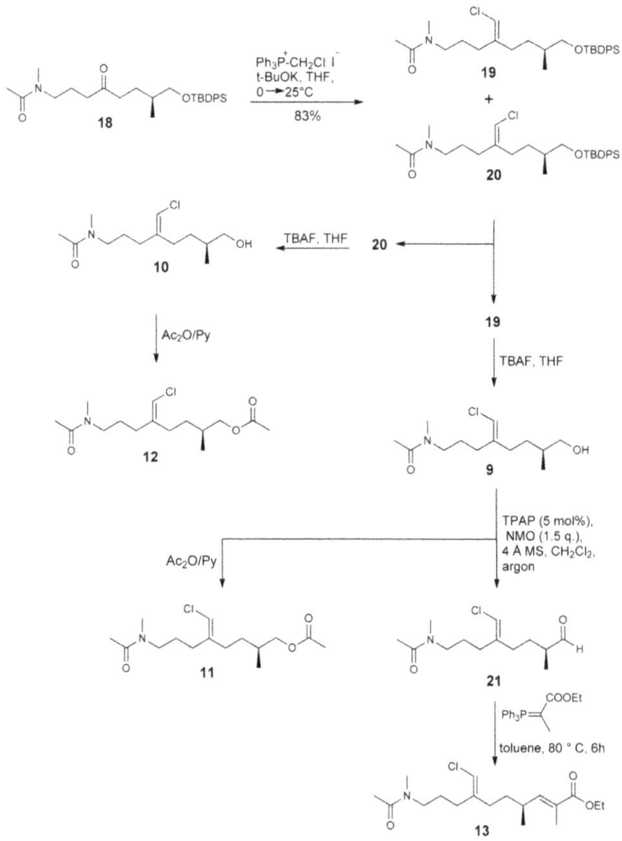

Figure 5. Preparation of compounds **9–13**.

Deprotection of both **19** and **20** with tetrabutylammonium fluoride (TBAF) in tetrahydrofuran (THF) afforded alcohols **9** and **10**, respectively, whose acetylation with Ac$_2$O/pyridine gave the corresponding acetyl derivatives **11** and **12**, respectively. In order to introduce the α,β-unsaturated ethyl ester function, the oxidation of **9** was accomplished with the Ley-Griffith method [tetrapropylammonium perruthenate (TPAP) (cat)/N-Methylmorpholine N-oxide (NMO)] [13–15] to give aldehyde **21** that was used in the subsequent Wittig reaction without further purification. Finally, the reaction with Ph$_3$P=CH(Me)-CO$_2$Et led to ethyl ester **13** in a 70% yield.

The methylene derivatives **14** and **15** were prepared by Wittig olefination of **18** using methylenetriphenylphosphorane (Figure 6). In particular, the first obtained product **22** was deprotected with TBAF in THF to give the desired alcohol **14** whose acetylation with Ac$_2$O/pyridine finally afforded the acetyl-derivative **15**.

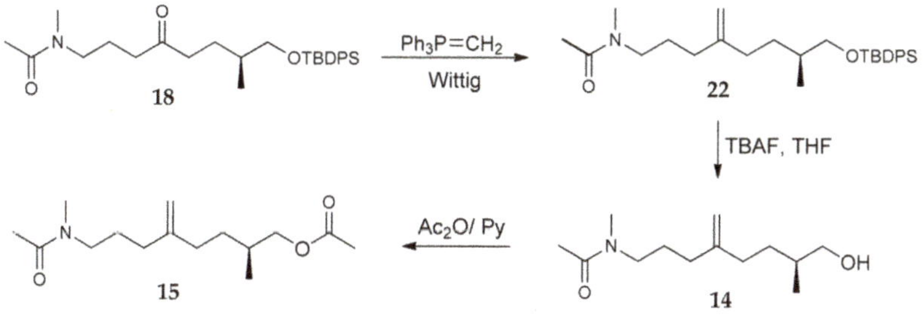

Figure 6. Preparation of methylene derivatives **14** and **15**.

All synthesized compounds were tested on RPMI-8226 cell lines, as described in Section 2.2. Compound **8**, lacking the great part of the polyketide moiety, was not active at all. As for the truncated polyketide compounds **9–15**, it was shown that only compound **13**, essentially lacking the pyrrolinone terminus, retained a certain degree of activity. In particular, a 1000-fold decreased EC50 value resulted, compared to the intact parent substance **7**. Equally, neither alcohols **9** and **10** nor the corresponding acetates **11** and **12**, not the dechlorinated analogues **14** and **15** showed significant activities. On the other hand, when the activity data of compounds **9–12** are compared with those of **13**, it is evident that the α,β-unsaturated ethyl ester function plays a role in the activity. In addition, even if it seems that the pyrrolinone terminus does not represent a crucial functional part of the molecule, its absence reduces the activity of **13** suggesting that it, or the entire C1–C15 unsaturated moiety, may be equally important for the full activity of smenamides, conferring rigidity to the molecule, possibly needed to exert the activity. However, these data alone do not allow us to speculate about the importance of the chlorine atom as well as of the configuration of the C20/C21 double bond on the activity.

2.2. In Vitro Evaluation of Activity on Multiple Myeloma Cell Lines

In order to study the in vitro effects of 16-*epi*-smenamide A (**7**) and its synthetic analogues **8–15**, MTS [3-(4,5-dimethylthiazol-2-yl)-5-(3-carboxymethoxyphenyl)-2-(4-sulfophenyl)-2H-tetrazolium, inner salt] assays were performed on SKM-M1 and RPMI-8226, MM cell lines, to evaluate their effects on cell viability. Compound **7**, tested at increasing concentrations (10–300 nM) for 48 h, was shown to reduce cell viability in both MM cell lines in a dose-dependent way (Figure 7). More than 50% of viability reduction was observed between 30 and 50 nM concentration. EC$_{50}$ for compound **7** was calculated as 44 nM in SKM-M1 cells, and 24 nM in RPMI-8226 cells, after 48 h of treatment.

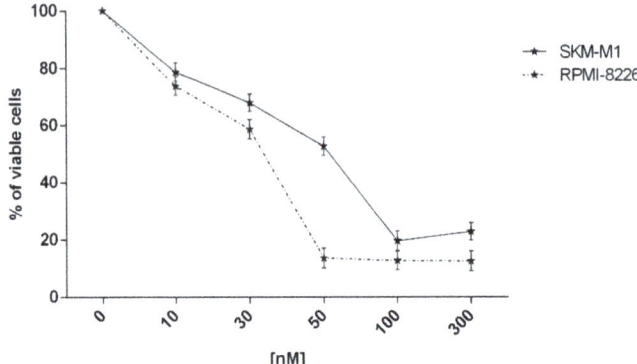

Figure 7. Viability of SKM-M1 and RPMI-8226 multiple myeloma (MM) cell lines was evaluated by MTS assay after treatment with compound **7** at different concentrations (10, 30, 50, 100 and 300 nM) for 48 h. Results are expressed as percent of cell viability normalized to dimethylsulfoxide (DMSO)-treated control cells. The line-graphs represent average with standard deviation (SD) from three independent experiments.

Likewise, compound **8** was used to treat SKM-M1 and RPMI-8226 cell lines at 50 nM, 100 nM, 1 µM, 5 µM and 10 µM concentrations, for 24, 48 and 72 h. MTS assays showed that compound **8** had no effect on cell viability on SKM-M1 cell line and negligible effect on RPMI-8226 cell viability (Figure 8). For this compound, EC_{50} was not calculated.

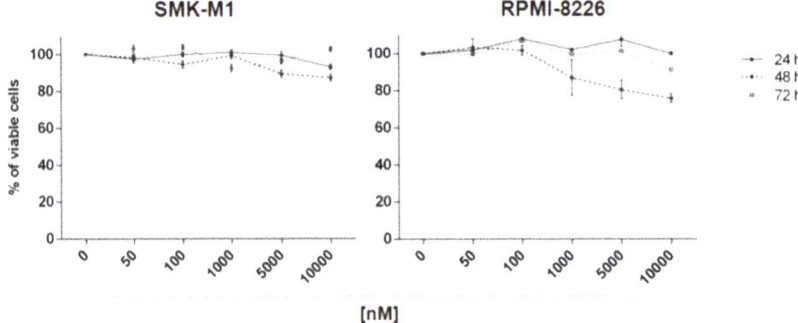

Figure 8. Cell viability was evaluated by MTS assay after treatment at different concentrations (50 nM, 100 nM, 1 µM, 5 µM, 10 µM) for 24, 48 and 72 h with compound **8** on SKM-M1 and RPMI-8226 cell lines. Results are expressed as percent of cell viability normalized to DMSO-treated cells. The line-graphs represent average with SD from three independent experiments.

Because compound **7** resulted more active on the RPMI-8226 cell line, its synthetic analogues **9–15** were tested on this cell line at increasing concentrations (50 nM, 100 nM, 1 µM, 5 µM) for all time points (24, 48 and 72 h). As shown in Figure 9, compound **9–12**, **14** and **15** have negligible effect on RPMI-8226 cell viability; while compound **13** was able to reduce cell viability reaching 80% of reduction at 5 µM, after 72 h of treatment. EC_{50} of compound **13** at 72 h was calculated as 1.1 µM.

Further investigation of the cell death mechanism was carried out using compound **13** (at 1 and 5 µM) to treat RPMI-8226 cells. Control experiments were carried out with dimethylsulfoxide (DMSO) as vehicle control, or with untreated cells. After 72 h of treatment, Annexin-V fluorescein isothiocyanate (FITC)/propidium iodide (PI) analyses were performed to evaluate whether the cytotoxic activity of compounds **13** was related to apoptosis induction. Data obtained showed that a significant increase of apoptotic cells at both concentrations occurred when cells are treated with compound **13** (5% of increase at 1 μM respect to control (* $p < 0.05$) and 66% at 5 μM (*** $p < 0.001$) (Figure 10a,b)). Moreover, compound **13** was able to significantly decrease the number of cell in G0/G1 phase and increase those in S phase at both concentrations (Figure 10c,d).

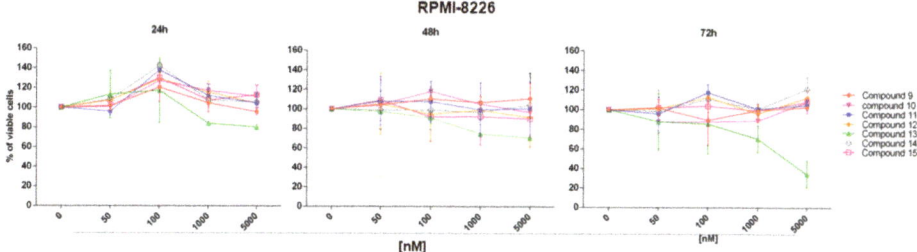

Figure 9. Cell viability was evaluated by MTS assay after treatment at different concentrations (50 nM, 100 nM, 1 μM, 5 μM) for 24, 48 and 72 h with compounds **9–15** on RPMI-8226 cell line. Results are expressed as percent of cell viability normalized to DMSO-treated cells. The line-graphs represent average with SD from three independent experiments.

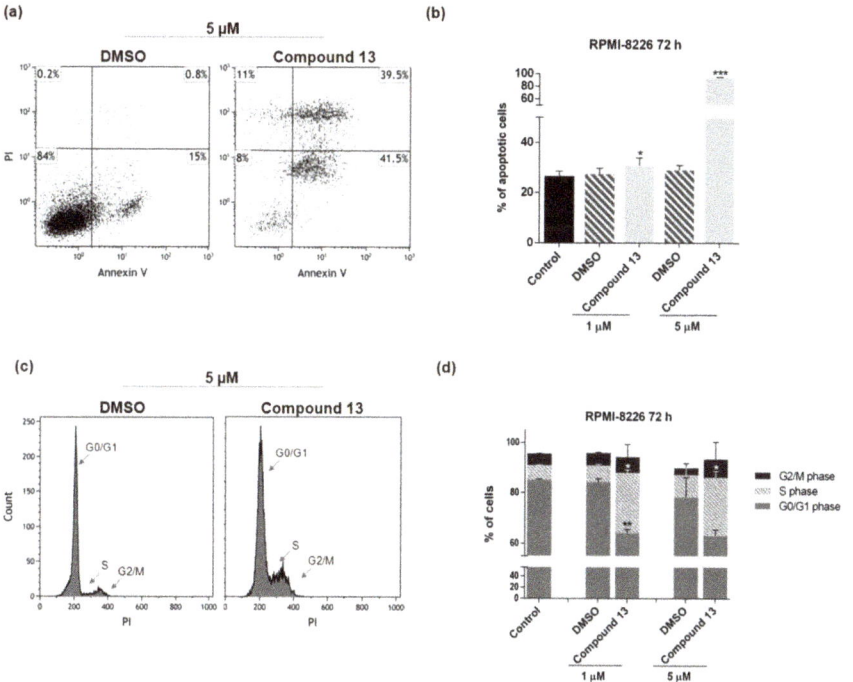

Figure 10. Compound **13**: cytofluorimetric evaluation of apoptosis/necrosis by the Annexin-V fluorescein isothiocyanate (FITC)/propidium iodide (PI) test (**a,b**) and cell cycle analysis by PI staining (**c,d**) on RPMI-8226 cell line, at 1 μM and 5 μM for 72 h. (**a**) Dot plots and (**c**) cell cycle histograms show a single representative experiment; (**b,d**) the bar-graphs represent average with S.D. (* $p < 0.05$, ** $p < 0.01$, *** $p < 0.001$).

3. Experimental Section

3.1. General Experimental Procedures

All reagents and anhydrous solvents were purchased (Aldrich and Fluka) at the highest commercial quality and used without further purification. Where necessary, flame-dried and argon-charged glassware was used. The reactions were monitored using thinlayer chromatography (TLC) carried out on precoated silica gel plates (Merck 60, F254, 0.25 mm thick). Merck silica gel (Kieselgel 40, particle size 0.063–0.200 mm) was used for the column chromatography. Na_2SO_4 was used as a drying agent for aqueous workup. Nuclear magnetic resonance (NMR) experiments were performed using Varian Unity Inova spectrometers at 400, 500, and 700 MHz in $CDCl_3$. Proton chemical shifts were referenced to the residual $CHCl_3$ signal (7.26 ppm). ^{13}C-NMR chemical shifts were referenced to the solvent (77.0 ppm). Abbreviations for signal coupling are as follows: s = singlet, d = doublet, t = triplet, q = quartet, m = multiplet, and b = broad. Optical rotations were measured using a JASCO P-2000 polarimeter at the sodium D line. High resolution mass spectra were recorded by infusion on a Thermo Linear Trap Quadrupole (LTQ) Orbitrap XL mass spectrometer equipped with an electrospray source in the positive mode using MeOH as the solvent.

See Supplementary Materials for all NMR spectra.

Compound 8

Compound 8. To a solution of 2,4-dimethyl-2-pentenoic acid (114 mg, 0.889 mmol) in EtOAc (4.0 mL), pentafluorophenol (188.2 mg, 1.02 mmol) and DCC (210.5 mg, 1.02 mmol) were added at 0 °C. The reaction mixture was stirred for 1 h at 0 °C and 3 h at room temperature and evaporated under reduced pressure to give 16 (185.9 mg, 0.632 mmol) that was used in the next step without further purification. ^{1}H-NMR: (400 MHz, $CDCl_3$): δ 6.90 (1H, d, J=9.75), 2.8–2.6 (1H, m), 1.95 (3H, s), 1.07 (6H, d, J = 6.6).

To a stirred solution of pyrrolinone 17 (126.6 mg, 0.624 mmol) [8] in THF (5.0 mL), nBuLi (0.390 mL, 0.632 mmol, 1.6 M soln in hexane) was added dropwise at −78 °C. After 15 min, a solution of pentafluorophenyl ester 16 (183.45 mg, 0.624 mmol) in THF (0.1 mL) was added via syringe. After 2 h, the reaction was quenched with a saturated aqueous NH_4Cl solution (5 mL) and extracted with EtOAc (3 × 15 mL). The organic phase was washed with water (15 mL) and brine (15 mL), dried, and concentrated in vacuo. The crude was purified by preparative TLC ($CHCl_3/CH_3OH$, 98:2) to give 8 (166.2 mg, 0.530 mmol, 85%) as colourless oil. $[\alpha]_D^{20}$ = +22.1 (c = 10, $CHCl_3$); ^{1}H-NMR: (400 MHz, $CDCl_3$): δ 7.23–7.17 (3H, m, ArH), 7.0–6.9 (2H, m, ArH), 5.62 (1H, d, J = 9.47), 5.01–4.96 (1H, m), 4.84 (1H, s), 3.87 (3H, s, OCH_3), 3.39 (1H, dd, J = 14.1, 5.4, H_a-7), 3.15 (1H, dd, J = 14.1, 2.0, H_b-7), 2.68–2.54 (1H, m), 1.8 (3H, s), 0.99 (6H, d, J = 6.5); ^{13}C-NMR (100 MHz, $CDCl_3$): δ 177.2, 171.3, 168.8, 145.2, 134.4, 129.8, 129.4, 128.1, 127.0, 94.8, 59.1, 58.3, 33.9, 27.4, 21.9, 21.5, 13.3; HRMS (ESI) m/z calcd. for $C_{13}H_{25}ClNO_2$ [M + H]$^+$ 262.1568, found 262.1566.

Compound 9

A mixture of compounds **19** and **20** was prepared as previously described [8]. Pure **19** and **20** were obtained by silica gel chromatography (hexane-EtOAc, 1:2). Deprotection of **19**, as reported [5] afforded alcohol **9** as colourless oil. $[\alpha]_D^{20}$ = −63.4 (c = 1.5, CHCl$_3$); ^{1}H-NMR: (400 MHz, CDCl$_3$, mixture of rotamers): δ 5.86 (0.4H, s, vinyl proton), 5.82 (0.6H, s, vinyl proton), 3.46 (2H, t, J = 5.3), 3.42–3.24 (2H, m's), 2.99 (1.8H, s, H$_3$-27), 2.89 (1.2H, s, H$_3$-27), 2.27–2.02 (7H, overlapped signals including two singlets at 2.09 and 2.07 for H$_3$-26), 1.78–1.52 (4H, m), 1.30–1.15 (1H, m), 0.93, 0.91 (overall 3H, overlapped d's, both J = 6.0, H$_3$-17); ^{13}C-NMR (100 MHz, CDCl$_3$): δ 170.6, 170.4, 142.0, 141.3, 113.2, 112.6, 67.8, 67.7, 50.5, 47.3, 36.1, 35.2, 33.2, 32.3, 32.2, 31.1, 31.0, 27.4, 27.3, 25.8, 24.6, 21.9, 21.2, 16.44, 16.38; HRMS (ESI) m/z calcd. for C$_{13}$H$_{25}$ClNO$_2$ [M + H]$^+$ 262.1568, found 262.1566.

Compound 10

To a solution of **20** (3.9 mg, 0.008 mmol) in THF (0.6 mL), TBAF (0.012 mL, 0.012 mmol, 1.0 M solution in THF) was added at 0 °C. The reaction mixture was allowed to reach room temperature and stirred for 1 h. Then, the reaction was quenched with a satd. aq. solution of NH$_4$Cl (0.5 mL). The phases were separated, and the aqueous layer was extracted with EtOAc (3 × 3 mL). The combined organic phases were dried and evaporated in vacuo. The crude was subjected to High Performance Liquid Chromatography (HPLC) separation [column Ascentis Si (Supelco), 25 cm × 4.6 mm, 5 μm; eluent: n-hexane/isopropanol 7:3, flow rate 1 mLmin^{-1}] to give alcohol **10** (1.0 mg, 48%, t$_R$ = 14.5 min) as colourless oil. $[\alpha]_D^{20}$ = +12.1 (c = 0.13; CHCl$_3$); ^{1}H-NMR (400 MHz, CDCl$_3$, mixture of rotamers): δ 5.83 (0.4H, s, vinyl proton), 5.81 (0.6H, s, vinyl proton), 3.50 (2H, bt, J = 5.7), 3.34, 3.26 (1H each, both t, J = 7.5, H$_2$-24), 2.98 (1.8H, s, H$_3$-27), 2.92 (1.2H, s, H$_3$-27), 2.31–2.17 (2H, m), 2.11–2.05 (5H, overlapped signals including a singlet at 2.08 for H$_3$-26); 1.75–1.53 (4H, overlapped multiplets); 1.29–1.19 (1H, m), 0.98, 0.96 (overall 3H, overlapped doublets, both J = 6.1, H$_3$-17); ^{13}C-NMR (100 MHz, CDCl$_3$): δ 170.7, 170.5, 142.0, 141.4, 113.0, 112.5, 67.9, 50.2, 47.4, 36.25, 36.0, 35.7, 35.6, 33.2, 32.2, 31.7, 30.33, 30.28, 27.6, 27.5, 26.2, 25.2, 22.0, 16.4; HRMS (ESI) m/z calcd. for C$_{13}$H$_{25}$ClNO$_2$ [M + H]$^+$ 262.1568; found 262.1566.

Compound 11

To a stirred solution of alcohol **9** (1.4 mg, 0.005 mmol) in pyridine (0.6 mL), excess acetic anhydride (0.4 mL) was added at rt. After 2 h the reaction mixture was evaporated under reduced pressure. The crude was subjected to HPLC separation [column Ascentis Si (Supelco), 25 cm × 4.6 mm, 5 μm; eluent: n-hexane/isopropanol 75:25, flow rate 1 mLmin^{-1}] to give acetyl derivative **11** as a colourless oil (1.5 mg, 0.0047 mmol, 95%). $[\alpha]_D^{20}$ = +5.1 (c = 0.12, CHCl$_3$); ^{1}H-NMR (400 MHz, CDCl$_3$, mixture of rotamers): δ 5.87 (0.4H, s, vinyl proton), 5.82 (0.6H, s, vinyl proton), 3.98–3.85 (2H, m), 3.39 (1.2H, t, J = 6.7, H$_2$-24), 3.29 (0.8H, t, J = 6.7, H$_2$-24), 3.00 (1.8H, s, H$_3$-27), 2.93 (1.2H, s, H$_3$-27), 2.27–2.03 (10H, overlapped signals including singlets at 2.10, 2.09 and 2.07 for acetates), 1.80–1.54 (4H, m), 1.57–1.47 (1H, m), 1.31–1.21 (1H, m), 0.95, 0.93 (overall 3H, overlapped d's, both J = 6.0, H$_3$-17); ^{13}C-NMR (100 MHz, CDCl$_3$): δ 141.9, 141.7, 141.3, 141.0, 113.5, 112.7, 68.92, 68.83, 50.5, 47.2, 36.0, 33.2, 32.12, 32.11, 32.09, 32.08, 31.31, 31.29, 31.27, 31.26, 27.45, 27.40, 27.38, 25.8, 24.7, 21.2, 20.9, 16.7; HRMS (ESI) m/z calcd. for C$_{15}$H$_{27}$ClNO$_3$ [M + H]$^+$ 304.1674, found 304.1669.

Compound 12

To a stirred solution of alcohol 10 (1.2 mg, 0.004 mmol) in pyridine (0.5 mL), excess acetic anhydride (0.4 mL) was added at room temperature. After 2 h the reaction mixture was evaporated under reduced pressure. The crude was subjected to HPLC separation [column Ascentis Si (Supelco), 25 cm × 4.6 mm, 5 μm; eluent: n-hexane/isopropanol 75:25, flow rate 1 mLmin^{-1}] to give acetyl derivative 12 as colourless oil (1.0 mg, 0.003 mmol, 75%). $[\alpha]_D^{20}$ = +12.88 (c = 0.06; CHCl$_3$); ^{1}H-NMR: (500 MHz, CDCl$_3$, mixture of rotamers): δ 5.83 (0.4H, s, vinyl proton), 5.82 (0.6H, s, vinyl proton), 3.99–3.88 (2H, m), 3.34 (1.2H, t, J = 7.6, H$_2$-24), 3.26 (0.8H, t, J = 7.6, H$_2$-24), 2.98 (1.8H, s, H$_3$-27), 2.91 (1.2H, s, H$_3$-27), 2.27–2.20 (3H, m,), 2.10–2.03 (7H, overlapped signals including singlets at 2.08, 2.07 and 2.06 for acetates), 1.85–1.45 (5H, m), 1.32–1.23 (1H, m), 0.99, 0.98 (overall 3H, overlapped d's, both J = 6.0, H$_3$-17); ^{13}C-NMR (100 MHz, CDCl$_3$): δ 171.4, 171.3, 170.6, 141.7, 141.0, 113.24, 112.7, 112.6, 69.0, 68.9, 50.2, 47.2, 36.2, 33.2, 32.44, 32.40, 31.7, 30.5, 27.5, 27.4, 26.1, 25.2, 22.0, 21.1 16.7; HRMS (ESI) m/z calcd. for C$_{15}$H$_{27}$ClNO$_3$ [M + H]$^+$ 304.1674; found 304.1671.

Compound 13

Compound 13 was prepared from alcohol 9 as previously described [8]. $[\alpha]_D^{20}$ = +127.4 (c = 0.5, CHCl$_3$); IR (neat) ν$_{max}$: 2957, 2927, 2858, 1707, 1651, 1596, 1459, 1424, 1373, 1262, 1122 cm^{-1}; ^{1}H-NMR (400 MHz, CDCl$_3$, mixture of rotamers): δ 6.49 (1H, d, J = 10.1, H-15), 5.82 (0.5H, s, vinyl proton), 5.76 (0.5H, s, vinyl proton), 4.18 (2H, q, J = 7.0, OCH2CH3), 3.37, 3.27 (1H each, both t, J = 7.6, H2-24), 2.99 (1.5H, s, H$_3$-27), 2.91 (1.5H, s, H$_3$-27), 2.46 (1H, m, H-16), 2.18 (2H, m), 2.09 (1.5H, s, H$_3$-26), 2.08 (1.5H, s, H$_3$-26), 2.01 (2H, t, J = 8.6), 1.83 (1.5H, d, J = 1.2, H3-14), 1.82 (1.5H, d, J = 1.2, H3-14), 1.30 (3H, t, J = 7.0, OCH$_2$CH$_3$), 1.02 (1.5H, d, J = 6.6, H$_3$-17), 1.00 (1.5H, d, J = 6.6, H$_3$-17); ^{13}C-NMR (100 MHz, CDCl$_3$) δ 170.5, 170.3, 168.3, 168.2, 146.9, 146.6, 141.6, 140.8, 132.1, 132.0, 131.94, 131.91, 128.5, 128.4, 127.2, 127.0, 113.4, 112.7, 60.6, 60.5, 50.4, 47.1, 36.0, 34.7, 34.6, 33.1, 32.7, 27.4, 27.3, 25.7, 24.6, 21.9, 21.3, 20.01, 19.98, 14.3, 12.63, 12.61; HRMS (ESI) m/z calcd. for C$_{18}$H$_{30}$ClNNaO$_3$ [M + Na]$^+$ 366.1812; found 366.1802.

Compound 22

To a stirred suspension of methylenetriphenylphosphorane (6.6 mg, 0.024 mmol) in THF (0.5 mL), nBuLi (0.015 mL, 0.024 mmol, 1.6 M sol. in hexane) was added dropwise at 0 °C under argon. After 30 min at 0 °C, a solution of ketone 18 (5.5 mg, 0.012 mmol) in dry THF (0.3 + 0.3 mL rinse) was added, and the mixture was allowed to reach room temperature. After 4 h, the reaction was quenched with a saturated aqueous NH$_4$Cl solution (2 mL) and extracted using Et$_2$O (3× 5 mL). The organic phase was washed with brine, dried, and evaporated under reduced pressure. The crude was purified by preparative TLC (chloroform/methanol 95:5) affording compound **22** colourless oil (4.5 mg, 0.096 mmol, 80%) as a colourless oil. ^{1}H-NMR (400 MHz, CDCl$_3$, mixture of rotamers): δ 7.66 (4H, J = 6.9, ArH), 7.44–7.35 (6H, m, ArH), 4.76 (0.5H, s, methylene proton), 4.72 (0.5H, s, methylene proton), 4.71 (1H, s, methylene protons), 3.53–3.44 (2H, m), 3.34, 3.23 (1H each, both t, J = 7.6, H$_2$-24), 2.96 (1.5H, s, H$_3$-27), 2.90 (1.5H, s, H$_3$-27), 2.07 (3H, s, H$_3$-26), 2.05–1.92 (4H, m), 1.74–1.56 (4H, m), 1.32–1.17 (1H, m), 1.05 (9H, s, C(CH$_3$)$_3$), 0.93 (3H, d, J = 6.5, H$_3$-17); ^{13}C-NMR (100 MHz, CDCl$_3$): δ 170.4, 149.2, 148.4, 135.6, 134.0, 133.9, 129.52, 129.48, 109.5, 108.9, 68.8, 68.7, 50.5, 47.4, 36.1, 35.4, 33.45, 33.38, 33.2, 32.8, 31.2, 29.7, 26.9, 26.1, 25.3, 21.9, 21.2, 19.3, 16.7; HRMS (ESI) m/z calcd. for C$_{29}$H$_{43}$NO$_2$Si [M + H]$^+$ 466.3136; found 466.3124.

Compound 14

To a solution of **22** (5.4 mg, 0.012 mmol) in THF (0.8 mL), TBAF (0.017 mL, 0.017 mmol, 1.0 M solution in THF) was added at 0 °C. The reaction mixture was allowed to reach rt and stirred for 1 h. Then, the reaction was quenched with a satd. aq. solution of NH$_4$Cl (1 mL). The phases were separated, and the aqueous layer was extracted with EtOAc (3 × 5 mL). The combined organic phases were dried and evaporated in vacuo. The crude was subjected to HPLC separation [column Ascentis Si (Supelco), 25 cm × 4.6 mm, 5 µm; eluent: ethyl acetate/isopropanol 9:1, flow rate 1 mLmin^{-1}] to give alcohol **14** (1.9 mg, 0.008 mmol, 70%) as colourless oil. [α]$_D^{20}$ = +7.24 (c = 0.07; CHCl$_3$); ^{1}H-NMR (400 MHz, CDCl$_3$, mixture of rotamers): δ 4.79 (0.5H, s, methylene proton), 4.75 (1.5H, bs, methylene protons), 3.54–3.43 (2H, m), 3.41–3.30 (1H, m, H$_2$-24), 3.27 (1H, t, J=7.4, H$_2$-24), 2.99 (1.5H, s, H$_3$-27), 2.92 (1.5H, s, H$_3$-27), 2.12 1.98 (overall 7H, including singlets at 2.09 and 2.07 for H$_3$-26), 1.75–1.50 (4H, m), 1.32–1.19 (1H, m), 0.95, 0.93 (overall 3H, overlapped d's, J = 6.5, H$_3$-17); ^{13}C-NMR (100 MHz, CDCl$_3$): δ 170.6, 150.8, 148.8, 148.3, 109.6, 109.2, 68.14, 68.10, 50.4, 47.5, 36.3, 35.4, 33.4, 33.2, 33.1, 33.0, 32.1, 31.08, 31.03, 29.7, 26.0, 25.1, 21.3, 16.6, 16.5; HRMS (ESI) m/z calcd. for C$_{13}$H$_{26}$NO$_2$ [M + H]$^+$ 228.1958; found 228.1956.

Compound 15

To a stirred solution of alcohol **14** (1.5 mg, 0.006 mmol) in pyridine (0.2 mL), excess acetic anhydride (0.2 mL) was added at rt. After 2 h the reaction mixture was evaporated under reduced pressure. The crude was subjected to HPLC separation [column Ascentis Si (Supelco), 25 cm × 4.6 mm, 5 µm; eluent: n-hexane/isopropanol 75:25, flow rate 1 mLmin^{-1}] to give acetyl derivative **15** as a colourless oil (1.0 mg, 0.004 mmol, 62%). [α]$_D^{20}$ = +13.63 (c = 0.07; CHCl$_3$); ^{1}H-NMR (400 MHz, CDCl$_3$, mixture of rotamers): δ 4.78 (0.5H, s, methylene proton), 4.75 (0.5H, s, methylene proton), 4.74 (1H, s, methylene protons), 3.99–3.84 (2H, m), 3.36, 3.26 (1H each, both t, J = 7.6, H$_2$-24), 2.98 (1.5H, s, H$_3$-27), 2.92 (1.5H, s, H$_3$-27), 2.12–1.96 (10H, overlapped signals including singlets at 2.09, 2.08 and 2.06 for acetates) 1.82–1.60 (4H, m), 1.34–1.22 (1H, m), 0.95, 0.94 (overall 3H, overlapped d's, J = 6.5, H$_3$-17); ^{13}C-NMR (175 MHz, CDCl$_3$): δ 170.42, 171.36, 170.6, 141.7, 141.05, 113.24, 112.6, 112,65, 69.0, 68.9, 50.2, 47.2, 36.2, 33.2, 32.43, 32.40, 31.9, 31.7, 30.5, 27.5, 27.4, 26.1, 25.2, 22.0, 21.4, 21.1, 16.7; HRMS (ESI) m/z calcd. for C$_{15}$H$_{27}$NO$_3$ [M + H]$^+$ 270.2063; found 270.2061.

3.2. Biological Activity

3.2.1. Cell Lines and Chemical

Human MM cell lines, SKM-M1 and RPMI-8226, were cultured in RPMI 1640 (Gibco, Life Technologies, Carlsbad, CA, USA) supplemented with 10% fetal bovine serum (FBS. Gibco, Life Technologies, Carlsbad, CA, USA), 1% of penicillin-streptomycin (Gibco) at 37 °C and 5% CO_2.

All chemical compounds were dissolved in DMSO (Sigma Aldrich, St. Louis, MO, USA) and diluted in FBS for cell treatments.

3.2.2. Cell Viability

SKM-M1 and RPMI-8226 cell lines were seeded into 96-well plates (3×10^4 cells/100 µL) and incubated with all compounds at increasing concentrations for different time points. In particular, compound **7** was used at concentrations 10–300 nM for 48 h; compound **8** at 50–10 µM for 24, 48 and 72 h; compounds **9–15** at 50–5 µM for 24, 48 and 72 h. Cells treated with the DMSO vehicle were used as control. Cell viability was determined using the CellTiter 96 Aqueous One Solution assay kit (MTS, Promega, Madison, WI, USA). The optical density was measured at 492 nm by plate reader (Das srl, Rome, Italy). Cellular viability was calculated as percentage of viable cells compared with DMSO control. All experiments were conducted in triplicate. EC_{50} values were obtained by GraphPad Prism (GraphPad Prism, San Diego, CA, USA).

3.2.3. Functional Tests

RPMI-8226 cell line was treated with 1 µM and 5 µM of compound **13** or with DMSO vehicle or not treated for 72 h (cell density 3×10^5 cells/mL) and used in:

- Apoptosis assay

Apoptosis of RPMI-8226 was evaluated by cytometric analysis of Annexin V and PI-stained cells using fluorescein isothiocyanate (FITC) Annexin V Apoptosis Detection kit I (Becton Dickinson, BD, Franklin, NJ, USA) [16]. Samples were prepared following the manufacturer's instructions; stained cells were acquired using NAVIOS flow cytometer (Beckman Coulter, Brea, CA, USA) and analyzed by Kaluza software (Beckman Coulter). 10,000 events were acquired for each samples; single positive for Annexin V and double positive for Annexin V and PI cells were interpreted as signs of early and late phases of apoptosis respectively. Percent of apoptotic cells was obtained from the sum of early and late apoptosis.

- Cell cycle analysis

After treatment RPMI-8226 cells were fixed in cold ethanol 70% for 1 h, then labeled with PI (Sigma Aldrich, St. Louis, MO, USA)/RNase A (EuroClone S.p.a., Pero, MI, Italy) staining solution for 30 min. Samples were acquired by NAVIOS flow cytometer and analyzed by Kaluza software (Beckman Coulter). 10,000 events were acquired for each sample.

3.2.4. Statistical Analysis

Statistical significance was determined using a paired t test by GraphPad Prism. All error bars represent the standard deviation (SD) of the average.

4. Conclusions

This study adds new knowledge about the antiproliferative activity and the possible role of smenamides, chlorinated peptide/polyketide substances originally isolated from the Caribbean sponge *Smenospongiaaurea*, as lead compounds in anticancer drug research. Our results have shown that the configuration at C-16 slightly affects the activity, since the 16-*epi*-analogue **7** was still active at nanomolar concentrations. Interestingly, it has been found that the truncated compound **8**, containing the pyrrolinone terminus, was not active while compound **13**, composed of the intact C12–C27 portion, retained the activity, even though its EC50 value was 1000 times smaller compared with the parent 16-*epi*-smenamide **7**. In addition, compound **13** was able to block the cell cycle at the G0/G1 phase. It is worth noting that smenothiazoles [17], biogenetically related but structurally different from smenamides, possess the same activity. This study provides the basic knowledge needed to design simplified and synthetically easily accessible analogues that could target MM cells.

Supplementary Materials: The following are available online at http://www.mdpi.com/1660-3397/16/6/206/s1, Figure S1: ^{1}H NMR spectrum of compound 16 (CDCl$_3$, 400 MHz), Figure S2: ^{13}C NMR spectrum of compound 16 (CDCl$_3$, 100 MHz), Figure S3: ^{1}H NMR spectrum of compound 8 (CDCl$_3$, 400 MHz), Figure S4: ^{13}C NMR spectrum of compound 8 (CDCl$_3$, 100 MHz), Figure S5: ^{1}H NMR spectrum of compound 10 (CDCl$_3$, 400 MHz), Figure S6: ^{13}C NMR spectrum of compound 10 (CDCl$_3$, 100 MHz), Figure S7: ^{1}H NMR spectrum of compound 11 (CDCl$_3$, 400 MHz), Figure S8: ^{13}C NMR spectrum of compound 11 (CDCl$_3$, 100 MHz), Figure S9: ^{1}H NMR spectrum of compound 12 (CDCl$_3$, 400 MHz), Figure S10: ^{13}C NMR spectrum of compound 12 (CDCl$_3$, 100 MHz), Figure S11: ^{1}H NMR spectrum of compound 22 (CDCl$_3$, 400 MHz), Figure S12: ^{13}C NMR spectrum of compound 22 (CDCl$_3$, 100 MHz), Figure S13: ^{1}H NMR spectrum of compound 14 (CDCl$_3$, 400 MHz), Figure S14: ^{13}C NMR spectrum of compound 14 (CDCl$_3$, 100 MHz), Figure S15: ^{1}H NMR spectrum of compound 15 (CDCl$_3$, 400 MHz), Figure S16: ^{13}C NMR spectrum of compound 15 (CDCl$_3$, 100 MHz).

Author Contributions: Conceptualization, V.P. and V.C.; Data curation, D.L. and S.T.; Funding acquisition, V.C.; Investigation, A.C., I.L. and G.E.; Supervision, V.P. and V.C.; Writing—original draft, A.C. and I.L.; Writing—review & editing, V.P. and V.C.

Funding: This research was funded by the European Union 7th Framework Programme (BlueGenics, FP7-KBBE-2012-6) under grant agreement No. 311848 and of the Università degli Studi di Napoli Federico II under the STAR project named SeaLEADS.

Conflicts of Interest: The authors declare no conflict of interest. The founding sponsors had no role in the design of the study; in the collection, analyses, or interpretation of the data; in the writing of the manuscript, and in the decision to publish the results.

References

1. Costantino, V.; Fattorusso, E.; Imperatore, C.; Mangoni, A. Glycolipids from sponges. Part 17.1 Clathrosides and isoclathrosides, unique glycolipids from the Caribbean sponge *Agelas clathrodes*. *J. Nat. Prod.* **2006**, *69*, 73–78. [CrossRef] [PubMed]
2. Costantino, V.; D'Esposito, M.; Fattorusso, E.; Mangoni, A.; Basilico, N.; Parapini, S.; Taramelli, D. Damicoside from *Axinella damicornis*: The Influence of a Glycosylated Galactose 4-OH Group on the Immunostimulatory Activity of α-Galactoglycosphingolipids. *J. Med. Chem.* **2005**, *48*, 7411–7417. [CrossRef] [PubMed]
3. Costantino, V.; Fattorusso, E.; Mangoni, A.; Perinu, C.; Teta, R.; Panza, E.; Ianaro, A. Tedarenes A and B: Structural and stereochemical analysis of two new strained cyclic diarylheptanoids from the marine sponge *Tedania ignis*. *J. Org. Chem.* **2012**, *77*, 6377–6383. [CrossRef] [PubMed]
4. Laurenzana, I.; Caivano, A.; La Rocca, F.; Trino, S.; De Luca, L.; D'Alessio, F.; Schenone, S.; Falco, G.; Botta, M.; Del Vecchio, L.; et al. A pyrazolo[3,4-*d*]pyrimidine compound reduces cell viability and induces apoptosis in different hematological malignancies. *Front. Pharmacol.* **2016**, *7*, 416. [CrossRef] [PubMed]
5. Teta, R.; Irollo, E.; Della Sala, G.; Pirozzi, G.; Mangoni, A.; Costantino, V. Smenamides A and B, chlorinated peptide/polyketide hybrids containing a dolapyrrolidinone unit from the Caribbean sponge *Smenospongia aurea*. Evaluation of their role as leads in antitumor drug research. *Mar. Drugs* **2013**, *11*, 4451–4463. [CrossRef] [PubMed]
6. Bai, R.; Friedman, S.J.; Pettit, G.R.; Hamel, E. Dolastatin 15, a potent antimitotic depsipeptide derived from *Dolabella auricularia*: Interaction with tubulin and effects on cellular microtubules. *Biochem. Pharmacol.* **1992**, *43*, 2637–2645. [CrossRef]
7. Edwards, D.J.; Marquez, B.L.; Nogle, L.M.; McPhail, K.; Goeger, D.E.; Roberts, M.A.; Gerwick, W.H. Structure and Biosynthesis of the Jamaicamides, New Mixed Polyketide-Peptide Neurotoxins from the Marine Cyanobacterium *Lyngbya majuscule*. *Chem. Biol.* **2004**, *11*, 817–833. [CrossRef] [PubMed]

8. Caso, A.; Mangoni, A.; Piccialli, G.; Costantino, V.; Piccialli, V. Studies toward the Synthesis of Smenamide A, an Antiproliferative Metabolite from *Smenospongia aurea*: Total Synthesis of ent-Smenamide A and 16-*epi*-Smenamide A. *ACS Omega* **2017**, *2*, 1477–1488. [CrossRef]
9. La Rocca, F.; Airoldi, I.; Di Carlo, E.; Marotta, P.; Falco, G.; Simeon, V.; Laurenzana, I.; Trino, S.; De Luca, L.; Todoerti, K.; et al. EphA3 targeting reduces in vitro adhesion and invasion and in vivo growth and angiogenesis of multiple myeloma cells. *Cell. Oncol.* **2017**, *40*, 483–496. [CrossRef] [PubMed]
10. Caivano, A.; La Rocca, F.; Laurenzana, I.; Annese, T.; Tamma, R.; Famigliari, U.; Simeon, V.; Trino, S.; De Luca, L.; Villani, O.; et al. Epha3 acts as proangiogenic factor in multiple myeloma. *Oncotarget* **2017**, *8*, 34298–34309. [CrossRef] [PubMed]
11. Esposito, G.; Bourguet-Kondracki, M.-L.; Mai, L.H.; Longeon, A.; Teta, R.; Meijer, L.; Van Soest, R.; Mangoni, A.; Costantino, V. Chloromethylhalicyclamine B, a Marine-Derived Protein Kinase CK1δ/ε Inhibitor. *J. Nat. Prod.* **2016**, *79*, 2953–2960. [CrossRef] [PubMed]
12. Esposito, G.; Della Sala, G.; Teta, R.; Caso, A.; Bourguet-Kondracki, M.-L.; Pawlik, J.R.; Mangoni, A.; Costantino, V. Chlorinated thiazole containing polyketide-peptides from the Caribbean sponge *Smenospongia conulosa*: Structure elucidation on microgram scale. *EJOC* **2016**, *16*, 2871–2875. [CrossRef]
13. Ley, S.V.; Norman, J.; Griffith, W.P.; Marsden, S.P. Tetrapropylammoniumperruthenate, $Pr^4N^+RuO4^-$, TPAP: A catalytic oxidant for organic synthesis. *Synthesis* **1994**, 639–666. [CrossRef]
14. Piccialli, V. Ruthenium tetroxide and perruthenate chemistry. Recent advances and related transformations mediated by other transition metal oxospecies. *Molecules* **2014**, *19*, 6534–6582. [CrossRef] [PubMed]
15. Zerk, T.J.; Moore, P.W.; Harbort, J.S.; Chow, S.; Byrne, L.; Koutsantonis, G.A.; Harmer, J.R.; Martínez, M.; Williams, C.M.; Bernhardt, P.V. Elucidating the mechanism of the Ley–Griffith (TPAP) alcohol oxidation. *Chem. Sci.* **2017**, *8*, 8435–8442. [CrossRef] [PubMed]
16. Laurenzana, I.; Caivano, A.; Trino, S.; De Luca, L.; La Rocca, F.; Simeon, V.; Tintori, C.; D'Alessio, F.; Teramo, A.; Zambello, R.; et al. A Pyrazolo[3,4-*d*]pyrimidine compound inhibits Fyn phosphorylation and induces apoptosis in natural killer cell leukemia. *Oncotarget* **2016**, *7*, 65171–65184. [CrossRef] [PubMed]
17. Esposito, G.; Teta, R.; Miceli, R.; Ceccarelli, L.S.; Della Sala, G.; Camerlingo, R.; Irollo, E.; Mangoni, A.; Pirozzi, G.; Costantino, V. Isolation and assessment of the in vitro anti-tumor activity of smenothiazole A and B, chlorinated thiazole-containing peptide/polyketides from the Caribbean sponge, Smenospongiaaurea. *Mar. Drugs* **2015**, *13*, 444–459. [CrossRef] [PubMed]

© 2018 by the authors. Licensee MDPI, Basel, Switzerland. This article is an open access article distributed under the terms and conditions of the Creative Commons Attribution (CC BY) license (http://creativecommons.org/licenses/by/4.0/).

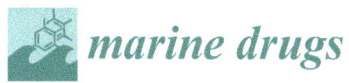

Article

Synthesis and Antitumor Activity Evaluation of Compounds Based on Toluquinol

Iván Cheng-Sánchez [1,†], José A. Torres-Vargas [2,3,†], Beatriz Martínez-Poveda [2,3], Guillermo A. Guerrero-Vásquez [1], Miguel Ángel Medina [2,3,4], Francisco Sarabia [1,*] and Ana R. Quesada [2,3,4,*]

1 Department of Organic Chemistry, Faculty of Sciences, University of Málaga, Campus de Teatinos s/n, 29071 Málaga, Spain
2 Department of Molecular Biology and Biochemistry, Faculty of Sciences, University of Málaga, Campus de Teatinos s/n, 29071 Málaga, Spain
3 IBIMA (Biomedical Research Institute of Málaga), 29071 Málaga, Spain
4 CIBER of Rare Diseases; Group U741 (CB06/07/0046), 29071 Málaga, Spain
* Correspondence: frsarabia@uma.es (F.S.); quesada@uma.es (A.R.Q.); Tel.: +34-952-134-258 (F.S.)
† Iván Cheng-Sánchez and José A. Torres-Vargas contributed equally to the execution of this work.

Received: 28 July 2019; Accepted: 18 August 2019; Published: 23 August 2019

Abstract: Encouraged by the promising antitumoral, antiangiogenic, and antilymphangiogenic properties of toluquinol, a set of analogues of this natural product of marine origin was synthesized to explore and evaluate the effects of structural modifications on their cytotoxic activity. We decided to investigate the effects of the substitution of the methyl group by other groups, the introduction of a second substituent, the relative position of the substituents, and the oxidation state. A set of analogues of 2-substituted, 2,3-disubstituted, and 2,6-disubstituted derived from hydroquinone were synthesized. The results revealed that the cytotoxic activity of this family of compounds could rely on the hydroquinone/benzoquinone part of the molecule, whereas the substituents might modulate the interaction of the molecule with their targets, changing either its activity or its selectivity. The methyl group is relevant for the cytotoxicity of toluquinol, since its replacement by other groups resulted in a significant loss of activity, and in general the introduction of a second substituent, preferentially in the para position with respect to the methyl group, was well tolerated. These findings provide guidance for the design of new toluquinol analogues with potentially better pharmacological properties.

Keywords: toluquinol; thymoquinone; marine hydroquinone; antitumor; natural compound analogues

1. Introduction

Hydroquinones and quinones are ubiquitous in nature, playing essential roles in oxidative metabolism, including in electron transport chains and photosynthesis, and are produced as primary or secondary metabolites by many organisms. A myriad of hydroquinones and quinones have been isolated from marine sources, including microbes, algae, and marine invertebrates, such as ascidians, sponges, cnidarians, and mollusks [1,2]. Some of them display a wide range of biological activities, including cytotoxicity to cancer cells, probably related to their involvement in redox cycling and/or Michael-1,4-addition reactions [3]. In many cases, the molecules responsible for the biological activities detected in some marine macroorganisms derive from the complex secondary metabolite relationship between the marine microorganisms and their hosts [4]. Marine fungi are a rich source of structurally diverse compounds with a high pharmaceutical potential [5]. In the course of our ongoing research program aimed at the search and characterization of new drug candidates of a marine origin, toluquinol (2-methylhydroquinone, compound **1**) was isolated from the culture broth of the marine fungus *Penicillium* sp. HL-85-ALS5-R004 [6]. The antitumoral, antiangiogenic, and antilymphangiogenic activities of toluquinol [6,7] make this compound a good example of the potential of marine-derived compounds in the treatment of cancer. Encouraged by these results, we decided to explore the effects of structural modifications of toluquinol on its antitumoral properties in order to establish a structure-activity relationship as a guide to identify and develop either more potent or more specific analogues based on this natural product. These structural modifications included the substitution of the methyl group of toluquinol by different substituents (derivatives **2–7**), the introduction of a second substituent (derivatives **8–11**), the effect of the position of this second substituent (derivatives **12–13**), and, finally the oxidation state of the hydroquinone, such as the case of toluquinol (**1**) and toluquinone (**14**), and thymoquinol (**15**) and thymoquinone (**16**) (Figure 1).

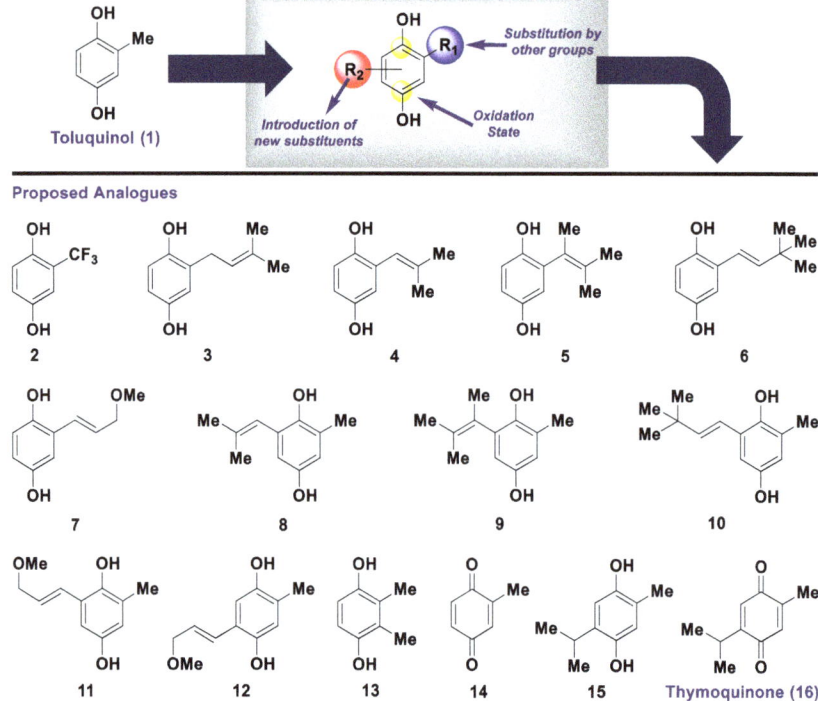

Figure 1. Structures of toluquinol (**1**) and programmed set of analogues **2–16**.

2. Results and Discussion

2.1. Synthesis of Compounds **2–15**

For the synthesis of analogues **2** and **3**, we used the procedures described in the literature [8,9], according to which the trifluoromethyl derivative **2** and the prenyl derivative **3** were prepared by direct treatment of 1,4-hydroquinone (**17**) with 5-(trifluoromethyl)-dibenzothiophenium trifluoromethanesulfonate (Umemoto's reagent) and prenol, respectively, under acidic conditions (Scheme 1). Whereas the preparation of **2** proceeded without further issues, the synthesis of **3** was more complicated due to the low yield of the coveted prenyl derivative **3**, obtained at a poor 15% yield, and the formation of sub-products that could be identified as the disubstituted derivative **18** and the benzopyrane **19**, obtained in 3% and 2.7% yields, respectively. The three compounds obtained from this reaction could be separated by flash column chromatography and sub-products **18** and **19** were considered for inclusion in the biological studies (Scheme 1).

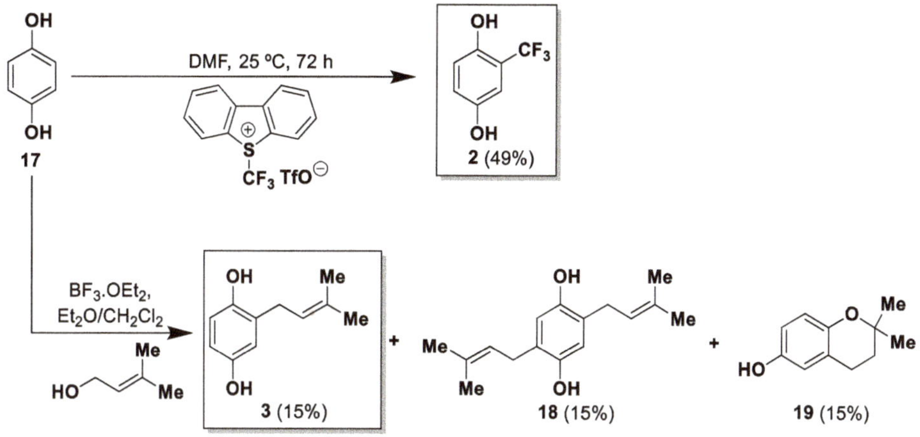

Scheme 1. Synthesis of analogues 2 and 3.

For the synthesis of analogues 4–7, we considered a Suzuki coupling reaction as a straightforward and powerful method [10] to install a vinyl-type substituent via direct coupling of the 2-bromo-1,4-hydroquinone **20**, prepared by bromination of **17** [11], with the corresponding pinacol boronic ester. The optimization of this coupling reaction led us to establish Pd[PPh$_3$]$_4$ and K$_2$CO$_3$ as the most suitable catalyst and base, respectively. On the other hand, the solvent, temperature, and reaction time depended on the boronic ester employed. Thus, when the reactions were undertaken using the solvent system 1,4-dioxane/H$_2$O at 80 °C, which are the usual reaction conditions for Suzuki couplings (Conditions A), we observed an important degree of degradation of the reaction mixture, detecting only small amounts of the corresponding coupling products. In light of these discouraging results, we found that reactions undertaken in THF instead of 1,4-dioxane produced better results in terms of the resulting yields of the coupling products. With this new solvent system, products **4** and **5** were obtained in 92 and 32% yields, requiring a reaction time for completion of 48 h (Conditions B), and products **6** and **7** were obtained in 79 and 56% yields, respectively, after 15 h for the completion of the coupling reactions (Conditions C) (Scheme 2).

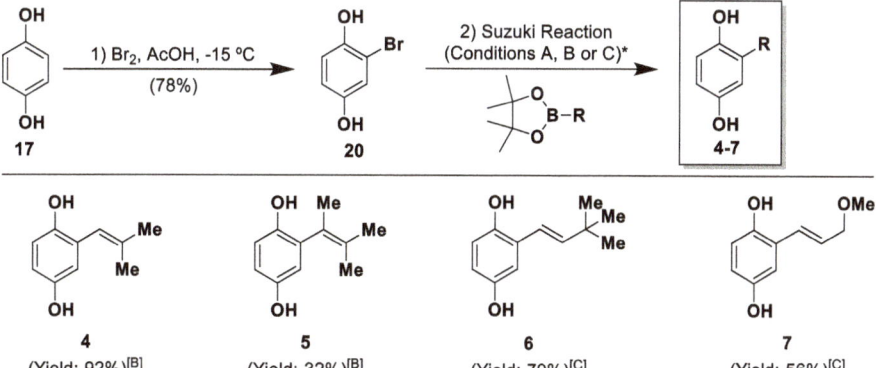

Scheme 2. Synthesis of analogues 4–7 via Suzuki couplings (* Conditions A: Pd[PPh$_3$]$_4$, solid K$_2$CO$_3$, dioxane, H$_2$O, 80 °C, 15 h; conditions B: Pd[PPh$_3$]$_4$, 2 M aq. K$_2$CO$_3$, THF, 80 °C, 48 h; conditions C: Pd[PPh$_3$]$_4$, 2 M aq. K$_2$CO$_3$, THF, 80 °C, 15 h).

For the cases of the 2,6-disubstituted 1,4-hydroquinone derivatives **8–11**, we devised their syntheses based again on a Suzuki coupling reaction as the most suitable method for rapid access to the targeted molecules. To this end, the bromo derivative of toluquinol **22** was prepared according to the procedures described in the literature [12] from *o*-cresol (**21**), and the corresponding Suzuki couplings were achieved following the modified conditions previously established for the synthesis of derivatives **4–7**. However, on this occasion we found that, for some cases (compounds **8** and **11**), the solvent system 1,4-dioxane/H_2O provided better results compared with the use of THF as solvent, whereas for compounds **9** and **10**, THF was the solvent of choice for the Suzuki coupling (Scheme 3).

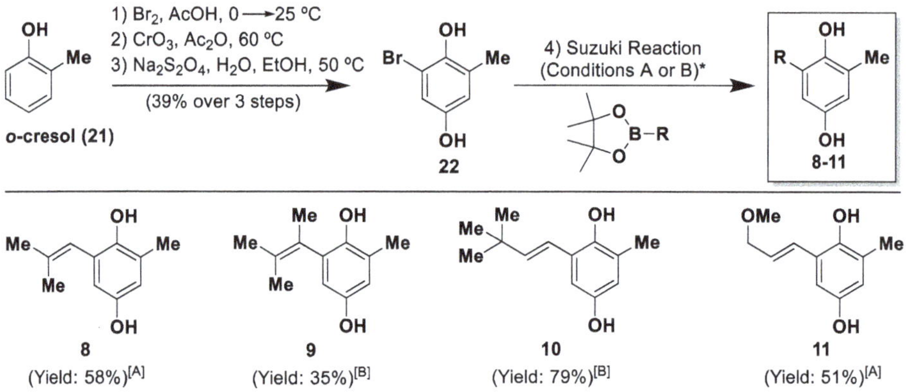

Scheme 3. Synthesis of disubstituted analogues **8–11** via Suzuki couplings (* Conditions A: Pd[PPh$_3$]$_4$, solid K$_2$CO$_3$, dioxane, H$_2$O, 80 °C, 15 h; conditions B: Pd[PPh$_3$]$_4$, 2 M aq. K$_2$CO$_3$, THF, 80 °C, 48 h).

As a continuation of the synthetic strategy based on a Suzuki reaction for the installation of new substituents, the synthesis of the corresponding 2,5-disubstituted analogues requires the bromo derivative **24** as the key starting material. The synthesis of this bromo derivative was achieved according to the procedure described in the literature [13], starting from toluquinol (**1**) and proceeding through bromo toluquinone **23**, prepared in three steps from **1**. The reduction of this bromo quinone by the action of sodium thiosulfate provided the bromo precursor **24** at a 44% yield. The Suzuki coupling reaction of **24** with the corresponding pinacol boronic ester afforded the desired 2,5-disubstituted **12** at a reasonable 50% yield (Scheme 4).

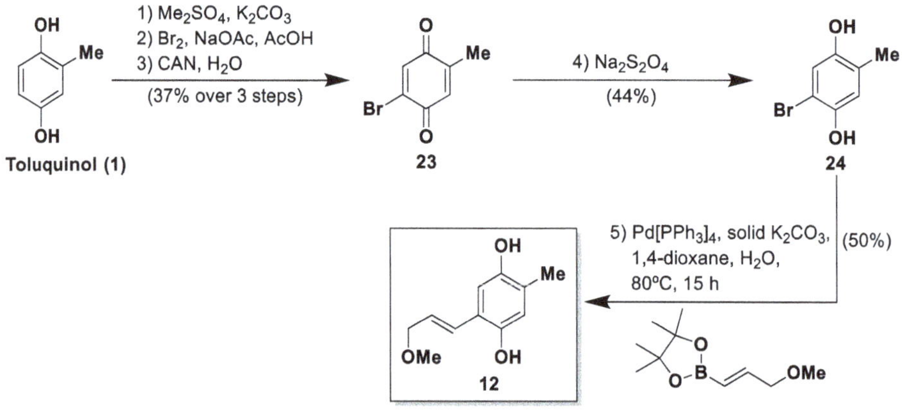

Scheme 4. Synthesis of the *p*-disubstituted analogue **12** via a Suzuki reaction.

Finally, compounds 2,3-dimethyl-1,4-hydroquinone (**13**) and toluquinone (**14**) were commercially available and, in the case of thymoquinol (**15**), its preparation was achieved from commercial thymoquinone (**16**) by reduction with sodium thiosulfate [14].

2.2. Antitumoral Properties of the Compounds

The synthesized 1,4-hydroquinone derivatives **2–12** and **15** and the commercially available compounds **13**, **14**, and **16** were subjected to biological evaluation with regard to their effect on cell growth against a panel of various human cancer cell lines. They included MDA-MB-231 (human breast adenocarcinoma), HL-60 (human promyelocytic leukemia), U87-MG (human glioblastoma), HT-1080 (human fibrosarcoma), and HT-29 (human colorectal adenocarcinoma). In these studies, toluquinol (**1**) was used as a control, for comparison purposes.

To elucidate the effect of the toluquinol analogs on the growth of tumors, logarithmically proliferating cells were treated with serial dilutions of the compounds for 72 h. Then, the number of viable cells was evaluated by the addition of MTT, and results were expressed as a percentage of viable cells versus the untreated controls. Representative dose-response curves are presented in the Supplementary Materials. In those figures each point represents the mean of quadruplicates, and SD values were typically lower than 10% of the mean values and were omitted for clarity. The half-maximal inhibitory concentration (IC_{50}) value was calculated from each dose-response curve as the concentration of compound yielding 50% of the control cells' survival. Table 1, containing the IC_{50} values (means ± SD of three independent experiments with quadruplicate samples each one), summarizes the results of these biological evaluations.

Table 1. In vitro antitumor activities of toluquinol and analogues (IC_{50}, µM) [a].

Structure	Compound	Tumor Cell Line				
		MDA-MB-231 [b]	HL-60 [c]	U87-MG [d]	HT-1080 [e]	HT-29 [f]
	Toluquinol (1)	2.3 ± 0.8	1.7 ± 0.5	5.6 ± 1.5	1.4 ± 0.6	4.1 ± 0.4
	Compound 2	14.5 ± 1.8	13.9 ± 1.1	31.7 ± 5.6	41.2 ± 11.4	29.7 ± 7.1
	Compound 3	>100	50.0 ± 3.4	>100	>100	>100
	Compound 18	>100	7.0 ± 1.2	>100	>100	>100
	Compound 4	4.1 ± 1.1	3.0 ± 0.7	10.4 ± 3.6	3.7 ± 1.8	7.9 ± 0.1
	Compound 5	3.9 ± 1.5	5.3 ± 2.0	29.7 ± 4.9	8.4 ± 1.4	15.5 ± 4.5
	Compound 6	6.7 ± 1.8	6.3 ± 1.3	15.9 ± 4.4	6.1 ± 2.5	12.3 ± 2.5

Table 1. Cont.

Structure	Compound	Tumor Cell Line				
		MDA-MB-231 [b]	HL-60 [c]	U87-MG [d]	HT-1080 [e]	HT-29 [f]
	Compound 7	4.2 ± 1.8	6.2 ± 1.7	8.8 ± 0.8	3.2 ± 1.9	9.8 ± 3.2
	Compound 8	2.2 ± 0.3	3.1 ± 1.7	10.0 ± 2.1	3.3 ± 0.1	8.1 ± 0.6
	Compound 9	2.6 ± 1.3	3.6 ± 1.5	15.8 ± 2.3	5.5 ± 1.9	14.2 ± 4.3
	Compound 10	3.2 ± 1.2	4.7 ± 0.8	16.0 ± 1.3	5.0 ± 1.5	15.6 ± 1.2
	Compound 11	2.4 ± 0.3	3.1 ± 1.3	9.6 ± 1.3	2.9 ± 1.0	7.7 ± 1.6
	Compound 12	1.6 ± 0.5	2.9 ± 1.4	5.2 ± 1.2	1.1 ± 0.2	7.9 ± 2.0
	Compound 13	2.0 ± 0.3	3.2 ± 1.6	5.1 ± 0.4	1.6 ± 0.3	6.5 ± 2.6
	Thymoquinol (15)	1.0 ± 0.1	1.6 ± 0.5	10.2 ± 2.0	2.0 ± 1.1	8.2 ± 1.4
	Thymoquinone (16)	1.0 ± 0.1	2.0 ± 0.9	15.1 ± 3.2	4.0 ± 0.9	12.9 ± 1.6
	Toluquinone (14)	3.4 ± 0.1	5.6 ± 1.9	8.8 ± 0.9	4.9 ± 1.7	9.5 ± 0.5
	Compound 19	>100	82.0 ± 5.9	>100	>100	>100

[a] Half-maximal inhibitory concentration (IC50) values calculated from dose-response curves as the concentration of compound yielding 50% of control cell survival. They are expressed as means ± SD of three independent experiments with quadruplicate samples each. [b] MDA-MB-231: Human breast adenocarcinoma. [c] HL-60: Human promyelocytic leukemia. [d] U87-MG: Human glioblastoma. [e] HT-1080: Human fibrosarcoma. [f] HT-29: Human colorectal adenocarcinoma.

2.2.1. Antitumor Properties with Structure-Activity Relationship (SAR) of 2-Substituted Hydroquinones 2–7

Relevant conclusions can be derived from the results presented in Table 1. At first sight, they clearly indicate a relevant role of the methyl group of toluquinol in the cytotoxic activity of this compound, since compounds lacking this methyl group (2–7) exhibited significantly increased IC$_{50}$ values for all the tested cell lines. In this regard, substitution of the methyl group of toluquinol by a trifluoromethyl group (compound 2) caused a 6- to 30-fold increase in the IC_{50} values for all the cell types, approaching the recently reported IC_{50} values for 1,4-hydroquinone in tumor cell lines [15]. These results are also in agreement with our previous results showing that substitution of the methyl group of toluquinol with either a carboxylic acid (as in gentisic acid) or a sulfonic acid (as in calcium dobesilate) provoked a notable decrease in the growth inhibitory activity of the compounds, as deduced from the higher IC_{50} values obtained for them in endothelial and tumor cells [6].

Many bioactive quinones and hydroquinones derived from marine organisms have one or more prenyl groups in their molecules [1–3]. Our results show that the substitution of a prenyl group (compound 3) for a toluquinol methyl group practically abrogated the generic antitumor activity of the compound that only exerted a moderate cytotoxic effect against the HL60 human leukemia cell line. This activity is consistent with that already described in P388 murine leukemia cells for this natural marine compound, first isolated from the tunicate *Aplidium californicum* [16,17]. Disubstituted prenyl hydroquinones are also frequently found in marine organisms. Although a correlation between their substitution pattern and the producing organism has been proposed, there is some evidence that the pharmacophore responsible for the cytotoxicity of these naturally occurring secondary metabolites could be the quinone, hydroquinone, or naphthoquinone nucleus [1,18]. As shown in Table 1, the inclusion of a second isoprenyl group in the molecule (compound 18, obtained as a sub-product in the synthesis of compound 3, as shown in Scheme 1) caused a 7-fold increase in the antileukemic activity of the new compound, which remained noncytotoxic for the other tumor cell lines. This suggests that the structural modification of the natural isoprenyl hydroquinone can effectively increase its activity, maintaining the interesting putative specificity of this compound to leukemia cells.

It is worth noting that, when substituted vinyl groups were introduced instead of the methyl group, their corresponding derivatives (compounds 4–7) retained some antitumor activities, with compound 7 being the most active in this series and compound 6 the least active, as an indication of the detrimental effect of the steric hindrance when either a bulky substituent is present, such as the *tert*-butyl group (compound 6), or an increased number of methyl groups are included in the aliphatic chain (compound 5). In any case, all of them showed significantly lower cytotoxicity than toluquinol, indicating that these structural changes are not well tolerated with regard to their antiproliferative properties and again suggesting the important role of the methyl group for the cytotoxicity of this compound.

2.2.2. Antitumor Properties with SAR of 2,6-Disubstituted Hydroquinones 8–11

Our results show that good tolerance was displayed after the inclusion of a second substituent in the biological properties of the resulting disubstituted 1,4-hydroquinones (compounds 8–13). All those toluquinol derivatives presented antitumoral activities in the same low μM range as the original molecule. The biological evaluation of the subset comprised by the 2,6-disubstituted-1,4-hydroquinones (compounds 8–11) revealed a number of intriguing findings. Although the resulting cytotoxicity values showed that the introduction of a second substituent in the toluquinol molecule was well tolerated, a significant decrease in the cytotoxic activity was only observed as the steric volume of the substituent increased (compounds 9 and 10). This is in agreement with the abovementioned results obtained with the monosubstituted vinyl derivatives. We analyzed the effect of the position of the second substituent in the 1,4-hydroquinone.

2.2.3. Antitumor Properties with SAR of 2,3-Disubstituted Hydroquinone 13 and 2,5-Disubstituted Hydroquinones 12 and 15

A comparison of the IC_{50} values obtained for 2,3-dimethyl-1,4-hydroquinone (13), the 2,5-disubstituted derivatives (compounds 12 and 15), and the 2, 6-disubstituted derivatives (compounds 8 and 11) indicates that, although no major differences were observed when non-bulky groups were included in any of those positions, in general, 2,5-disubstituted compounds seemed to exhibit higher cytotoxic activity. In this regard, compound 12 proved to be one of the most potent analogues, exhibiting cytotoxic activity higher than that of the 2,6-disubstituted counterpart (compound 11).

Special mention should be made of thymoquinol (compound **15**), which in our assays demonstrated very similar activity to that of toluquinol. Several thymoquinol glycosides have been isolated from plants used in folk medicine to treat infections [19,20]. The main reason that we included thymoquinol in this study is that it is the reduced form of thymoquinone (compound **16**), the major active ingredient of *Nigella sativa*, known as black seed or black cumin, which has been used as a traditional remedy to treat a variety of diseases for more than 2000 years [21]. Known as "the miracle herb of the century," its impressive biological activities include antibacterial, antifungal, antiviral, antihelminthic, anti-inflammatory, immunomodulatory, and anticancer, as well as curative properties against cardiovascular diseases, diabetes, asthma, and oral or kidney diseases [22]. Thymoquinone, also found in many other medicinal plants, presents a wide range of biological activities of pharmacological value, including an interesting antitumor activity derived from its antiproliferative, anti-oxidant, cytotoxic, apoptogenic, and antimetastatic effects [21,23]. Thymoquinone has been recently identified as a potent anticancer compound capable of inducing apoptotic cell death by upregulating the expression of apoptotic genes p53 and caspase 9 and downregulating the expression of anti-apoptotic genes such as Bcl2 [24]. The antiangiogenic activity of thymoquinone may also contribute to enhancing the pharmacological potential of this compound in oncology [25,26].

2.2.4. Antitumor Properties with SAR of Benzoquinones **14**, **16**, and Benzopyrane **19**

To shed light on the effect of the oxidation state of the toluquinol derivatives on their biological properties, we compared the activities of toluquinol (**1**) and thymoquinol (**15**) with those of their respective quinones, toluquinone (**14**) and thymoquinone (**16**). Our results show that the reduced compounds have better activities than those of their corresponding quinones, although these differences were not very significant. Although this contradicts the previous statement that the keto form of thymoquinone could be responsible for the pharmacological properties of the compound [27], it is in agreement with recent reported data showing that the reduction of thymoquinone, toluquinone, and other quinones to their respective hydroquinones increased their cytotoxic potency and selectivity on four cell lines of ovarian cancer [28]. In any case, it cannot be ruled out that both species might play a role in the toxicity of the compounds, which could generate a redox cycle in the tumor cell, responsible for the ROS production leading to cell death, in a similar mechanism to that proposed to explain the cytotoxic activities of marine terpenoquinones [3]. Supporting this hypothesis, the cytotoxic activity of thymoquinone has been related to the induction of oxidative damage in cancer cells, resulting in apoptosis [29]. Thymoquinone has a dual effect, with antioxidant properties at low concentration, but pro-oxidant ones at higher concentrations, derived from ROS generation [30]. Acting as a redox-cycler, the quinone can be metabolized by enzymatic or non-enzymatic reactions to hydroquinone or semiquinone, generating superoxide anion radicals [31]. The relevance of the cyclic interconversion of quinones and hydroquinones in the activity of these compounds might also explain the negligible cytotoxic activity of compound **19** (obtained as a subproduct in the synthesis of compound **3**, as shown in Scheme 1), in which this interconversion between the two forms is prevented.

3. Experimental Section

3.1. General Techniques

All reactions were carried out under an argon atmosphere with dry, freshly distilled solvents under anhydrous conditions, unless using aqueous reagents or otherwise noted. All solvents used in reactions were dried and distilled using standard procedures. Tetrahydrofuran (THF) was distilled from sodium benzophenone, and methylene chloride (CH_2Cl_2) from calcium hydride. Yields refer to chromatographically and spectroscopically (^{1}H NMR) homogeneous materials, unless otherwise stated. All solutions used in workup procedures were saturated unless otherwise noted. All reagents were purchased at highest commercial quality and used without further purification unless otherwise stated. All reactions were monitored by thin-layer chromatography (TLC) using 0.25-mm silica gel plates (60F-254), using UV light (254 nm) as the visualizing agent and acidic ceric ammonium molybdate/phosphomolybdic acid or potassium permanganate solutions and heat as the developing agents. Flash column chromatography (FCC) was performed using silica gel (60 Å, particle size 230–400 mesh) under air pressure. All solvents used for chromatographic purifications were distilled prior to use. ^{1}H and ^{13}C NMR spectra were recorded on a Bruker DPX-400 MHz instrument (Fällanden, Switzerland) and calibrated using residual undeuterated solvent as an internal reference. Chemical shifts are reported in ppm, with the resonance resulting from incomplete deuteration of the solvent as the internal standard (^{13}CDCl$_3$: 7.26 ppm, s and 77.0 ppm, t; ^{13}CD$_3$OD: 4.87 ppm, s, 3.31 ppm, quin and 49.1 ppm, sep; ^{13}C$_2$D$_6$OS: 2.49 ppm, quin and 39.52 ppm, sep). Data are reported as follows: chemical shift δ/ppm (multiplicity, coupling constants J (Hz) and integration (^{1}H only)). The following abbreviations were used to explain the multiplicities: s = singlet; d = doublet; t = triplet; q = quartet; quin = quintet; b = broad; m = multiplet or combination thereof. ^{13}C signals are singles, unless otherwise stated. High-resolution mass spectrometry (HRMS) was performed on a Thermo Fisher Scientific H-ESI and APCI mass spectrometer (Waltham (MA), USA) in positive mode and using an ion trap (Orbitrap) as the mass analyzer type. HRMS signals are reported to four decimal places and are within ± 5 ppm of theoretical values. Melting points were collected using a Gallenkamp melting point apparatus (London, UK), using a gradient of 0.5 °C per min.

3.2. Biological Material and Methods

All the cancer cell lines used in this study were obtained from the American Type Culture Collection (ATCC, Manassas, Virginia, USA). Human fibrosarcoma HT-1080 and human glioblastoma U87-MG cells were maintained in Eagle's Minimum Essential Medium (EMEM), supplemented with 10% FBS. Human colon adenocarcinoma HT-29 cells were maintained in DMEM containing glucose (4.5 g/L) supplemented with 10% FBS. Human breast cancer carcinoma MDA-MB-231 cells were maintained in a RPMI1640 medium supplemented with 10% FBS. Acute promyelocytic leukemia HL-60 cells were maintained in a RPMI1640 medium supplemented with 20% FBS. All culture media contained glutamine (2 mM), penicillin (50 IU/mL), streptomycin (50 μg/mL), and amphotericin (1.25 μg/mL), and all cell lines were grown at 37 °C in a humidified 5% CO$_2$ atmosphere.

3.3. Synthesis

3.3.1. 2-(Trifluoromethyl)benzene-1,4-diol (**2**)

Hydroquinone **17** (50 mg, 0.45 mmol, 1.0 equiv.), 5-(Trifluoromethyl) dibenzothiophenium trifluoromethanesulfonate (362 mg, 0.9 mmol, 2.0 equiv.) and pyridine (0.04 mL, 0.45 mmol, 1.0 equiv.) were dissolved in DMF (2 mL) and the reaction mixture was stirred for 72 h at 25 °C. After this time, the reaction mixture was diluted with water and the aqueous phase was extracted with Et$_2$O twice. The combined organic phases were washed sequentially with a saturated aqueous CuSO$_4$ solution and brine, dried over MgSO$_4$, filtered, and the solvent removed under reduced pressure. The crude mixture was purified by flash column chromatography (silica gel, 5% EtOAc in hexanes → 20% EtOAc in hexanes) to obtain **2** (39 mg, 49%) as a yellow oil [8]: R_f = 0.23 (silica gel, 30% EtOAc in hexanes); ^{1}H NMR (400 MHz, CD$_3$OD) δ 6.88 (d, J = 2.9 Hz, 1 H), 6.81 (ddd, J = 8.8, 2.9, 0.6 Hz, 1 H), 6.76 (dd, J = 4.9, 4.4 Hz, 1 H); ^{19}F NMR (400 MHz, CD$_3$OD) δ −63.78; HRMS (H-ESI) *m/z*: [M + H]$^+$ calculated for C$_7$H$_6$F$_3$O$_2$ 179.0320; found 179.0318.

3.3.2. 2-(3-Methylbut-2-en-1-yl)benzene-1,4-diol (**3**), 2,5-bis-(3-Methylbut-2-en-1-yl)benzene-1,4-diol (**18**) and 2,2-dimethyl-6-chromanol (**19**): Reaction of **17** with Prenol

Hydroquinone **17** (300 mg, 2.72 mmol, 1.0 equiv.) and 3-methyl-2-buten-1-ol (0.55 mL, 5.45 mmol, 2.0 equiv.) were dissolved in a 1:1 mixture of Et$_2$O:CH$_2$Cl$_2$ (10 mL). Then, BF$_3$•OEt$_2$ (0.1 mL, 0.54 mmol, 0.2 equiv.) was added at 0 °C and the reaction mixture was stirred for 48 h at 25 °C. After this time, cold water was added and the aqueous phase was extracted with EtOAc. The organic phase was washed with brine, dried over MgSO$_4$, filtered, and the solvent removed under reduced pressure. The residue was purified by flash column chromatography (silica gel, 15% EtOAc in hexanes → 25% EtOAc in hexanes) to obtain **3** (72 mg, 15%), together with side products **18** (21 mg, 3%) and **19** (13 mg, 2.7%) [9]. [**3**]: white solid; R$_f$ = 0.30 (silica gel, 50% EtOAc in hexanes); m.p. = 101–103 °C; ^{1}H NMR (400 MHz, CDCl$_3$) δ 6.68 (d, J = 8.3 Hz, 1 H), 6.63–6.54 (m, 2 H), 5.29 (t, J = 7.3 Hz, 1 H), 3.29 (d, J = 7.0 Hz, 2 H), 1.77 (s, 3 H), 1.76 (s, 3 H); ^{13}C NMR (100 MHz, CDCl$_3$) δ 149.7, 147.5, 131.6, 128.8, 122.6, 115.7, 115.1, 112.4, 27.8, 24.5, 16.4; HRMS (H-ESI) *m/z*: [M + H]$^+$ calculated for C$_{11}$H$_{15}$O$_2$ 179.1072; found 179.1064. [**18**]: white solid; ^{1}H NMR (400 MHz, CDCl$_3$) δ 6.70–6.45 (m, 4 H), 5.29 (t, J = 7.9 Hz, 1 H), 3.31–3.24 (m, 1 H), 2.71 (dd, J = 13.0, 6.4 Hz, 1 H), 1.82–1.69 (m, 12 H); ^{13}C NMR (100 MHz, CDCl$_3$) δ 147.2, 131.4, 125.8, 122.9, 115.6, 27.5, 24.6, 16.5; HRMS (H-ESI) *m/z*: [M + H]$^+$ calculated for C$_{16}$H$_{23}$O$_2$ 247.1698; found 247.1708. [**19**]: red oil; ^{1}H NMR (400 MHz, CDCl$_3$) δ 6.65 (d, J = 8.6 Hz, 1 H), 6.62–6.53 (m, 2 H), 2.72 (t, J = 6.8 Hz, 2 H), 1.77 (t, J = 6.8 Hz, 2 H), 1.31 (s, 6 H); ^{13}C NMR (100 MHz, CDCl$_3$) δ 149.8, 146.9, 121.3, 117.1, 114.8, 113.9, 73.2, 32.5, 25.6, 22.2; HRMS (H-ESI) *m/z*: [M + H]$^+$ calculated for C$_{11}$H$_{15}$O$_2$ 179.1072; found 179.1071.

3.3.3. Synthesis of Compounds **20** and **22**

2-Bromobenzene-1,4-diol (**20**). Bromine (0.56 mL, 10.90 mmol, 1.2 equiv.) was added dropwise to a solution of 1,4-hydroquinone (**17**) (1.0 g, 9.08 mmol, 1.0 equiv.) in ^{t}BuOMe (20 mL) at -15 °C and the reaction mixture was stirred for 2 h. After this time, the reaction mixture was quenched by the addition of 10% aqueous sodium thiosulfate solution and extracted with Et$_2$O twice. The combined organic phases were washed with brine, dried over MgSO$_4$, filtered, and the solvent removed under reduced pressure. The residue was purified by flash column chromatography (silica gel, 10% EtOAc in hexanes) to obtain **20** (1.3 g, 78%) as a colorless solid [11]: R$_f$ = 0.35 (silica gel, 30% EtOAc in hexanes); ^{1}H NMR (400 MHz, CD$_3$OD) δ 6.89 (d, J = 2.8 Hz, 1 H), 6.72 (d, J = 8.7 Hz, 1 H), 6.60 (dd, J = 8.7, 2.9 Hz, 1 H); ^{13}C NMR (100 MHz, CD$_3$OD) δ 152.0, 148.2, 120.3, 117.7, 116.4, 110.7.

2-Bromo-6-methylbenzene-1,4-diol (**22**). Bromine (2.8 mL, 55.48 mmol, 2.0 equiv.) was added dropwise over 15 min to a solution of *o*-cresol (**21**) (2.9 mL, 27.74 mmol, 1.0 equiv.) in AcOH (30 mL) at 0 °C and the reaction mixture was stirred at 25 °C for 1 h. After this time, cold water was added and the resulting white precipitate was filtered and washed with cold water to obtain 2,4-dibromo-6-methyl phenol (S1) (5.8 g, 80%) as a colorless solid that did not require further purification [12]: R$_f$ = 0.60 (20% EtOAc in hexanes); m.p. = 56–57 °C; ^{1}H NMR (400 MHz, CDCl$_3$) δ 7.43 (dd, J = 2.3, 0.6 Hz, 1 H), 7.21–7.19 (m, 1 H), 2.27 (t, J = 0.7 Hz, 3 H); ^{13}C NMR (100 MHz, CDCl$_3$) δ 149.8, 133.1, 131.3, 127.7, 112.0, 110.4, 16.5. A solution of CrO$_3$ (1.5 g, 15.31 mmol, 1.1 equiv.) in H$_2$O (4 mL) was added to a solution of 2,4-dibromo-6-methyl phenol (3.7 g, 13.91 mmol, 1.0 equiv.) in Ac$_2$O (7 mL)/CH$_3$CN (3.5 mL) and the resulting mixture was heated at 60 °C for 1.5 h. After this time, the reaction mixture was cooled to 25 °C and diluted with water. Then, the aqueous phase was extracted with CH$_2$Cl$_2$ three times, and the combined organic phases were washed with brine, dried over MgSO$_4$, filtered, and the solvent removed under reduced pressure to obtain 2-bromo-6-methyl-*p*-benzoquinone (S2) (2.3 g, 85%) as an orange solid that did not require further purification: R$_f$ = 0.45 (silica gel, 20% EtOAc in hexanes); m.p. = 92–93 °C; ^{1}H NMR (400 MHz, CDCl$_3$) δ 7.23 (d, J = 2.4 Hz, 1 H), 6.65 (dq, J = 2.4, 1.6 Hz, 1 H), 2.14 (d, J = 1.6 Hz, 3 H); ^{13}C NMR (100 MHz, CDCl$_3$) δ 184.8, 179.9, 145.7, 138.1, 137.3, 133.4, 16.8. The resulting *p*-benzoquinone derivative (1.0 g, 4.97 mmol, 1.0 equiv.) was dissolved in a mixture of EtOH (10 mL)/H$_2$O (2 mL) and the mixture was heated at 50 °C. Then, Na$_2$S$_2$O$_4$ (1 g, 5.97 mmol, 1.2 equiv.) was added and the reaction mixture was heated at 50 °C for 1.5 h. After this time, EtOH was removed under reduced pressure, the crude mixture was diluted with water, and the aqueous phase was extracted with EtOAc. The organic phase was washed with brine, dried over MgSO$_4$, filtered, and the solvent removed under reduced pressure to obtain a solid that was washed with cold CH$_2$Cl$_2$ to obtain **22** (585 mg, 57%) as a pale yellow solid that did not require further purification: R$_f$ = 0.25 (silica gel, 20% EtOAc in hexanes); ^{1}H NMR (400 MHz, CDCl$_3$) δ 6.82 (dd, J = 2.9, 0.5 Hz, 1 H), 6.60 (dd,

J = 2.9, 0.7 Hz, 1 H), 2.25 (t, J = 0.5 Hz, 3 H); ^{13}C NMR (100 MHz, CDCl$_3$) δ 148.8, 144.8, 126.5, 117.7, 115.7, 109.6, 16.9; HRMS (H-ESI) m/z: [M + H]$^+$ calculated for C$_7$H$_8$BrO$_2$ 202.9708; found 202.9726.

3.3.4. General Procedures for Suzuki Couplings: Synthesis of the 2-Substituted and 2,6-Disubstituted Hydroquinones 4–11

Condition A: To a solution of boronic acid pinacol ester derivative (2.0 equiv.), bromo derivative (1.0 equiv.), Pd[PPh$_3$]$_4$ (0.2 equiv.), and K$_2$CO$_3$ (3.6 equiv.) in 1,4-dioxane was added a drop of water and the reaction mixture was heated at 80 °C for 15 h. After this time, a saturated aqueous NH$_4$Cl solution was added and the aqueous phase was extracted with EtOAc three times. The combined organic phases were washed with brine, dried over MgSO$_4$, filtered, and the solvent removed under reduced pressure. The residue was purified by flash column chromatography (silica gel) to obtain the corresponding product. Condition B: Boronic acid pinacol ester derivative (1.1 equiv.), bromo derivative (1.0 equiv.), Pd[PPh$_3$]$_4$ (0.05 equiv.), and K$_2$CO$_3$ (2.0 M aqueous solution, 6.6 equiv.) were dissolved in THF and the reaction mixture was heated at 80 °C for 48 h. After this time, a saturated aqueous NH$_4$Cl solution was added and the aqueous phase was extracted with EtOAc three times. The combined organic phases were washed with brine, dried over MgSO$_4$, filtered, and the solvent removed under reduced pressure. The residue was purified by flash column chromatography (silica gel) to obtain the corresponding product. Conditions C: Boronic acid pinacol ester derivative (1.1 equiv.), bromo derivative (1.0 equiv.), Pd[PPh$_3$]$_4$ (0.05 equiv.), and K$_2$CO$_3$ (2.0 M aqueous solution, 6.6 equiv.) were dissolved in THF and the reaction mixture was heated at 80 °C for 15 h. After this time, a saturated aqueous NH$_4$Cl solution was added and the aqueous phase was extracted with EtOAc three times. The combined organic phases were washed with brine, dried over MgSO$_4$, filtered, and the solvent removed under reduced pressure. The residue was purified by flash column chromatography (silica gel) to obtain the corresponding product.

2-(2-Methylprop-1-en-1-yl)benzene-1,4-diol (4). Compound 4 was prepared from bromohydroquinone 20 (50 mg, 0.29 mmol, 1.0 equiv.) by treatment with 2-methyl-1-propenylboronic acid pinacol ester (0.06 mL, 0.29 mmol, 1.1 equiv.), Pd[PPh$_3$]$_4$ (15 mg, 0.01 mmol, 0.05 equiv.), and K$_2$CO$_3$ (0.9 mL, 2.0 M aqueous solution, 1.72 mmol, 6.6 equiv.) in THF (2 mL), according to the general procedure for Suzuki couplings (conditions B), as described above. Purification by flash column chromatography (silica gel, 20% EtOAc in hexanes) afforded 4 (39 mg, 92%) as a pale yellow oil: R_f = 0.48 (silica gel, 50% EtOAc in hexanes); ^{1}H NMR (400 MHz, MeOD) δ 6.60 (d, J = 8.6 Hz, 1 H), 6.56 (d, J = 3.0 Hz, 1 H), 6.49 (ddd, J = 8.6, 3.0, 0.4 Hz, 1 H), 6.21–6.14 (m, 1 H), 1.88 (d, J = 1.4 Hz, 3 H), 1.76 (d, J = 1.1 Hz, 3 H); ^{13}C NMR (100 MHz, MeOD) δ 150.7, 148.7, 136.3, 127.6, 121.9, 117.7, 116.8, 114.9, 26.5, 19.6; HRMS (H-ESI) m/z: [M + H]$^+$ calculated for C$_{10}$H$_{13}$O$_2$ 165.0916; found 165.0938.

2-(3-Methylbut-2-en-2-yl)benzene-1,4-diol (5). Compound 5 was prepared from bromohydroquinone 20 (50 mg, 0.26 mmol, 1.0 equiv.) by treatment with 3-Methyl-2-buten-2-ylboronic acid pinacol ester (0.06 mL, 0.29 mmol, 1.1 equiv.), Pd[PPh$_3$]$_4$ (15 mg, 0.01 mmol, 0.05 equiv.), and K$_2$CO$_3$ (0.9 mL, 2.0 M aqueous solution, 1.72 mmol, 6.6 equiv.) in THF (2 mL), according to the general procedure for Suzuki coupling (conditions B). Purification by flash column chromatography (silica gel, 5% EtOAc in hexanes → 15% EtOAc in hexanes) gave 5 (15 mg, 32%) as a pale yellow oil: R_f = 0.40 (silica gel, 50% EtOAc in hexanes); ^{1}H NMR (400 MHz, CD$_3$OD) δ 6.61 (d, J = 8.7 Hz, 1 H), 6.50 (dd, J = 8.6, 3.0 Hz, 1 H), 6.37 (d, J = 2.9 Hz, 1 H), 1.86 (dd, J = 1.4, 1.0 Hz, 3 H), 1.79 (d, J = 0.5 Hz, 3 H), 1.50 (dd, J = 2.7, 1.3 Hz, 3 H); ^{13}C NMR (100 MHz, CD$_3$OD) δ 149.7, 146.1, 132.4, 128.1, 126.2, 115.7, 115.6, 113.4, 20.7, 18.7, 18.6; HRMS (H-ESI) m/z: [M + H]$^+$ calculated for C$_{11}$H$_{15}$O$_2$ 179.1072; found 179.1065.

(E)-2-(3,3-Dimethylbut-1-en-1-yl)benzene-1,4-diol (6). Compound 6 was prepared from bromohydroquinone 12 (100 mg, 0.53 mmol, 1.0 equiv.) by treatment with 2-t-Butyl-E-vinylboronic acid pinacol ester (0.14 mL, 0.58 mmol, 1.1 equiv.), Pd[PPh$_3$]$_4$ (31 mg, 0.03 mmol, 0.05 equiv.), and K$_2$CO$_3$ (1.75 mL, 2.0 M aqueous solution, 3.49 mmol, 6.6 equiv.) in THF (4 mL), according to the general procedure for Suzuki coupling (conditions C). Purification by flash column chromatography (silica gel, 15% EtOAc in hexanes) afforded 6 (80 mg, 79%) as a pale yellow oil: R_f = 0.33 (silica gel, 50% EtOAc in hexanes); ^{1}H NMR (400 MHz, CD$_3$OD) δ 6.81 (t, J = 3.0 Hz, 1 H), 6.58 (dd, J = 12.4, 3.9 Hz, 2 H), 6.47 (dd, J = 8.6, 2.9 Hz, 1 H), 6.14 (d, J = 16.3 Hz, 1 H), 1.11 (s, 9 H); ^{13}C NMR (100 MHz, CD$_3$OD) δ 151.2, 148.6, 141.9, 127.2, 120.8, 117.3, 115.5, 112.9, 34.3, 30.1; HRMS (H-ESI) m/z: [M + H]$^+$ calculated for C$_{12}$H$_{17}$O$_2$ 193.1229; found 193.1238.

(*E*)-2-(3-Methoxyprop-1-en-1-yl) benzene-1,4-diol (**7**). Compound **7** was prepared from bromohydroquinone **20** (50 mg, 0.26 mmol, 1.0 equiv.) by treatment with *trans*-3- Methoxy-1-propenylboronic acid pinacol ester (0.06 mL, 0.29 mmol, 1.1 equiv.), Pd[PPh$_3$]$_4$ (15 mg, 0.01 mmol, 0.05 equiv.), and K$_2$CO$_3$ (0.90 mL, 2.0 M aqueous solution, 1.72 mmol, 6.6 equiv.) in THF (2 mL), according to the general procedure for Suzuki coupling (conditions C). Purification by flash column chromatography (silica gel, 25% EtOAc in hexanes) gave **7** (26 mg, 56%) as a pale yellow oil: R$_f$ = 0.30 (silica gel, 50% EtOAc in hexanes); ^{1}H NMR (400 MHz, CD$_3$OD) δ 6.88–6.82 (m, 2 H), 6.62 (d, J = 8.5 Hz, 1 H), 6.54 (dd, J = 8.6, 2.9 Hz, 1 H), 6.22 (dt, J = 16.0, 6.3 Hz, 1 H), 4.07 (dd, J = 6.3, 1.4 Hz, 2 H), 3.36 (s, 3 H); ^{13}C NMR (100 MHz, CD$_3$OD) δ 151.2, 149.2, 129.4, 126.1, 125.6, 117.5, 116.7, 113.6, 74.7, 57.9; HRMS (H-ESI) m/z: [M + H]$^+$ calculated for C$_{10}$H$_{13}$O$_3$ 181.0865; found 181.0884.

2-Methyl-6-(2-methylprop-1-en-1-yl)benzene-1,4-diol (**8**). Compound **8** was prepared from bromo derivative **22** (58 mg, 0.29 mmol, 1.0 equiv.) by treatment with 2-methyl-1-propenylboronic acid pinacol ester (0.12 mL, 0.58 mmol, 2.0 equiv.), Pd[PPh$_3$]$_4$ (66 mg, 0.06 mmol, 0.2 equiv.), and K$_2$CO$_3$ (142 mg, 1.03 mmol, 3.6 equiv.) in 1,4-dioxane (1.5 mL), according to the general procedure for Suzuki coupling (conditions A). Purification by flash column chromatography (silica gel, 20% EtOAc in hexanes) afforded **8** (29 mg, 58%) as a yellow oil: R$_f$ = 0.50 (silica gel, 30% EtOAc in hexanes); ^{1}H NMR (400 MHz, CD$_3$OD) δ 6.44 (dd, J = 3.0, 0.5 Hz, 1 H), 6.38–6.36 (m, 1 H), 6.17 (s, 1 H), 2.14 (s, 3 H), 1.89 (d, J = 1.2 Hz, 3 H), 1.73 (d, J = 1.0 Hz, 3 H); ^{13}C NMR (100 MHz, CD$_3$OD) δ 149.1, 145.0, 135.9, 126.4, 125.7, 120.5, 115.3, 113.6, 24.9, 18.2, 15.4; HRMS (H-ESI) m/z: [M + H]$^+$ calculated for C$_{11}$H$_{15}$O$_2$ 179.1072; found 179.1081.

2-Methyl-6-(3-methylbut-2-en-2-yl)benzene-1,4-diol (**9**). Compound **9** was prepared from bromo derivative **22** (50 mg, 0.24 mmol, 1.0 equiv.) by treatment with 3-methyl-2-buten-2-ylboronic acid pinacol ester (0.06 mL, 0.26 mmol, 1.1 equiv.), Pd[PPh$_3$]$_4$ (14 mg, 0.01 mmol, 0.05 equiv.) and K$_2$CO$_3$ (0.8 mL, 2.0 M aqueous solution, 1.72 mmol, 6.6 equiv.) in THF (2 mL), according to the general procedure for Suzuki coupling (conditions B). Purification by flash column chromatography (silica gel, 10% EtOAc in hexanes) gave **9** (16 mg, 35%) as a pale yellow oil: R$_f$ = 0.60 (silica gel, 30% EtOAc in hexanes); ^{1}H NMR (400 MHz, CDCl$_3$) δ 6.52 (dd, J = 3.0, 0.7 Hz, 1 H), 6.33 (dd, J = 3.1, 0.5 Hz, 1 H), 2.21 (t, J = 0.6 Hz, 3 H), 1.89 (dd, J = 1.5, 1.0 Hz, 3 H), 1.85 (d, J = 0.7 Hz, 3 H), 1.55 (q, J = 1.4 Hz, 3 H); ^{13}C NMR (100 MHz, CDCl$_3$) δ 148.4, 143.8, 132.1, 130.7, 124.7, 124.6, 116.1, 112.2, 21.7, 20.1, 20.0, 16.3; HRMS (H-ESI) m/z: [M + H]$^+$ calculated for C$_{12}$H$_{17}$O$_2$ 193.1229; found 193.1234.

(*E*)-2-(3,3-Dimethylbut-1-en-1-yl)-6-methylbenzene-1,4-diol (**10**). Compound **10** was prepared from bromo derivative **22** (100 mg, 0.53 mmol, 1.0 equiv.), by treatment with 2-*t*-Butyl-*E*-vinylboronic acid pinacol ester (0.14 mL, 0.58 mmol, 1.1 equiv.), Pd[PPh$_3$]$_4$ (31 mg, 0.03 mmol, 0.05 equiv.), and K$_2$CO$_3$ (1.75 mL, 2.0 M aqueous solution, 3.50 mmol, 6.6 equiv.) in THF (4 mL), according to the general procedure for Suzuki coupling (conditions B). Purification by flash column chromatography (silica gel, 15% EtOAc in hexanes) gave **10** (40 mg, 79%) as a pale yellow oil: R$_f$ = 0.40 (silica gel, 30% EtOAc in hexanes); ^{1}H NMR (400 MHz, CDCl$_3$) δ 6.67–6.65 (m, 1 H), 6.52 (dd, J = 3.0, 0.6 Hz, 1 H), 6.43 (d, J = 16.2 Hz, 1 H), 6.16 (d, J = 16.2 Hz, 1 H), 2.20 (t, J = 0.6 Hz, 3 H), 1.12 (s, 9 H); ^{13}C NMR (100 MHz, CDCl$_3$) δ 148.8, 144.9, 144.9, 125.6, 125.2, 118.8, 116.3, 110.9, 33.7, 29.5, 16.1; HRMS (H-ESI) m/z: [M + H]$^+$ calculated for C$_{13}$H$_{19}$O$_2$ 207.1385; found 207.1367.

(*E*)-2-(3-Methoxyprop-1-en-1-yl)-6-methylbenzene-1,4-diol (**11**). Compound **10** was prepared from bromo derivative **22** (50 mg, 0.25 mmol, 1.0 equiv.) by treatment with *trans*-3-methoxy-1-propenylboronic acid pinacol ester (0.10 mL, 0.49 mmol, 2.0 equiv.), Pd[PPh$_3$]$_4$ (57 mg, 0.05 mmol, 0.2 equiv.), and K$_2$CO$_3$ (122 mg, 0.89 mmol, 3.6 equiv.) in 1,4-dioxane (1.5 mL), according to the general procedure for Suzuki coupling (conditions A). Purification by flash column chromatography (silica gel, 25% EtOAc in hexanes) afforded **11** (24 mg, 51%) as a pale yellow oil: R$_f$ = 0.30 (silica gel, 50% EtOAc in hexanes); ^{1}H NMR (400 MHz, CD$_3$OD) δ 6.97–6.90 (m, 1 H), 6.71 (d, J = 3.0 Hz, 1 H), 6.50 (dd, J = 3.0, 0.7 Hz, 1 H), 6.16 (dt, J = 15.9, 6.3 Hz, 1 H), 4.08 (dd, J = 6.3, 1.4 Hz, 2 H), 3.37 (s, 3 H), 2.15 (s, 3 H); ^{13}C NMR (100 MHz, CD$_3$OD) δ 150.1, 145.2, 128.2, 127.1, 125.6, 124.9, 116.9, 109.3, 73.2, 56.6, 15.5; HRMS (H-ESI) m/z: [M + H]$^+$ calculated for C$_{11}$H$_{15}$O$_3$ 195.1021; found 195.1023.

3.3.5. Synthesis of Compounds 23, 24, and 2,5-Disubstituted Hydroquinones 12 and 15

2-Bromo-5-methylcyclohexa-2,5-diene-1,4-dione (23). To a solution of toluquinol (1) (2.5 g, 20.14 mmol, 1.0 equiv.) in acetone (15 mL) was added K$_2$CO$_3$ (14 g, 100.70 mmol, 5.0 equiv.) and Me$_2$SO$_4$ (5.7 mL, 60.41 mmol, 3.0 equiv.) and the reaction mixture was stirred for 3 h. After this time, the reaction mixture was diluted with water and the aqueous phase was extracted with Et$_2$O. The organic phase was washed with brine, dried over MgSO$_4$, filtered, and the solvent removed under reduced pressure to obtain the corresponding dimethoxy derivative (~20 mmol), which was used in the next steps without purification. To a solution of the dimethoxy derivative obtained above (~20 mmol) and NaOAc (3.3 g, 40.28 mmol, 2.0 equiv.) in AcOH (20 mL) was added bromine (1.2 mL, 2.15 mmol, 1.1 equiv.) over 25 min and, after the addition, the reaction mixture was stirred for 1 h. Then, the reaction mixture was quenched by a slow addition of a saturated aqueous NaHCO$_3$ solution at 0 °C. The aqueous phase was then extracted with EtOAc and the organic phase washed with brine, dried over MgSO$_4$, filtered, and the solvent removed under reduced pressure to obtain the corresponding bromo derivative (~20 mmol), which was used in the next step without purification. The bromo derivative obtained above (~20 mmol) was dissolved in CH$_3$CN (35 mL). Then, CAN (28 g, 50.34 mmol, 2.5 equiv.) and H$_2$O (20 mL) were added and the reaction mixture was stirred for 1 h at 25 °C. After this time, the reaction mixture was diluted with water and the aqueous phase was extracted with Et$_2$O twice. The combined organic phases were washed with brine, dried over MgSO$_4$, filtered, and the solvent removed under reduced pressure. The residue was purified by flash column chromatography (silica gel, 1% EtOAc in hexanes) to obtain compound 23 (1.5 g, 37% over 3 steps) as an orange solid [13]: R_f = 0.45 (silica gel, 20% EtOAc in hexanes); ^{1}H NMR (400 MHz, CDCl$_3$) δ 7.29 (s, 1 H), 7.26 (s, 2 H), 2.08 (d, J = 1.6 Hz, 3 H); ^{13}C NMR (100 MHz, CDCl$_3$) δ 185.1, 179.5, 146.5, 138.1, 137.5, 132.6, 15.7.

2-Bromo-5-methylbenzene-1,4-diol (24). Quinone 23 (264 mg, 1.31 mmol, 1.0 equiv.) was dissolved in a mixture of EtOH/H$_2$O (3/0.5 mL) and heated to 50 °C. Then, Na$_2$S$_2$O$_4$ (264 mg, 1.57 mmol, 1.2 equiv.) was added and the reaction mixture was stirred at 50 °C for 1.5 h. After this time, the reaction mixture was cooled to 25 °C and the EtOH was removed under reduced pressure. The resulting residue was diluted with water and extracted with EtOAc twice and the combined organic phases washed with brine, dried over MgSO$_4$, filtered, and the solvent removed under reduced pressure to obtain a yellow solid. This solid was washed with cold CH$_2$Cl$_2$ to afford pure compound 24 (118 mg, 44%) as a pale yellow solid that did not require further purification: R_f = 0.52 (silica gel, 50% EtOAc in hexanes); ^{1}H NMR (400 MHz, CD$_3$OD) δ 6.83 (s, 1 H), 6.64 (d, J = 0.7 Hz, 1 H), 2.08 (s, 3 H); ^{13}C NMR (100 MHz, CD$_3$OD) δ 148.7, 146.4, 124.9, 117.9, 117.8, 105.6, 14.6; HRMS (H-ESI) m/z: [M + H]$^+$ calculated for C$_7$H$_8$BrO$_2$ 202.9708; found 202.9715.

(E)-2-(3-Methoxyprop-1-en-1-yl)-5-methylbenzene-1,4-diol (12). Compound 12 was prepared from bromo derivative 24 (113 mg, 0.56 mmol, 1.0 equiv.) by treatment with $trans$-3-Methoxy-1-propenylboronic acid pinacol ester (0.24 mL, 1.11 mmol, 2.0 equiv.), Pd[PPh$_3$]$_4$ (129 mg, 0.11 mmol, 0.2 equiv.), and K$_2$CO$_3$ (277 mg, 2.00 mmol, 3.6 equiv.) in 1,4-dioxane (3 mL), according to the general procedure for Suzuki coupling (conditions A). Purification by flash column chromatography (silica gel, 5% EtOAc in hexanes → 20% EtOAc in hexanes) gave compound 12 (54 mg, 50%) as a pale yellow oil: R_f = 0.50 (silica gel, 50% EtOAc in hexanes); ^{1}H NMR (400 MHz, CD$_3$OD) δ 6.85–6.78 (m, 2 H), 6.52 (d, J = 0.6 Hz, 1 H), 6.15 (dt, J = 15.9, 6.5 Hz, 1 H), 4.06 (dd, J = 6.4, 1.3 Hz, 2 H), 3.35 (s, 3 H), 2.11 (s, 3 H); ^{13}C NMR (100 MHz, CD$_3$OD) δ 147.9, 147.5, 128.2, 125.4, 123.4, 121.4, 117.6, 111.7, 73.5, 56.5, 14.8; HRMS (H-ESI) m/z: [M + H]$^+$ calculated for C$_{11}$H$_{15}$O$_3$ 195.1021; found 195.1017.

Thymoquinol 15. To a solution of thymoquinone (16) (100 mg, 0.61 mmol, 1.0 equiv.) in MeOH (2 mL) was added a solution of Na$_2$S$_2$O$_4$ (225 mg, 1.29 mmol, 2.1 equiv.) in H$_2$O (2 mL). The reaction mixture was stirred for 2 h at 25 °C and, after this time, the organic solvent was removed under reduced pressure. Then, the crude mixture was diluted with water and the aqueous phase was extracted with EtOAc. The organic phase was washed with brine, dried over MgSO$_4$, filtered, and the solvent removed under reduced pressure. The residue was purified by flash column chromatography (silica gel, 20% EtOAc in hexanes) to obtain **15** (50 mg, 49%) as a pale brown solid [14]: R_f = 0.50 (silica gel, 30% EtOAc in hexanes); ^{1}H NMR (400 MHz, CD$_3$OD) δ 6.56 (s, 1 H), 6.48 (s, 1 H), 3.17 (dt, J = 13.8, 6.9 Hz, 1 H), 1.17 (s, 3 H), 1.15 (s, 3 H); ^{13}C NMR (100 MHz, CD$_3$OD) δ 147.8, 146.6, 132.8, 121.6, 116.9, 112.1, 26.3, 21.8, 14.5; HRMS (H-ESI) m/z: [M + H]$^+$ calculated for C$_{10}$H$_{15}$O$_2$ 167.1072; found 167.1058.

3.4. Cell Growth Assay

The 3-(4,5-dimethylthiazol-2-yl)-2,5-diphenyltetrazolium bromide or MTT dye reduction assay in 96-well microplates was used [32]. This assay is dependent on the reduction of MTT by mitochondrial dehydrogenases of a viable cell to a blue formazan product, which can be measured spectrophotometrically. 3 × 10^3 HL-60, and 2 × 10^3 HT-1080, HT-29, MDA-MB-231, and U87MG cells in a total volume of 100 μL of their respective growth medium were incubated with serial dilutions 1:1 of the tested compounds. After three days of incubation (37 °C and 5% CO$_2$ in a humid atmosphere), 10 μL of MTT (5 mg/mL in phosphate-buffered saline) were added to each well, and the plate was incubated for a further 4 h at 37 °C. The resulting formazan was dissolved in 150 μL of 0.04 N HCl/2-propanol and read at 550 nm. IC$_{50}$ values were calculated from semi-logarithmic dose-response plots as those concentrations of the compound yielding 50% cell survival, taking the values obtained for the control to be 100%. IC$_{50}$ results are expressed as means ± S.D. of at least three independent experiments.

4. Conclusions and Future Perspectives

Bioactive marine compounds can serve as the basis for the synthesis of derivatives with improved pharmacological properties. The synthesis of a set of analogues of the natural product toluquinol has been described and their in vitro cytotoxicity against a panel of cancer cell lines was compared. Our results indicate that the cytotoxic activity of this family of compounds could rely on the hydroquinone part of the molecule, probably due to its capability to undergo redox cycling. Although the hydroquinones seemed to be more cytotoxic than their quinone counterparts, the differences between them were not very significant. Substituents in the ring may modulate the interaction of the molecule with their targets, changing either the activity or the selectivity. Tolerance for biological activity was much more restricted for the methyl group of the molecule, whose replacement by other groups resulted in a significant loss of cytotoxic activity. An increased selectivity was obtained when prenyl groups were used as substituents. The inclusion of a second substituent group in the toluquinol molecule was well tolerated and originated a series of derivatives with cytotoxic activities that were similar to or even higher than that of the natural product. These findings provide guidance for the design of new toluquinol analogues with potentially better pharmacological properties. Two of the compounds studied here (toluquinol and thymoquinone) have been reported to inhibit angiogenesis in vitro and in vivo. Further optimization and development of the new compounds and biochemical studies to determine the mechanism of the biological actions of this family of compounds, with an emphasis on their putative antiangiogenic activity and their undesired toxic effects, are currently in progress.

Supplementary Materials: The following are available online at http://www.mdpi.com/1660-3397/17/9/492/s1.

Author Contributions: Conceptualization, A.R.Q., F.S., M.Á.M., B.M.-P.; Methodology, J.A.T.-V., I.C.-S., G.A.G.-V.; Validation and Analysis, A.R.Q., F.S., J.A.T.-V., I.C.-S., M.Á.M., B.M.-P.; Writing—Original Draft Preparation, A.R.Q., F.S.; Writing—Review and Editing, A.R.Q., F.S., M.Á.M., B.M.-P.; Funding Acquisition, A.R.Q., M.Á.M., F.S., B.M.-P.

Funding: Supported by grants BIO2014-56092-R, CTQ2014-60223-R (MINECO and FEDER), P12-CTS-1507, and UMA18-FEDERJA-220 (Andalusian Government and FEDER) and funds from group BIO-267 (Andalusian Government). The "CIBER de enfermedades raras" is an initiative of the ISCIII (Spain). The funders had no role in the study design, data collection and analysis, decision to publish, or preparation of the manuscript.

Acknowledgments: J.A.T.-V. and I.C.-S. thank the Ministerio de Educación, Cultura y Deporte for their predoctoral fellowships (FPU programme).

Conflicts of Interest: The authors declare no conflict of interest. The funders had no role in the design of the study; in the collection, analyses, or interpretation of data; in the writing of the manuscript, or in the decision to publish the results.

References

1. Sunassee, S.N.; Davies-Coleman, M.T. Cytotoxic and antioxidant marine prenylated quinones and hydroquinones. *Nat. Prod. Rep.* **2012**, *29*, 513–535. [CrossRef] [PubMed]
2. García, P.A.; Hernández, Á.P.; San Feliciano, A.; Castro, M.A. Bioactive Prenyl- and Terpenyl-Quinones/Hydroquinones of Marine Origin. *Mar. Drugs* **2018**, *16*, 292. [CrossRef] [PubMed]
3. Gordaliza, M. Cytotoxic terpene quinones from marine sponges. *Mar. Drugs* **2010**, *8*, 2849–2870. [CrossRef] [PubMed]
4. Waters, A.L.; Hill, R.T.; Place, A.R.; Hamann, M.T. The expanding role of marine microbes in pharmaceutical development. *Curr. Opin. Biotechnol.* **2010**, *21*, 780–786. [CrossRef] [PubMed]
5. Bhatnagar, I.; Kim, S.K. Immense essence of excellence: Marine microbial bioactive compounds. *Mar. Drugs* **2010**, *8*, 2673–2701. [CrossRef] [PubMed]
6. García-Caballero, M.; Marí-Beffa, M.; Cañedo, L.; Medina, M.A.; Quesada, A.R. Toluquinol, a Marine Fungus Metabolite, is a New Angiosuppresor that Interferes the Akt Pathway. *Biochem. Pharmacol.* **2013**, *85*, 1727–1740. [CrossRef] [PubMed]
7. García-Caballero, M.; Blacher, S.; Paupert, J.; Quesada, A.R.; Medina, M.A.; Noël,, A. Novel Application Assigned to Toluquinol: Inhibition of Lymphangiogenesis by Interfering with VEGF-C/VEGFR-3 Signalling Pathway. *Br. J. Pharmacol.* **2016**, *173*, 1966–1987. [CrossRef] [PubMed]
8. Yang, J.-J.; Kirchmeier, R.L.; Shreeve, J.M. New Electrophilic Trifluoromethylating Agents. *J. Org. Chem.* **1998**, *63*, 2656–2660. [CrossRef]
9. Osorio, M.; Aravena, J.; Vergara, A.; Taborga, L.; Baeza, E.; Catalán, K.; González, C.; Carvajal, M.; Carrasco, H.; Espinoza, L. Synthesis and DPPH Radical Scavenging Activity of Prenylated Phenol Derivatives. *Molecules* **2012**, *17*, 556–570. [CrossRef]
10. Nicolaou, K.C.; Bulger, P.G.; Sarlah, D. Palladium-Catalyzed Cross-Coupling Reactions in Total Synthesis. *Angew. Chem. Int. Ed.* **2005**, *44*, 4442–4489. [CrossRef]
11. Viault, G.; Grée, D.; Das, S.; Yadav, J.S.; Grée, R. Synthesis of a Focused Chemical Library Based on Derivatives of Embelin, a Natural Product with Proapoptotic and Anticancer Properties. *Eur. J. Org. Chem.* **2011**, *2011*, 1233–1241. [CrossRef]
12. Löbermann, F.; Mayer, P.; Trauner, D. Biomimetic Synthesis of (−)-Pycnanthuquinone C through the Diels-Alder Reaction of a Vinyl Quinone. *Angew. Chem. Int. Ed.* **2010**, *49*, 6199–6202. [CrossRef] [PubMed]
13. Kutz, S.K.; Schmidt, A.; Knölker, H.-J. Palladium-Catalyzed Synthesis of Pyrayaquinones, Murraya-quinones, and Murrayafoline-B. *Synthesis* **2017**, *49*, 275–292.
14. Johnson-Ajinwo, O.R.; Li, E.-W. Stable Isotope Dilution Gas Chromatography-Mass Spectrometry for Quantification of Thymoquinone in Black Cumin Seed Oil. *J. Agric. Food Chem.* **2014**, *62*, 5466–5471. [CrossRef] [PubMed]
15. Byeon, S.E.; Yi, Y.S.; Lee, J.; Yang, W.S.; Kim, J.H.; Kim, J.; Hong, S.; Kim, J.H.; Cho, J.Y. Hydroquinone Exhibits In Vitro and In Vivo Anti-Cancer Activity in Cancer Cells and Mice. *Int. J. Mol. Sci.* **2018**, *19*, 903. [CrossRef] [PubMed]
16. Howard, B.M.; Clarkson, K.; Bernstein, R.L. Simple prenylated hydroquinone derivatives from the marine Urochordate Aplidium californicum. Natural anticancer and antimutagenic agents. *Tetrahedron Lett.* **1979**, *20*, 4449–4452. [CrossRef]
17. Bertanha, C.S.; Januário, A.H.; Alvarenga, T.A.; Pimenta, L.P.; Silva, M.L.; Cunha, W.R.; Pauletti, P.M. Quinone and hydroquinone metabolites from the ascidians of the genus Aplidium. *Mar. Drugs* **2014**, *12*, 3608–3633. [CrossRef] [PubMed]

18. Fisch, K.M.; Böhm, V.; Wright, A.D.; König, G.M. Antioxidative meroterpenoids from the brown alga Cystoseira crinita. *J. Nat. Prod.* **2003**, *66*, 968–975. [CrossRef] [PubMed]
19. Kamel, M.S.; Assaf, M.H.; Hasanean, H.A.; Ohtani, K.; Kasai, R.; Yamasaki, K. Monoterpene glucosides from Origanum syriacum. *Phytochemistry* **2001**, *58*, 1149–1152. [CrossRef]
20. Sevindik, H.G.; Ozgen, U.; Atila, A.; Er, H.O.; Kazaz, C.; Duman, H. Phtytochemical Studies and Quantitative HPLC Analysis of Rosmarinic Acid and Luteolin 5-*O*-β-D-Glucopyranoside on *Thymus praecox* subsp. *grossheimii* var. *grossheimii*. *Chem. Pharm. Bull.* **2015**, *63*, 720–725. [CrossRef]
21. Darakhshan, S.; Bidmeshki Pour, A.; Hosseinzadeh Colagar, A.; Sisakhtnezhad, S. Thymoquinone and its therapeutic potentials. *Pharmacol. Res.* **2015**, *95–96*, 138–158. [CrossRef] [PubMed]
22. Ahmad, A.; Husain, A.; Mujeeb, M.; Khan, S.A.; Najmi, A.K.; Siddique, N.A.; Damanhouri, Z.A.; Anwar, F. A Review on Therapeutic Potential of *Nigella sativa*: A Miracle Herb. *Asian Pac. J. Trop. Biomed.* **2013**, *3*, 337–352. [CrossRef]
23. Majdalawieh, A.F.; Fayyad, M.W.; Nasrallah, G.K. Anti-cancer properties and mechanisms of action of thymoquinone, the major active ingredient of Nigella sativa. *Crit. Rev. Food Sci. Nutr.* **2017**, *57*, 3911–3928. [CrossRef] [PubMed]
24. Alaufi, O.M.; Noorwali, A.; Zahran, F.; Al-Abd, A.M.; Al-Attas, S. Cytotoxicity of Thymoquinone Alone or in Combination with Cisplatin (CDDP) against Oral Squamous Cell Carcinoma in Vitro. *Sci. Rep.* **2017**, *7*, 13131. [CrossRef] [PubMed]
25. Yi, T.; Cho, S.G.; Yi, Z.; Pang, X.; Rodriguez, M.; Wang, Y.; Sethi, G.; Aggarwal, B.B.; Liu, M. Thymoquinone inhibits tumor angiogenesis and tumor growth through suppressing AKT and extracellular signal-regulated kinase signaling pathways. *Mol. Cancer. Ther.* **2008**, *7*, 1789–1796. [CrossRef] [PubMed]
26. Peng, L.; Liu, A.; Shen, Y.; Xu, H.Z.; Yang, S.Z.; Ying, X.Z.; Liao, W.; Liu, H.X.; Lin, Z.Q.; Chen, Q.Y.; et al. Antitumor and anti-angiogenesis effects of thymoquinone on osteosarcoma through the NF-κB pathway. *Oncol. Rep.* **2013**, *29*, 571–578. [CrossRef]
27. Alkharfy, K.M.; Al-Daghri, N.M.; Al-Attas, O.S.; Alokail, M.S. The protective effect of thymoquinone against sepsis syndrome morbidity and mortality in mice. *Int. Immunopharmacol.* **2011**, *11*, 250–254. [CrossRef]
28. Johnson-Ajinwo, O.R.; Ullah, I.; Mbye, H.; Richardson, A.; Horrocks, P.; Li, W.W. The synthesis and evaluation of thymoquinone analogues as anti-ovarian cancer and antimalarial agents. *Bioorg. Med. Chem. Lett.* **2018**, *28*, 1219–1222. [CrossRef]
29. Koka, P.S.; Mondal, D.; Schultz, M.; Abdel-Mageed, A.B.; Agrawal, K.C. Studies on molecular mechanisms of growth inhibitory effects of thymoquinone against prostate cancer cells: Role of reactive oxygen species. *Exp. Biol. Med.* **2010**, *235*, 751–760. [CrossRef]
30. Mahmoud, Y.K.; Abdelrazek, H.M.A. Cancer: Thymoquinone antioxidant/pro-oxidant effect as potential anticancer remedy. *Biomed. Pharmacother.* **2019**, *115*, 108783. [CrossRef]
31. Zubair, H.; Khan, H.Y.; Sohail, A.; Azim, S.; Ullah, M.F.; Ahmad, A.; Sarkar, F.H.; Hadi, S.M. Redox cycling of endogenous copper by thymoquinone leads to ROS mediated DNA breakage and consequent cell death: Putative anticancer mechanism of antioxidants. *Cell Death Dis.* **2013**, *4*, e660. [CrossRef] [PubMed]
32. Cárdenas, C.; Quesada, A.R.; Medina, M.Á. Evaluation of the anti-angiogenic effect of aloe-emodin. *Cell. Mol. Life Sci.* **2006**, *63*, 3083–3089. [CrossRef] [PubMed]

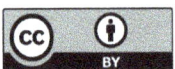 © 2019 by the authors. Licensee MDPI, Basel, Switzerland. This article is an open access article distributed under the terms and conditions of the Creative Commons Attribution (CC BY) license (http://creativecommons.org/licenses/by/4.0/).

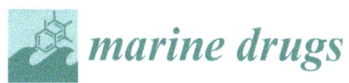

Communication

Hybrid Polyketides from a *Hydractinia*-Associated *Cladosporium sphaerospermum* SW67 and Their Putative Biosynthetic Origin

Seoung Rak Lee [1], Dahae Lee [1], Hee Jeong Eom [1], Maja Rischer [2], Yoon-Joo Ko [3], Ki Sung Kang [4], Chung Sub Kim [5,6], Christine Beemelmanns [2,*] and Ki Hyun Kim [1,*]

1. School of Pharmacy, Sungkyunkwan University, Suwon 16419, Korea; davidseoungrak@gmail.com (S.R.L.); pjsldh@naver.com (D.L.); itprthj44@gmail.com (H.J.E.)
2. Leibniz Institute for Natural Product Research and Infection Biology e.V., Hans-Knöll-Institute (HKI), 07745 Jena, Germany; Maja.Rischer@hki-jena.de
3. Laboratory of Nuclear Magnetic Resonance, National Center for Inter-University Research Facilities (NCIRF), Seoul National University, Gwanak-gu, Seoul 08826, Korea; yjko@snu.ac.kr
4. College of Korean Medicine, Gachon University, Seongnam 13120, Korea; kkang@gachon.ac.kr
5. Department of Chemistry, Yale University, New Haven, CT 06520, USA; chungsub.kim@yale.edu
6. Chemical Biology Institute, Yale University, West Haven, CT 06516, USA
* Correspondence: Christine.beemelmanns@hki-jena.de (C.B.); khkim83@skku.edu (K.H.K.); Tel.: +49-3641-532-1525 (C.B.); +82-31-290-7700 (K.H.K.)

Received: 22 August 2019; Accepted: 20 October 2019; Published: 24 October 2019

Abstract: Five hybrid polyketides (**1a**, **1b**, and **2**–**4**) containing tetramic acid core including a new hybrid polyketide, cladosin L (**1**), were isolated from the marine fungus *Cladosporium sphaerospermum* SW67, which was isolated from the marine hydroid polyp of *Hydractinia echinata*. The hybrid polyketides were isolated as a pair of interconverting geometric isomers. The structure of **1** was determined based on 1D and 2D NMR spectroscopic and HR-ESIMS analyses. Its absolute configuration was established by quantum chemical electronic circular dichroism (ECD) calculations and modified Mosher's method. Tetramic acid-containing compounds are reported to be derived from a hybrid PKS-NRPS, which was also proved by analyzing our ^{13}C-labeling data. We investigated whether compounds **1**–**4** could prevent cell damage induced by cisplatin, a platinum-based anticancer drug, in LLC-PK1 cells. Co-treatment with **2** and **3** ameliorated the damage of LLC-PK1 cells induced by 25 µM of cisplatin. In particular, the effect of compound **2** at 100 µM (cell viability, 90.68 ± 0.81%) was similar to the recovered cell viability of 88.23 ± 0.25% with 500 µM *N*-acetylcysteine (NAC), a positive control.

Keywords: hybrid polyketides; tetramic acid; *Cladosporium sphaerospermum*; hybrid PKS-NRPS; LLC-PK1 cells

1. Introduction

Marine invertebrates host a diverse assemblage of mostly beneficial microbes that play important roles in host development, fitness, and protection [1,2]. To ensure propagation within these often extreme and highly competitive host-specific microenvironments, microorganisms have developed unique metabolic and physiological capabilities that aid in their survival [3,4]. Amongst many other important biochemical traits, marine microorganisms are well known to produce structurally diverse and unique secondary metabolites, which often show important pharmacological activities, such as antioxidant, antibiotic, anticancer, or anti-inflammatory activities [5–9]. Previous reports have shown interesting marine natural products, e.g., hypochromins A and B were isolated from *Hypocrea vinisa*; penicillinolide

A, a 10-membered lactone, was purified from *Penicillium* sp., and *p*-hydroxyphenopyrrozin was identified from *Chromocleista sphaerospermum* [10–12].

As a part of our continuing endeavor to discover novel bioactive natural products from various natural sources [13–17], we recently analyzed the marine fungus *Cladosporium sphaerospermum* sp. SW67, which was obtained from the polyp surface of the marine invertebrate *Hydractinia echinata* (Cnidaria). Subsequent co-culture assays and comparative metabolomics studies led to the isolation and characterization of three novel spirocyclic natural products containing a tetramic acid core—namely, cladosporicin A and cladosporiumins I and J—as well as the isolation of previously reported stereoisomers [18]. Based on our acquired whole genome sequence of *C. sphaerospermum* sp. SW67 and gene expression studies, we proposed a putative PKS-NRPS hybrid gene cluster (*cls*) as a genetic basis for the tetramic acid-derived metabolites [18].

Intriguingly, a previous study exploring the metabolites of the related deep-sea-derived fungus *C. sphaerospermum* sp. 2005-01-E3 led to the characterization of structurally-related hybrid polyketides containing 2,4-pyrrolidinedione (tetramic acid) derivatives, named cladosins A-E [19]. In addition, cladosins H-K, featuring tetramic acid derivatives with aniline moiety, were identified from the deep-sea-derived fungus *C. sphaerospermum* L3P3 [20]. These studies and the intriguing HPLC-UV profiles of our fungal extract prompted us to re-analyze our culture extracts resulting in the isolation of five hybrid polyketides (**1a**, **1b**, and **2–4**) containing tetramic acid core including a new fungal hybrid polyketide named cladosin L (**1**). Herein, we describe the isolation and structural characterization of the hybrid polyketides and their plausible biogenetic pathway, as well as their bioactivity screening.

2. Results and Discussions

2.1. Isolation and Structural Characterization

C. sphaerospermum SW67 was cultivated on a large scale on PDA and MEA agar plates for 14 days at 25 °C. Mycelium-covered plates were then extracted with MeOH and then filtered and evaporated to afford the crude culture extract. Subsequent solvent-partitioning of the extract and LC/MS-guided chemical analysis of the fractions combined with semi-preparative C18 reverse-phase HPLC yielded five hybrid polyketides (**1a**, **1b**, and **2–4**) with a very similar NMR signal pattern (Figure 1).

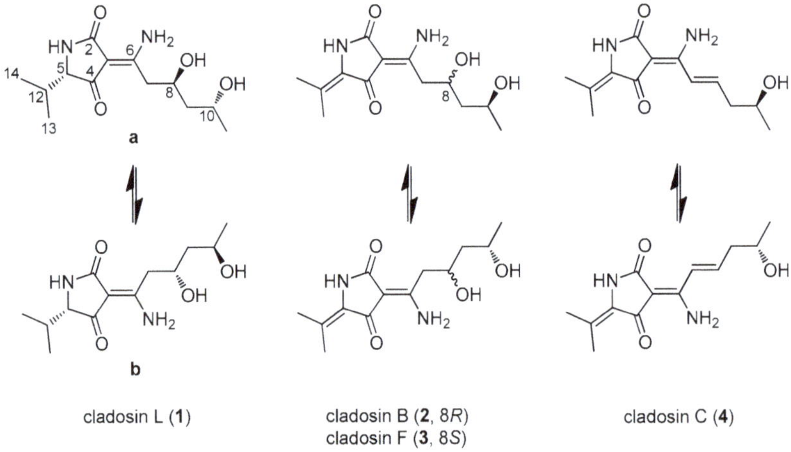

Figure 1. Chemical structures of compounds **1–4** from *C. sphaerospermum* SW67.

Compound **1** was isolated as a yellowish oil with a negative optical rotation, $[\alpha]_D^{25}$ −25.5 (*c* 0.05, MeOH) and as an inseparable mixture of two geometric isomers (**1a**:**1b**) present in an approximate ratio of 1:1. The mixture (**1a/1b**) was determined to have the same molecular formula of $C_{13}H_{22}N_2O_4$, requiring five degrees of unsaturation by the adduct ion of m/z 271.1658 [M+H]$^+$ (calcd. for $C_{13}H_{23}N_2O_4$, 271.1658) detected in HR-ESI-MS. The IR spectrum showed absorption bands for the hydroxyl groups at 3435 cm^{-1} and carbonyl groups at 1634 cm^{-1}. The ^{1}H and ^{13}C NMR data (Table 1) exhibited three methyls, two methylenes, and four methines including two oxygenated methines, an amide-like carbonyl, an α/β-unsaturated ketone, and two non-protonated sp^2 carbons. Its NMR spectral features were very similar to those of the previously described cladosins B (**2**) and F (**3**), which were also isolated in the present work, except for the apparent difference in the chemical shifts of the methyl groups and one additional methine signal set at $δ_H$ 3.59/3.66 and $δ_C$ 68.0/67.0. The gross structure of **1a** was assembled by extensive 2D NMR analysis (Figure 2). The COSY correlations from H$_2$-7 ($δ_H$ 2.85 and 3.17)/H-8 ($δ_H$ 4.14)/H$_2$-9 ($δ_H$ 1.59 and 1.60)/H-10 ($δ_H$ 3.99)/H$_3$-11 ($δ_H$ 1.18) unambiguously established the spin system from C-7 to C-11 with the oxygen attached to C-8 and C-10. This partial structure was connected to the $Δ^{3(6)}$ double bond as evidenced by the key HMBC correlations from H-7 ($δ_H$ 2.85 and 3.17) to C-3 ($δ_C$ 99.1) and C-6 ($δ_C$ 172.3). The HMBC correlations from H$_3$-13 ($δ_H$ 0.77) and H$_3$-14 ($δ_H$ 1.01) to C-5 ($δ_C$ 68.0) and C-12 ($δ_C$ 32.1) led to the identification of an isobutyl moiety in the molecule. That the isobutyl unit was linked to the 2,4-pyrrolidinedione (tetramic acid) scaffold was based on the HMBC correlations from H-5 ($δ_H$ 3.59) to the amide carbonyl (C-2, $δ_C$ 178.3), olefinic carbon (C-3, $δ_C$ 99.1), and α/β-unsaturated ketone carbon (C-4, $δ_C$ 199.8). Finally, the amino group was placed on C-6 as deduced by the molecular formula of $C_{13}H_{22}N_2O_4$. Comparison of the NMR data of **1a** and **1b** suggested that they had a similar planar structure. The only significant differences between **1a** and **1b** were the chemical shifts of carbons attributable to the 2,4-pyrrolidinedione scaffold (Table 1), indicating that **1** existed as a pair of interconverting geometric isomers in solution [19]. The probability of the geometric isomers of **1** could be explained by the interconversion of keto-enamine and enol-imine forms [21,22]. However, the isomers **1a/1b** existed only in the keto-enamine form (Figure 1), which was explained through a conversion via tautomerism of the 3-acyltetramic acids. The geometric forms of **1a** and **1b** were determined as exo-form A ($Δ^{3(6)}$: Z) and exo-form B ($Δ^{3(6)}$: E) since the chemical shift of a carbonyl group forming the hydrogen-bond with amine group, is more downshifted when compared to that of the corresponding free carbonyl group in ^{13}C NMR data [21,22].

Table 1. ^{1}H (800 MHz) and ^{13}C (200 MHz) NMR data of **1** in CD$_3$OD.

Position	1			
	Exo-Form A (a)		Exo-Form B (b)	
	$δ_H$ (J in Hz)	$δ_C$, typ	$δ_H$ (J in Hz)	$δ_C$, typ
2		178.3, CO		176.5, CO
3		99.1, C		97.7, C
4		199.8, CO		202.0, CO
5	3.59, d (3.0)	68.0, CH	3.66 d (3.0)	67.0, CH
6		172.3, C		172.7, C
7	2.85, m; 3.17, dd (13.0, 4.0)	41.1, CH$_2$	2.82 m; 3.13 dd (13.5, 4.5)	42.1, CH$_2$
8	4.14, m	69.6, CH	4.13 m	69.2, CH
9	1.59, m; 1.60, m	48.0, CH$_2$	1.59 m; 1.60 m	47.8, CH$_2$
10	3.99, m	66.1, CH	3.99 m	66.1, CH
11	1.18, d (6.0)	25.0, CH$_3$	1.18 d (6.0)	25.1, CH$_3$
12	2.13, m	32.1, CH	2.12 m	32.1, CH
13	0.77, d (7.0)	16.4, CH$_3$	0.78 d (7.0)	16.7, CH$_3$
14	1.01, d (7.0)	20.7, CH$_3$	1.01 d (7.0)	20.6, CH$_3$

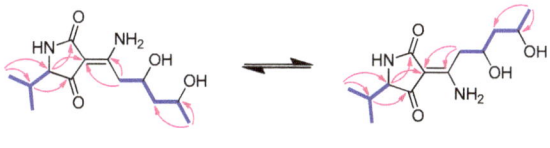

Exo-form A   Exo-form B

Figure 2. Key COSY (—) and HMBC (→) correlations for **1**.

The relative configuration of the stereogenic carbons of the pentan-1,3-diol (C-8 and C-10) of **1** was determined based on the characteristic signals for C-9 methylene protons (methylene group between the 1,3-diol), which were overlapped in *anti*-1,3-diols whereas, they appeared as two sets of multiplets in *syn*-1,3-diols [19,23]. Since the signals of the methylene protons of C-9 in **1** were overlapped at δ_H 1.58–1.60, the 1,3-diol was determined as *anti*. The absolute configuration of the *anti*-1,3-diol system was determined by the modified Mosher's method. A detailed analysis of ^{1}H NMR and TOCSY spectra of the (*R*)- and (*S*)-di-MTPA ester derivatives of **1** indicated that the distributed Δδ values were negative ($\Delta\delta_L$), negative ($\Delta\delta_C$), and negative ($\Delta\delta_R$), which implied that the absolute configurations of both C-8 and C-10 were (*R*) (Figure 3A) [24]. To establish the absolute configuration of C-5 in **1**, the experimental ECD spectrum of **1** was compared to the calculated ECD spectra of two possible epimers (**1A**, 5(*R*); **1B**, 5(*S*), Figure 3B). Since **1** exists as 1:1 mixture of two geometric isomers, total four ECD spectra of **1Aa**, **1Ab**, **1Ba**, and **1Bb** were simulated (Figure S22) and the ECD spectra of the two geometric isomers (**1Aa** and **1Ab**; **1Ba** and **1Bb**) were averaged to generate two ECD spectra of **1A** and **1B** (Figure 3C). The experimental ECD spectrum of **1** showed two negative Cotton effects at 241 and 297 nm, which corresponded to two negative Cotton effects at 235 and 277 nm of **1B** spectrum whereas **1A** spectrum exhibited two positive Cotton effects at 230 and 274 nm. Therefore, the C-5 configuration was assigned as (*S*), which is in agreement with previously reported structures of cladosporiumins G and H; both were reported to be built up by L-valine. Accordingly, the complete structure of **1**, named cladosin L, is shown in Figure 1.

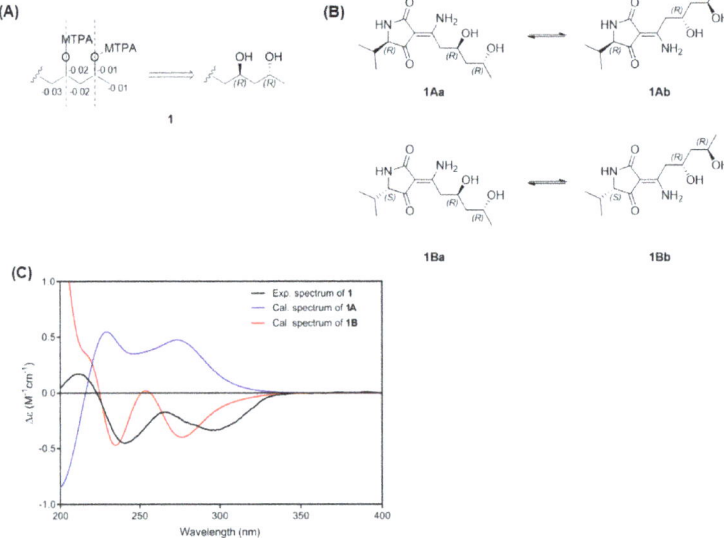

Figure 3. (**A**) Analysis of the modified Mosher's method for **1**. Δδ (δ_S–δ_R) values are shown. (**B**) Four diastereomers of **1**. (**C**) Experimental ECD spectrum of **1** and calculated ECD spectra of **1A/1B**.

The known hybrid polyketides, isolated from *C. sphaerospermum* SW67, were identified as cladosin B (**2**), cladosin F (**3**), and cladosin C (**4**) by comparison of their NMR data with those reported in the literature [19,25].

2.2. Proposed Biogenesis of **1–4**

It is generally assumed that tetramic acid-containing compounds, such as cladosins and structurally related natural products [26], are built up by polyketide synthases (PKS)–non ribosomal peptide synthetases (NRPS) hybrid megaenzymes, which catalyze the formation and condensation of a tetraketide or a related unsaturated or reduced polyketide unit and an activated amino acid to yield the 1,3-dione-5,7-diol conjugate (Figure 4) [27–29].

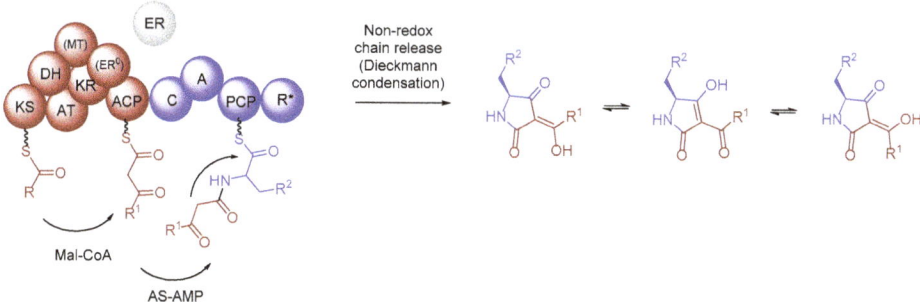

Figure 4. Fungal iterative hybrid PKS–NRPS megaenzymes are responsible for the formation of tetramic acid derivatives and often require a discrete ER to be completely functional. The R-domain catalyzes a non-reductive Dickmann condensation to release the product from the enzyme. Tetramic acids exists often as mixture of rapidly interconverting tautomers in solution arising from C–C bond rotation of the acyl side chain.

In fungi, these PKS/NRPS hybrid gene clusters generally consist of a single iterative PKS module (incorporating acetate building blocks), which is followed by a single NRPS module (attaching the polyketide chain to an amino acid) and an offloading domain. The domain architecture of the iterative PKS module closely resembles the mammalian fatty acid synthases (FAS) with the following domain organization: KS (ketosynthase), AT (acyltransferase), DH (dehydratase), CMeT (C-methyltransferase), *KR (a structural domain variant of a ketoreductase), ER (enoylreductase), KR (ketoreductase), and ACP (acyl carrier protein). In contrast to FAS, modules of an iterative PKS within hybrid organizations are more promiscuous and produce individual and diverse polyketide chains with different reduction and methylation patterns [27–29]. In particular, enoyl reduction carried out by the ER domain in polyketide biosynthesis adds diversity to the growing PKS chain. However, sequence alignments of fungal ER domains in iterative PKS–NRPSs showed that almost all ERs are predicted to be inactive (ER^0) due to a variety of significant sequence differences, e.g., missing a typical GGVG motif for NADPH binding. In most cases, *trans*-acting ERs were found to be necessary for the respective product formation [27–29]. The NRPS modules of iterative NRPS/PKS hybrids have the general domain organization of C (condensation), A (adenylation) and T (thiolation, also known as PCP peptide carrier protein). Different release mechanisms are responsible for offloading from PKS, NRPS or their respective hybrids, which are catalyzed by the respective enzymatic domains such as R (reductase), DKC (Dieckmann cyclase) or TE (thioesterase) [30].

A previous genome mining approach of the cladosin producing organism *Cladosporium* sp. SW67 and the related strain *Cladosporium* sp. UM843 revealed a putative PKS-NRPS cluster (*clsA-clsL*), which is proposed to be responsible for the formation of cladosins, cladosporiumins and cladosporicins. The region of the gene cluster *cls* encodes for five genes: a siderophore esterase (*clsA*), an AMP dependet synthetase/ligase (*clsD*), a γ-glutamyl transferase (*clsF*), a cytochrome P450 (*clsK*) and a PKS-NRPS hybrid gene (*clsI*), of which, only the cytochrome P450 (*clsK*) and the PKS-NRPS hybrid (*clsI*) gene appear to be necessary for tetramic acid formation. The possible roles of *clsA-F* remain unclear.

The domains of the putative PKS-NRPS were predicted as KS-AT-X-Y-KR-C-A-PCP-TD using PKS/NRPS analysis predictor [31], Blast searches [32] and Antismash [33]. Here, two domains (X, Y) located between the AT and the KS domain of the PKS-NRPS hybrid enzyme ClsI could not be assigned despite intensive manual database analyses of the three most similar genes using e.g., MIBig [34] and UniProt [35]. Here, it needs to be acknowledged that until today only limited numbers of fungal

PKS/NRPS domains have been fully characterized, which clearly limits the assignments based on homology searches.

To identify possible conserved motifs within the unknown domains, the corresponding areas were extracted by using ClustalW implemented in Bioedit 7.2.0 [36] and aligned against each other (Table 2). Based on different motif alignments, we found that the first unidentified domain (X) within *clsI* shows weak homologies to known dehydratase (DH) domains. In general, dehydratase (DH) domains carry a characteristic catalytic proline and aspartic acid residues within a characteristic conserved H**P**ALL**D** motif [37]. Alignment of the unknown domain within ClsI and a related domain in CluI detected in *Cladosporium* sp. UM843 revealed a T**P**MAA**D** motif, which is in weak accordance with so far reported homologous (Table S8).

Table 2. Sequence alignment of the first unknown domain of *Cladosporium* SW67 and *Cladosporium* sp. UM843 with DH-domains of known NRPS-PKSs with high identities (Tables S8 and S9). Red marked lines indicate conserved DH motif. Accession numbers are derived from the UniProt database.

	Amino Acid Sequence
SW67_clsI_unknown_1	R E W E T Q F Q L T **P** M A A **D** S R Y N F R L M I C G P S E S
UM843_cluI_unknown_1	R E W E T Q F Q L T **P** M A A **D** S R Y N F R L M I C G P S E S
ACLA_078660_DH	F N H S Q P L L I H **P** A T L **D** A A I Q S I M L A Y C Y P G D
A0A0C6E017_DH	D M Q I D N Y V V N **P** G F L **D** V A F Q S V Y T A F S S P A S
ANIA_08412_DH	V P D A D E L L V H **P** I D L **D** A A F Q S V M L A Y S Y P G D
A0A0C6E0I7_DH	P V S W T H T L T H **P** A P I **D** T A V Q G L L T A F S F P G D
FFUJ_12239_DH	F N H S Q P L L I H **P** A T L **D** A A I Q S I M L A Y C Y P G D
ACLA_078660_DH	C L S D T G L L V H **P** A F L **D** M T L H A T L A A F A S P G D
B1GVX7_DH	P V S W T H T L T H **P** A P I **D** T A V Q G L L T A F S F P G D
A0JJU1_DH	A D L N D C Y L V H **P** A I L **D** V A F Q T I F V A R A H P D S
S0EET5_DH	V V P D F P A M I H **P** A L I **D** G A F Q S I F A A Y C Q P D D

Subsequently, we analyzed the second unknown domain by different motif alignments. Genes with the highest identities for already described PKS-NRPSs mainly contained methyltransferase (C-MT) domains at the corresponding sites. Regions of sequence similarities within SAM dependent MTs are divided into three different motifs (I, II and II) [38,39] and comparative alignments between the unknown second domains (Y) and known C-MT domains showed that neither Motif I [(L/I/V)(V/L)(E/D)(V/I)G(C/G)G(P/T/G)] nor Motif III [(G/P)(T/Q)(A/Y/F)DA(Y/V/I)(I/F)(L/V/C)] was detectable within the second domain (Y). However, weak homologies to Motif II [LL(K/R)PGG(L/I/R)(I/L)(V/I/F/L)(L/I)] could be detected in both unknown domains (Y) of *Cladosporium* sp. SW67 and UM843 (Table 3).

Table 3. Sequence alignment of the second unknown domain of *Cladosporium* sp. SW67 and *Cladosporium* sp. UM843 and C-MT-domains of known NRPS-PKSs with high identities (Tables S8 and S9). Colored lines indicate conserved MT-domain motif II. Accession numbers are derived from the UniProt database.

	Amino Acid Sequence
SW67_clsI_unknown_2	- - - - - - - F D Q E N H R **V** S **P G G** C **I** C **V L** H S R T - -
UM843_cluI_unknown_2	- - - - - - - F D Q E N H R **V** S **P G G** C **I** C **V L** H S R T - -
ACLA_078660_C-MT	T R D L A Q T V R N V R R **L L** K **P G G** Y **L L L L** E I T E N -
A0A0C6E017_C-MT	C A R L D E A V A N **L** R K **L L** K **P G G L L** V **L** G E G A S D G
ANIA_08412_C-MT	T H S L E N T L R Q C R K **L L** R **P G G** R **L** V **L L** E I T R - -
A0A0C6E0I7_C-MT	T R D L A Q T V R N V R R **L L** K **P G G** Y **L L L L** E I T E N -
FFUJ_12239_C-MT	T E F L E K T M R N V R T **L L** K **P G G** Y **L** C **L L** E C T G - -
ACLA_078660_C-MT	T H S L E N T L R Q C R K **L L** R **P G G** R **L** V **L L** E I T R - -
B1GVX7_C-MT	T R N L G V T L G N V R S **L L** K **P G G** Y **L L L L** N E K T G P -
A0JJU1_C-MT	T K S L T V T M R N T R K **L L** K **P G G** Q **L L L** L E V T S - -
S0EET5_C-MT	T P D L E K T M A H A R S **L L** K **P G G** Q **M** V **I L** E I T H K -

In a last step, we analyzed the catalytic domain responsible for product-release from the PKS-NRPS enzyme. The formation of the 1,3-dione-5,7-diol conjugate requires a Dieckmann-type condensation/cyclization of a polyketide unit and a valine residue (Figure 5). To analyze if the proposed PKS-NRPS enzymes harbors the necessary release domain [30,40]. Thus, amino acid sequences of NR-PKSs enzymes with known product release mechanisms were again collected from NCBI and UniProt databases [35] and closest homologues were obtained by identity search in the MiBIG database [34] and the first three matches were individually evaluated by BLAST. The product-release enzyme domains of *clsI* and *cluI* were extracted by PKS/NRPS Analyzer and manually aligned using the ClustalW tool implemented in Bioedit 7.2.0 and partial sequences were manually compiled, assembled and trimmed (Tables S8 and S9). Initial tree(s) for the heuristic search were obtained automatically by applying neighbor joining approach. The robustness of branches was assessed by bootstrap analysis with 1000 replicates. The tree is drawn to scale with branch lengths measured in the number of substitutions per site and evolutionary analyses were conducted in MEGA7 [41].

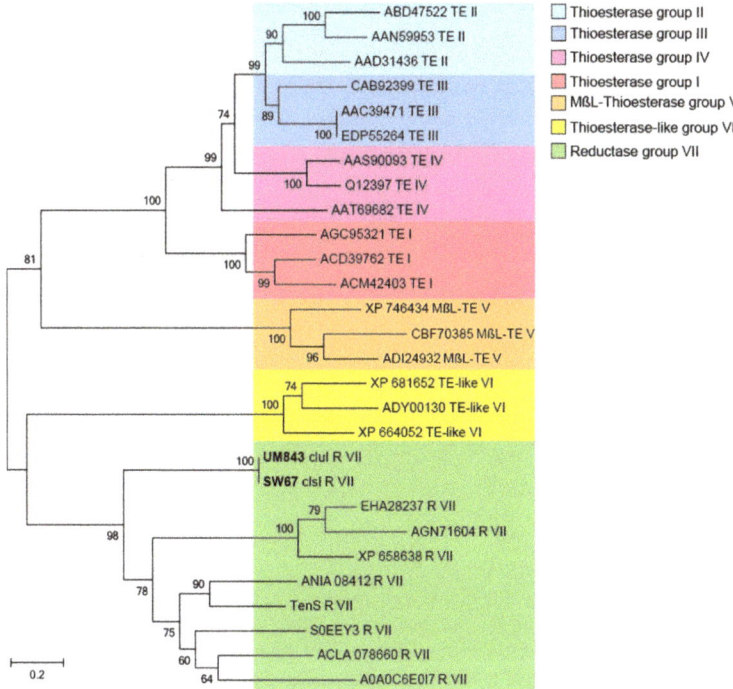

Figure 5. Phylogenetic tree of different fungal product-releasing and their functional classification. The different types of product-releasing enzyme domains in NR-PKSs have been highlighted with different color code [42]. Phylogenetic analysis was conducted using neighbor joining method [43,44]. Bold text represents the *Cladosporium* sp. SW67 and UM843 group (accession number/gene name, type of release reaction, group of product-release enzyme). Probability values > 50% are shown at the nodes based on 1000 bootstraps. The tree is drawn to scale with branch lengths measured in the number of substitutions per site.

Due to similarities and cluster grouping, the product release domain of *Cladosporium* SW67 and UM843 can be classified as reductase (R) domain (Figure 4). This domain was initially found to catalyze an NAD(P)H-dependent reductive release of fungal iterative PKS–NRPSs products based on sequence homology to SDR (shortchain dehydrogenase/reductase) family proteins. Detailed studies on tenellin [45,46] and aspyridone A [47] biosynthesis showed that R domains also catalyze non-reductive Dieckmann-type condensation reactions yielding the tetramic acids derivatives peraspyridone A and pretenellin A (Figure 6A) [48]. In case of peraspyridone A, subsequent oxidation by an additional P450 monooxygenase yields aspyridone A; a similar mechanism was proposed for the biosynthesis of tenellin A.

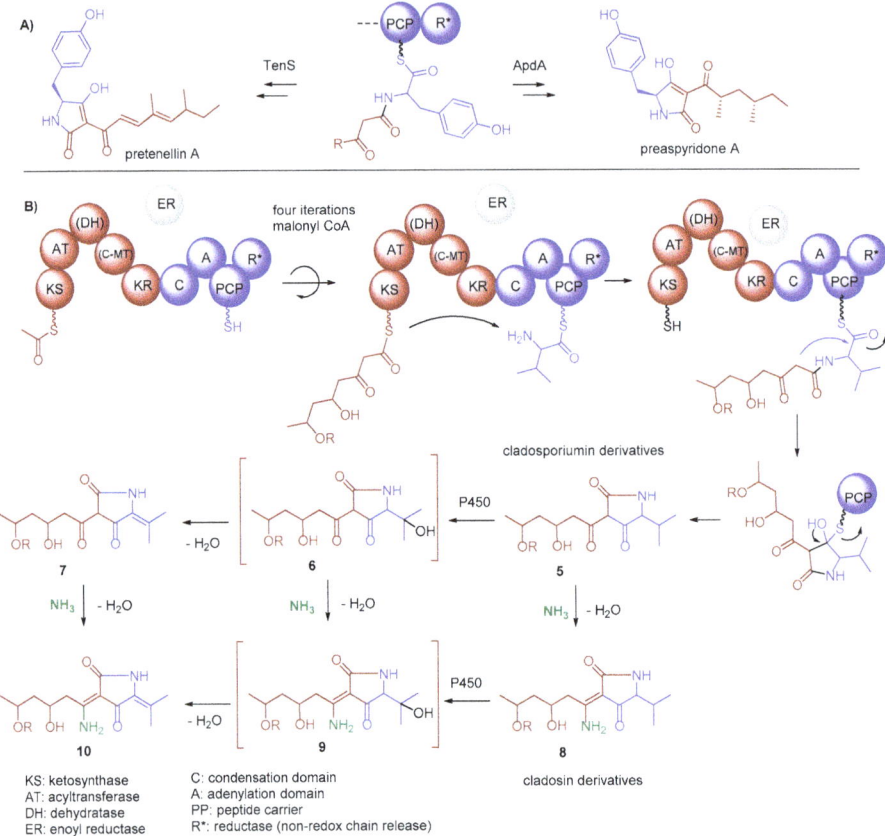

Figure 6. (**A**) TenS and ApDA as examples of fungal iterative hybrid PKS–NRPS that include a non-reductive Dieckmann-type condensation reactions yielding peraspyridone A and pretenellin A, respectively. (**B**) Proposed biosynthetic pathway of the core structure formation of cladosporiumin and cladosin-type natural products. Domains of PKS-NRPS are putatively assigned as KS-AT-(*DH)-(*C-MT)-KR-C-A-PCP-TE (* weak homologies).

In summary, we propose the following domain arrangement of the putative PKS-NRPS (KS-AT-*DH-*cMT-KR-C-A-PCP-R) (Figure 6B). Whether or not the poorly assigned domains (-*DH-*cMT-) are fully functional, cannot be deduced at this stage. Here, we also propose that the identified terminal reductase (R) domain in *clsI* and *cluI* performs a non-reductive Dieckmann-type cyclisation to yield the 2,4-pyrrolidinedione skeleton, which after oxidation of the valine unit (cytochrome P450 *clsK*) and (spontaneous) elimination of H_2O results in derivative **7** bearing a thermodynamically stable tetra-substituted double bond (Figure 6B). Whether or not the cytochrome P450 *clsK* [49] is also responsible for the elimination of H_2O cannot be deduced at this stage.

Tetramic acids of types **5** and **7** exist in both, keto and enol form, which allows for the (spontaneous) reaction with NH_3 yielding enamines **8** and **10**, respectively. Due to a tautomeric equilibrium, enols and imines were found as interconverting *E/Z*-mixtures. To confirm the biosynthetic origin, we re-analyzed our ^{13}C-labeling data (addition of ^{13}C-valine and ^{13}C-acetate to a growth medium, Figure 7). As expected, an LC/MS based analysis of the enriched ^{13}C-labeled compound mixture revealed the incorporation of one valine residue and a PKS-typical CH_3CO_2-dependent pattern (incorporation of four acetate units) into **1** (Figure S15) confirming once more the biosynthetic proposal.

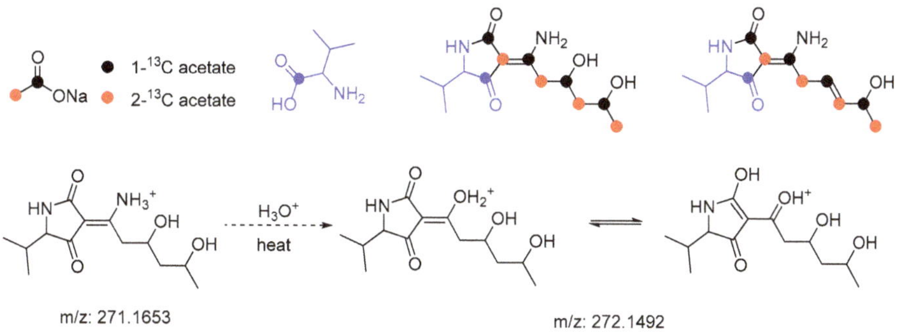

Figure 7. The proposed ^{13}C-labeling pattern of **1–4** based on a hybrid PKS-NRPS assembly line.

2.3. Biological Evaluation of 1–4

In our ongoing studies to explore biologically active unique natural products, we particularly focused on the discovery of renoprotective natural products for protection against cisplatin-induced nephrotoxicity [50–52], which is a major issue in the clinical use of cisplatin in cancer patients [53–55]. It has been reported in the literatures that some natural products exhibit effective protection against cisplatin-induced nephrotoxicity [55–57]. In our recent studies, it was found that 1-*O*-(2-aminobenzoyl)-α-L-rhamnopyranoside from a termite-associated *Streptomyces* sp. RB1 [50], dehydroeburicoic acid monoacetate from *Poria cocos* [51], and sterols, (22*E*,24*S*)-ergosta-7,22-diene-3β,5α,6β-triol and (22*E*,24*R*)-ergosta-8(14),22-diene-3β,5α,6β,7α-tetrol from *Pleurotus cornucopiae* [52] showed the renoprotective effects. Despite the continued publications of these effects, these studies failed to achieve clinical success. Therefore, there is an urgent need to develop effective agents to save the lives of cancer patients having impaired renal functions.

To identify active compounds having protective effects against cell damage caused by cisplatin, the LLC-PK1 cells were pre-treated with **1–4** for 2 h before treatment with 25 µM of cisplatin. After treatment with cisplatin, the cell viability was 63.01 ± 2.47% when compared to the control. The reduction in cell viability in response to cisplatin-induced cell death was recovered to 80.14 ± 4.16% and 90.68 ± 0.81% after pretreatment with 50 µM and 100 µM of **2**, respectively (Figure 8B). Cell viability was reduced by 61.93 ± 0.72% after treatment with 25 µM of cisplatin, whereas it was increased by 77.65 ± 2.43% and 85.6 ± 2.47% after treatment with 50 µM and 100 µM of **3**, respectively (Figure 8C). Although the protective effects of **2** and **3** were similar, **2** showed a better effect. In addition, the effect of **2** at 100 µM was similar to the recovered cell viability of 88.23 ± 0.25% with 500 µM N-acetylcysteine (NAC), a positive control (Figure 8E). Compound **4** showed no protective effect and **1** showed minor but insignificant protective effect (Figure 8A,D). In the structure activity relationship (SAR), the comparison of protective effects of active compounds (**1**, **2** and **3**) vs inactive compounds (**4**) suggested that the presence of hydroxy group at C-8 may be essential for the renoprotective effect against cisplatin-induced nephrotoxicity in LLC-PK1 cells. Therefore, there is a need to further evaluate the mechanisms of action of **2** and **3** against cisplatin-induced damage to LLC-PK1 cells.

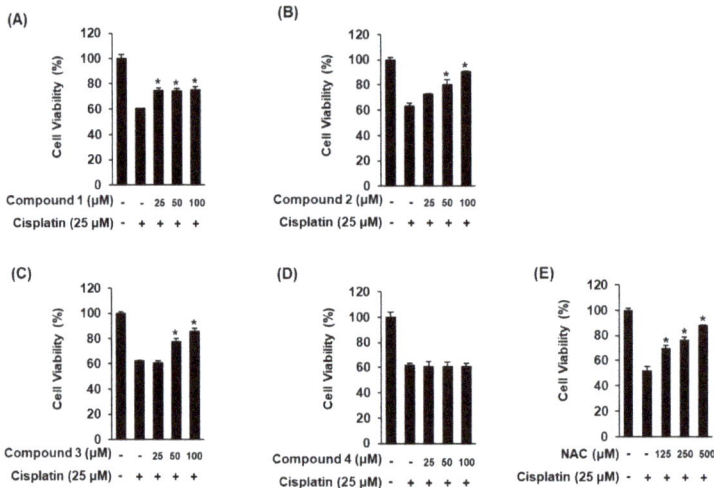

Figure 8. Comparison of the protective effects of **1–4** (**A**–**D**) and NAC (**E**, positive control) on the viability of LLC-PK1 cells exposed to 25 µL of cisplatin for 24 h by MTT assay. The control cells were treated with the vehicle only (mean ± SD, * $p < 0.05$ vs. control).

3. Materials and Methods

3.1. General Experimental Procedures

Optical rotations were measured using a Jasco P-1020 polarimeter (Jasco, Easton, MD, USA). The IR spectra were recorded on a Bruker IFS-66/S FT-IR spectrometer. The ESI and HR-ESI mass spectra were recorded on an SI-2/LCQ DecaXP Liquid chromatography (LC)-mass spectrometer. The experimental ECD spectra in MeOH were acquired in a quartz cuvette of 1 mm optical path length on a JASCO J-1500 spectropolarimeter (Tokyo, Japan). NMR, including COSY, HSQC, and HMBC, experiments were conducted utilizing a Varian UNITY INOVA 800 NMR spectrometer operating at 800 MHz (^{1}H) and 200 MHz (^{13}C) with chemical shifts given in ppm (δ). The preparative high-performance liquid chromatography (HPLC) utilized a Waters 1525 Binary HPLC pump with Waters 996 Photodiode Array Detector (Waters Corporation, Milford, CT, USA). Semi-preparative HPLC was carried out using a Shimadzu Prominence HPLC System with SPD-20A/20AV Series Prominence HPLC UV-Vis Detectors (Shimadzu, Tokyo, Japan). LC/MS analysis was carried out on an Agilent 1200 Series HPLC system (Agilent Technologies, Santa Clara, CA, USA) equipped with a diode array detector and a 6130 Series ESI mass spectrometer using an analytical Kinetex (4.6 × 100 mm, 3.5 µm). Merck precoated Silica gel F254 plates and RP-18 F254s plates were used for thin-layer chromatography (TLC). The spots were detected on TLC under UV light or by heating after spraying with anisaldehyde-sulfuric acid.

3.2. Biological Material

The fungus was obtained as previously described [18]. In brief, polyps of *H. echinata* (Alfred Wegener Institute, Sylt, Germany) were aseptically homogenized, diluted with sterile filtered seawater, and plated onto potato dextrose agar (PDA) plates. The plates were incubated for 1–3 weeks at room temperature, and colonies showing fungal morphologies were selected. The isolate SW67 was identified as *C. sphaerospermum* based on the analysis of the internal transcribed spacer (ITS) gene sequence.

3.3. Extraction and Isolation

Overall, approximately 400 PDA and 400 MEA plates were inoculated with a 100 µL aliquot of a turbid fungal spore suspension of *C. sphaerospermum* SW67 in sterile PBS. The suspension was evenly distributed over the agar surface, and the plates were incubated at 25 °C in the dark for 14 days. The agar was then cut into squares, consolidated, and macerated overnight in MeOH. The MeOH solution was filtered and removed under reduced pressure to obtain the crude MeOH extract. The MeOH extract (6 g) was dissolved in distilled water (700 mL) and then partitioned with EtOAc (700 mL), yielding 0.25 g of EtOAc-soluble fraction. The EtOAc-soluble fraction was fractionated by preparative reversed-phase HPLC (Phenomenex Luna C18, 250 × 21.2 mm i.d., 5 µm) using CH_3CN-H_2O (1:9–3:2, v/v, gradient system, flow rate: 5 mL/min) to afford six subfractions (A–F). Compound **1** (2.0 mg, t_R = 29.0 min) was purified from subfraction B (15 mg) by semi-preparative reversed-phase HPLC (Phenomenex Luna C18, 250 × 10.0 mm i.d., 5 µm) with an isocratic solvent system of 29% MeOH. The subfraction C (14 mg) was purified by semi-preparative reversed-phase HPLC (Phenomenex Luna C18, 250 × 10.0 mm i.d., 5 µm) with an isocratic solvent system of 31% MeOH to afford **2** (3.0 mg, t_R = 36.0 min) and **3** (7.4 mg, t_R = 40.0 min). Compound **4** (1.7 mg, t_R = 39.0 min) was isolated from subfraction D (8 mg) by semi-preparative reversed-phase HPLC (Phenomenex Luna C18, 250 × 10.0 mm i.d., 5 µm) with an isocratic solvent system of 38% MeOH.

Cladosin L (**1**)

Yellowish oil; $[\alpha]_D^{25}$ −25.5 (c 0.05, MeOH); IR (KBr) ν_{max} 3435, 2966, 2843, 1634, 1521, and 1060 cm^{-1}; UV (MeOH) λ_{max} (log ε) 198 (2.5), 236 (1.9), and 296 (3.9) nm; ECD (MeOH) λ_{max} (Δε) 211 (1.7), 241 (−3.2), 266 (−1.6), and 297 (−2.5) nm; ^{1}H (800 MHz) and ^{13}C NMR (200 MHz), see Table 1; (+)-HRESIMS m/z 271.1658 $[M + H]^+$ (calcd. for $C_{13}H_{23}N_2O_4$, 271.1658).

3.4. Preparation of Mosher Ester Derivatives from Cladosin L (1)

Cladosin L (**1**) (0.5 mg) was dissolved in deuterated pyridine (0.25 mL) and transferred to a clean NMR tube and then a small quantity of 4-(dimethylamino)pyridine was added. (S)-(+)-α-methoxy-α-(trifluoromethyl) phenylacetyl (MTPA) chloride (5 µL) was added into the NMR tubes under an N_2 gas stream and the NMR tube was shaken carefully to mix the sample with added reagents. The NMR tube was stored at room temperature overnight, which afforded the (R)-MTPA ester derivative of **1**. The (S)-MTPA ester derivative of **1** was also prepared using (R)-MTPA chloride according to the procedure described above. The ^{1}H NMR and TOCSY spectra were directly obtained from the Mosher's ester derivatives of **1** in NMR tube.

(R)-MTPA Ester of **1**. ^{1}H NMR (Pyridine-d_5, 800 MHz): δ 3.44 (H-7), 4.99 (H-8), 2.04 (H-9), 4.59 (H-10), 1.37 (H-11); ESIMS m/z 725.2 $[M + Na]^+$.

(S)-MTPA Ester of **1**. ^{1}H NMR (Pyridine-d_5, 800 MHz): δ 3.41 (H-7), 4.97 (H-8), 2.02 (H-9), 4.58 (H-10), 1.36 (H-11); ESIMS m/z 725.2 $[M + Na]^+$.

3.5. Computational Analysis

All conformers of **1Aa**, **1Ab**, **1Ba**, and **1Bb** used in this study were found using the Macromodel (version 2015-2, Schrödinger LLC, New York, NY, USA) module with "Mixed torsional/Low-mode sampling" in the MMFF force field. The searches were implemented in the gas phase with a 5 kJ/mol energy window limit and 10,000 maximum number of steps to explore all potential conformers. The Polak–Ribiere Conjugate Gradient (PRCG) method was utilized to minimize conformers with 10,000 iterations and a 0.001 kJ $(mol\ Å)^{-1}$ convergence threshold on the Root Mean Square (RMS) gradient. All the conformers were subjected to geometry optimization using the Gaussian 16 package (Gaussian Inc., Wallingford, CT, USA) in the gas phase at B3LYP/6-31+G(d,p) level and proceeded to calculation of excitation energies, oscillator strength, and rotatory strength at B3LYP/6-31+G(d,p) level in the Polarizable Continuum Model (PCM, methanol). The ECD spectra were Boltzmann-averaged based on the calculated Gibbs free energy of each conformer (Tables S2–S5) and visualized with SpecDis software (Version 1.71) [58] with a σ/γ value of 0.30 eV. The calculated ECD spectra of **1A** and **1B** were obtained by averaging those of **1Aa** and **1Ab,** and **1Ba** and **1Bb**, respectively, since the compound **1** exists as a 1:1 mixture of two geometric isomers (**1a** and **1b**) as described in the Section 2.1 above.

3.6. Isotope Labeling

For ^{13}C labeling experiments, 2 g/L of sodium [1-^{13}C] acetate, sodium [2-^{13}C] acetate, or [1-^{13}C] valine was each added separately to 1 L of PDA medium (6.6 g/L). Each plate was inoculated with 100 µL of a spore suspension (SW67) in sterile PBS, and the plates were incubated for 14 d at room temperature in the dark. The plates were cut into pieces and extracted with 100% MeOH (if not mentioned otherwise, mixtures refer to MeOH in ddH$_2$O) at 4 °C overnight. The extracts were filtrated and the solvent was evaporated under reduced pressure. The remaining extract was re-dissolved in 10% MeOH and loaded on a pre-activated and equilibrated C18 cartridge (100 mg C18, 10% MeOH). The loaded SPE column was washed with 20% MeOH, and then the metabolites were eluted using 100% MeOH. The extracts were then concentrated under reduced pressure. Finally, the organic extract was dissolved with 100% MeOH to yield a 1.0 mg/mL stock solution for the UHPLC-MS analysis.

For compound **1** (m/z = 271.15 [M − H]$^-$), feeding with [1-^{13}C] sodium acetate and [2-^{13}C] sodium acetate, respectively, resulted in the detection of the corresponding mass shift of up to +4 m/z. Similar, addition of [1-^{13}C] valine resulted in the detection of the corresponding mass shift of +1 m/z. However, it needs to be noted that a dominant signal (m/z 270) of the closely related cladosporiumin F overlapped with the respective signal of compound **1** due to their similar retention times. If the high detection level of cladosporiumin F was due to heat/acid-induced hydrolysis during measurement, it could not be excluded at this stage. Both the signal sets showed the same ^{13}C incorporation pattern.

3.7. Renoprotective Effects against Cisplatin-Induced Kidney Cell Damage

The protective effects of compounds **1–4** against cisplatin-induced renal cell death were determined by Ez-Cytox cell viability assay kit (DOGEN, Seoul, Korea) using LLC-PK1 pig kidney epithelium cells (American Type Culture Collection, Rockville, MD, USA). The LLC-PK1 cells were cultured in Dulbecco's modified Eagle medium (Manassas, VA, USA) supplemented with 10% FBS, 1% penicillin/streptomycin, and 4 mM L-glutamine at 37 °C with 5% CO$_2$ in a humidified incubator and with 5% CO2 in air at 37 °C. The cells were seeded onto 96-well culture plates at 1×10^4 cells per/well and incubated for 24 h to adhere. Thereafter, the cells were pre-treated with 25, 50, and 100 µM of compounds **1–4**, and then 25 µM of cisplatin was added to the wells. After 24 h, the medium containing the compounds **1–4** and/or cisplatin was removed, and a serum-free medium containing Ez-Cytox reagent was added to the wells. After incubation for 2 h at 37 °C, the cell viability was measured by absorbance at 450 nm using a microplate reader (PowerWave XS; Bio-Tek Instruments, Winooski, VT, USA). N-acetyl cysteine (NAC) was used as a positive control.

3.8. Statistical Analyses

All data described in this study were repeated at least three times and are represented as the mean ± S.E.M. The statistical significance was determined by one-way analysis of variance (ANOVA). p-values of < 0.05 were considered statistically significant.

4. Conclusions

Marine invertebrates host a diverse assemblage of mostly beneficial microbes that can produce novel natural products. Herein, we isolated the marine fungus *C. sphaerospermum* SW67 from the hydroid polyp of *H. echinata*. LC/MS-guided chemical analysis of the marine fungus *C. sphaerospermum* SW67 led to the isolation and characterization of five hybrid polyketides (**1a**, **1b**, and **2–4**) containing tetramic acid core including a previously unreported cladosin L (**1**), which was isolated as a pair of interconverting geometric isomers. As indicated by biosynthetic gene cluster analysis and ^{13}C-labeling studies, compounds **1–4** are formed via the generally assumed biosynthesis of microbial tetramic acids. Although the timing of the putative oxygenation and dehydration of the valine residue is unknown, the compound **1** could be regarded as a putative precursor of previously and herein reported cladosin F (**3**). Compounds **2** and **3** ameliorated the damage of LLC-PK1 cells induced by 25 µM of cisplatin. In particular, **2** at 100 µM (cell viability, 90.68 ± 0.81%) exhibited a significant protective effect against cell damage, which was similar to that of the positive control, 500 µM NAC (cell viability, 88.23 ± 0.25%). These findings provide experimental evidence that **2** could be an adjunct candidate to treat cisplatin-induced adverse effects and/or to prevent anticancer drug-induced nephrotoxicity.

Supplementary Materials: The following are available online at http://www.mdpi.com/1660-3397/17/11/606/s1, Figure S1: The HR-ESIMS data of **1**; Figure S2: The ^{1}H NMR spectrum of **1** (CD$_3$OD, 800 MHz); Figure S3: The ^{13}C NMR spectrum of **1** (CD$_3$OD, 200 MHz); Figure S4: The ^{1}H-^{1}H COSY spectrum of **1** (CD$_3$OD); Figure S5: The HSQC spectrum of **1** (CD$_3$OD); Figure S6: The HMBC spectrum of **1** (CD$_3$OD); Figure S7: The ROESY spectrum of **1** (CD$_3$OD); Figure S8: The ^{1}H NMR spectrum of the (*R*)-MTPA esterification of compound **1**; Figure S9: The TOCSY spectrum of the (*R*)-MTPA esterification of compound **1**; Figure S10: The ^{1}H NMR spectrum of the (*S*)-MTPA esterification of compound **1**; Figure S11: The TOCSY spectrum of the (*S*)-MTPA esterification of compound **1**; Figure S12: Media compositions for *C. sphaerospermum* SW67; Figure S13: Comparative total ion chromatogram (positive mode) of culture extracts obtained from SW67; Figure S14: Comparative selected ion chromatogram (*m/z* 271.15) of culture extracts obtained from SW67; Figure S15: LC/MS analysis of extracts obtained from ^{13}C-sublemented cultures; Figure S16: The ^{1}H NMR spectrum of **2** (CD$_3$OD, 800 MHz); Figure S17: The LC/MS data of **2**; Figure S18: The ^{1}H NMR spectrum of **3** (CD$_3$OD, 800 MHz); Figure S19: The LC/MS data of **3**; Figure S20: The ^{1}H NMR spectrum of **4** (CD$_3$OD, 800 MHz); Figure S21: The LC/MS data of **4**; Figure S22: Calculated ECD spectra of **1Aa**, **1Ab**, **1Ba**, and **1Bb** and experimental ECD spectrum of **1**; Table S1: Structures of reported hybrid polyketides containing the tetramic acid moiety; Table S2: Gibbs free energies and Boltzmann distribution of conformers **1Aa**; Table S3: Gibbs free energies and Boltzmann distribution of conformers **1Ab**; Table S4: Gibbs free energies and Boltzmann distribution of conformers **1Ba**; Table S5: Gibbs free energies and Boltzmann distribution of conformers **1Bb**; Table S6: Coordinates of the conformers; Table S7: Detailed analysis of the gene NRPS/PKS hybdrid gene cluster; Table S8: List of NR-PKSs used for alignment of unknown ClsI and CluI domains; Table S9: List of NR-PKSs related to known polyketides used for phylogenetic analysis of fungal product-release enzymes.

Author Contributions: Conceptualization, C.B. and K.H.K.; methodology, C.B., K.S.K., and K.H.K.; validation, C.B. and K.H.K.; formal analysis, S.R.L., D.L., H.J.E., Y.-J.K., C.S.K., and M.R.; investigation, S.R.L., D.L., H.J.E., C.S.K., and M.R.; resources, C.B.; data curation, S.R.L., Y.-J.K., K.S.K., C.S.K., C.B., and K.H.K.; writing—original draft preparation, S.R.L., K.S.K., C.B. and K.H.K.; writing—review and editing, C.B. and K.H.K.; supervision, K.H.K.; project administration, C.B. and K.H.K.; funding acquisition, K.H.K.

Funding: This work was supported by the National Research Foundation of Korea (NRF) grant funded by the Korean government (MSIT) (2018R1A2B2006879 and 2019R1A5A2027340). This work was also supported by the Nano Convergence Industrial Strategic Technology Development Program (20000105, Development of Cosmeceutical Material Platform using Organo-Nano Complexes based on Natural Active Compounds) funded By the Ministry of Trade, Industry & Energy (MOTIE, Korea).

Acknowledgments: We would like to thank Young Hye Kim (KBSI) for the ESIMS analysis.

Conflicts of Interest: The authors declare no conflict of interest.

References

1. Shnit-Orland, M.; Kushmaro, A. Coral mucus-associated bacteria: A possible first line of defense. *FEMS Microbiol. Ecol.* **2009**, *67*, 371–380. [CrossRef] [PubMed]
2. Olson, J.B.; Kellogg, C.A. Microbial ecology of corals, sponges, and algae in mesophotic coral environments. *FEMS Microbiol. Ecol.* **2010**, *73*, 17–30. [CrossRef] [PubMed]
3. Piel, J. Metabolites from symbiotic bacteria. *Nat. Prod. Rep.* **2004**, *21*, 519–538. [CrossRef] [PubMed]
4. Rohwer, F.; Seguritan, V.; Azam, F.; Knowlton, N. Diversity and distribution of coral-associated bacteria. *Mar. Ecol. Prog. Ser.* **2002**, *243*, 1–10. [CrossRef]
5. Lan, W.J.; Fu, S.J.; Xu, M.Y.; Liang, W.L.; Lam, C.K.; Zhong, G.H.; Xu, J.; Yang, D.P.; Li, H.J. Five new cytotoxic metabolites from the marine fungus *Neosartorya Pseudofischeri*. *Mar. Drugs* **2016**, *14*, 18. [CrossRef] [PubMed]
6. Wang, C.; Guo, L.; Hao, J.; Wang, L.; Zhu, W. α-glucosidase inhibitors from the marine-derived fungus *Aspergillus flavipes* HN4-13. *J. Nat. Prod.* **2016**, *79*, 2977–2981. [CrossRef] [PubMed]
7. Julianti, E.; Oh, H.; Jang, K.H.; Lee, J.K.; Lee, S.K.; Oh, D.C. Acremostrictin, a highly oxygenated metabolite from the marine fungus *Acremonium strictum*. *J. Nat. Prod.* **2011**, *74*, 2592–2594. [CrossRef]

8. Abdel-Lateff, A.; König, G.M.; Fisch, K.M.; Höller, U.; Jones, P.G.; Wright, A.D. New antioxidant hydroquinone derivatives from the algicolous marine fungus *Acremonium* sp. *J. Nat. Prod.* **2002**, *65*, 1605–1611. [CrossRef]
9. Kim, K.S.; Cui, X.; Lee, D.S.; Sohn, J.H.; Yim, J.H.; Kim, Y.C.; Oh, H. Anti-inflammatory effect of neoechinulin A from the marine fungus *Eurotium* sp. SF-5989 through the suppression of NF-κB and p38 MAPK pathways in lipopolysaccharide-stimulated RAW264.7 macrophages. *Molecules* **2013**, *18*, 13245–13259. [CrossRef]
10. Ohkawa, Y.; Miki, K.; Suzuki, T.; Nishio, K.; Sugita, T.; Kinoshita, K.; Takahashi, K.; Koyama, K. Antiangiogenic metabolites from a marine-derived fungus, *Hypocrea vinosa*. *J. Nat. Prod.* **2010**, *73*, 579–582. [CrossRef]
11. Lee, D.S.; Ko, W.; Quang, T.H.; Kim, K.S.; Sohn, J.H.; Jang, J.H.; Ahn, J.S.; Kim, Y.C.; Oh, H. Penicillinolide A: A new anti-inflammatory metabolites from the marine fungus Penicillium sp. SF-5292. *Mar. Drugs* **2013**, *11*, 4510–4526. [CrossRef] [PubMed]
12. Park, Y.C.; Gunasekera, S.P.; Lopez, J.V.; McCarthy, P.J.; Wright, A.E. Metabolites from the marine-derived fungus *Chromocleista* sp. Isolated from a deep-water sediment sample collected in the gulf of Mexico. *J. Nat. Prod.* **2006**, *69*, 580–584. [CrossRef] [PubMed]
13. So, H.M.; Eom, H.J.; Lee, D.; Kim, S.; Kang, K.S.; Lee, I.K.; Baek, K.H.; Park, J.Y.; Kim, K.H. Bioactivity evaluations of betulin identified from the bark of *Betula platyphylla* var. *japonica for cancer therapy*. *Arch. Pharm. Res.* **2018**, *41*, 815–822. [PubMed]
14. Yu, J.S.; Roh, H.S.; Baek, K.H.; Lee, S.; Kim, S.; So, H.M.; Moon, E.; Pang, C.; Jang, T.S.; Kim, K.H. Bioactivity-guided isolation of ginsenosides from Korean Red Ginseng with cytotoxic activity against human lung adenocarcinoma cells. *J. Ginseng Res.* **2018**, *42*, 562–570. [CrossRef] [PubMed]
15. Baek, S.C.; Choi, E.; Eom, H.J.; Jo, M.S.; Kim, S.; So, H.M.; Kim, S.H.; Kang, K.S.; Kim, K.H. LC/MS-based analysis of bioactive compounds from the bark of *Betula platyphylla* var. *japonica* and Their Effects on Regulation of Adipocyte and Osteoblast Differentiation. *Nat. Prod. Sci.* **2018**, *24*, 235–240.
16. Lee, S.R.; Park, Y.J.; Han, Y.B.; Lee, J.C.; Lee, S.; Park, H.J.; Lee, H.J.; Kim, K.H. Isoamericanoic acid B from *Acer tegmentosum* as a potential phytoestrogen. *Nutrients* **2018**, *10*, 1915. [CrossRef]
17. Kang, H.R.; Yun, H.S.; Lee, T.K.; Lee, S.; Kim, S.H.; Moon, E.; Park, K.M.; Kim, K.H. Chemical characterization of novel natural products from the roots of Asian rice (*Oryza sativa*) that control adipocyte and osteoblast differentiation. *J. Agric. Food Chem.* **2018**, *66*, 2677–2684. [CrossRef]
18. Rischer, M.; Lee, S.R.; Eom, H.J.; Park, H.B.; Vollmers, J.; Kaster, A.K.; Shin, Y.H.; Oh, D.C.; Kim, K.H.; Beemelmanns, C. Spirocyclic cladosporicin A and cladosporiumins I and J from a *Hydractinia*-associated *Cladosporium sphaerospermum* SW67. *Org. Chem. Front.* **2019**, *6*, 1084–1093. [CrossRef]
19. Wu, G.; Sun, X.; Yu, G.; Wang, W.; Zhu, T.; Gu, Q.; Li, D. Cladosins A−E, Hybrid polyketides from a deep-sea-derived fungus, *Cladosporium sphaerospermum*. *J. Nat. Prod.* **2014**, *77*, 270–275. [CrossRef]
20. Zhang, Z.; He, X.; Wu, G.; Liu, C.; Lu, C.; Gu, Q.; Che, Q.; Zhu, T.; Zhang, G.; Li, D. Aniline-tetramic acids from the deep-sea-derived fungus *Cladosporium sphaerospermum* L3P3 cultured with the HDAC Inhibitor SAHA. *J. Nat. Prod.* **2018**, *81*, 1651–1657. [CrossRef]
21. Jeong, Y.C.; Moloney, M.G. Synthesis of and tautomerism in 3-acyltetramic acids. *J. Org. Chem.* **2011**, *76*, 1342–1354. [CrossRef] [PubMed]
22. Aoki, S.; Higuchi, K.; Ye, Y.; Satari, R.; Kobayashi, M. Melophlins A and B, novel tetramic acids reversing the phenotype of ras-transformed cells, from the marine sponge *Melophlus sarassinorum*. *Tetrahedron* **2000**, *56*, 1833–1836. [CrossRef]
23. Liang, X.; Huang, Z.H.; Ma, X.; Qi, S.H. Unstable tetramic acid derivatives from deep-sea-derived fungus *Cladosporium sphaerospermum* EIODSF 008. *Mar. Drugs* **2018**, *16*, 448. [CrossRef] [PubMed]
24. Freire, F.; Seco, J.M.; Quinoa, E.; Riguera, R. Determining the absolute stereochemistry of secondary/secondary diols by ^{1}H NMR: Basis and applications. *J. Org. Chem.* **2005**, *70*, 3778–3790. [CrossRef]
25. Yu, G.H.; Wu, G.W.; Zhu, T.J.; Gu, Q.Q.; Li, D.H. Cladosins F and G, two new hybrid polyketides from the deep-sea-derived *Cladosporium sphaerospermum* 2005-01-E3. *J. Asian Nat. Prod. Res.* **2015**, *17*, 120–124. [CrossRef]
26. Mo, X.; Li, Q.; Ju, J. Naturally occurring tetramic acid products: Isolation, structure elucidation and biological activity. *RSC Adv.* **2014**, *4*, 50566–50593. [CrossRef]
27. Fisch, K.M. Biosynthesis of natural products by microbial iterative hybrid PKS–NRPS. *RSC Adv.* **2013**, *3*, 18228–18247. [CrossRef]
28. Boettger, D.; Hertweck, C. Molecular Diversity Sculpted by Fungal PKS–NRPS Hybrids. *ChemBioChem* **2013**, *14*, 28–42. [CrossRef]

29. Miyanaga, A.; Kudo, F.; Eguchi, T. Protein–protein interactions in polyketide synthase–nonribosomal peptide synthetase hybrid assembly lines. *Nat. Prod. Rep.* **2018**, *35*, 1185–1209. [CrossRef]
30. Du, L.; Lou, L. PKS and NRPS release mechanisms. *Nat. Prod. Rev.* **2010**, *27*, 255–278. [CrossRef]
31. Bachmann, B.O.; Ravel, J. Chapter 8. Methods for in silico prediction of microbial polyketide and nonribosomal peptide biosynthetic pathways from DNA sequence data. *Methods Enzymol.* **2009**, *458*, 181–217. [PubMed]
32. BLAST: Basic Local Alignment Search Tool—NCBI-NIH. Available online: https://blast.ncbi.nlm.nih.gov/Blast.cgi (accessed on 7 October 2019).
33. Blin, K.; Shaw, S.; Steinke, K.; Villebro, R.; Ziemert, N.; Lee, S.Y.; Medema, M.H.; Weber, T. AntiSMASH 5.0: Updates to the secondary metabolite genome mining pipeline. *Nucleic Acids Res.* **2019**, *47*, W81–W87. [CrossRef] [PubMed]
34. MIBiG: Minimum Information about a Biosynthetic Gene Cluster. Available online: https://mibig.secondarymetabolites.org/ (accessed on 7 October 2019).
35. Online Resource of Protein Sequence and Functional Information. Available online: https://www.uniprot.org/ (accessed on 7 October 2019).
36. Hall, T.A. Bioedit: A user-friendly biological sequences alignment editor and analysis program for windows 95/98/nt. *Nucleic Acids Symp. Ser.* **1999**, *41*, 95–98.
37. Li, Y.; Dodge, G.J.; Fiers, W.D.; Fecik, R.A.; Smith, J.L.; Aldrich, C.C. Functional characterization of a dehydratase domain from the pikromycin polyketide synthase. *J. Am. Chem. Soc.* **2015**, *137*, 7003–7006. [CrossRef]
38. Kagan, R.M.; Clarke, S. Widespread occurrence of three sequence motifs in diverse S-adenosylmethionine-dependent methyltransferases suggests a common structure for these enzymes. *Arch. Biochem. Biophys.* **1994**, *310*, 417–427. [CrossRef]
39. Ansari, M.Z.; Sharma, J.; Gokhale, R.S.; Mohanty, D. In silico analysis of methyltransferase domains involved in biosynthesis of secondary metabolites. *BMC Bioinform.* **2008**, *9*, 454. [CrossRef]
40. Liu, L.; Zhang, Z.; Shao, C.-L.; Wang, C.-Y. Analysis of the Sequences, Structures, and Functions of Product-Releasing Enzyme Domains in Fungal Polyketide Synthases. *Front. Microbiol.* **2017**, *8*, 1685. [CrossRef]
41. Kumar, S.; Stecher, G.; Tamura, K. Mega7: Molecular evolutionary genetics analysis version 7.0 for bigger datasets. *Mol. Biol. Evol.* **2016**, *33*, 1870–1874. [CrossRef]
42. Felsenstein, J. Evolutionary trees from DNA sequences: A maximum likelihood approach. *J. Mol. Evol.* **1981**, *17*, 368–376. [CrossRef]
43. Saitou, N.; Nei, M. The neighbor-joining method: A new method for reconstructing phylogenetic trees. *Mol. Biol. Evol.* **1987**, *4*, 406–425.
44. Kimura, M. A simple method for estimating evolutionary rates of base substitutions through comparative studies of nucleotide sequences. *J. Mol. Evol.* **1980**, *16*, 111–120. [CrossRef] [PubMed]
45. Eley, K.L.; Halo, L.M.; Song, Z.; Powles, H.; Cox, R.J.; Bailey, A.M.; Lazarus, C.M.; Simpson, T.J. Biosynthesis of the 2-pyridone tenellin in the insect pathogenic fungus *Beauveria bassiana*. *ChemBioChem* **2007**, *8*, 289–297. [CrossRef] [PubMed]
46. Halo, L.M.; Marshall, J.W.; Yakasai, A.A.; Song, Z.; Butts, C.P.; Crump, M.P.; Heneghan, M.; Bailey, A.M.; Simpson, T.J.; Lazarus, C.M.; et al. Authentic heterologous expression of the tenellin iterative polyketide synthase nonribosomal peptide synthetase requires coexpression with an enoyl reductase. *ChemBioChem* **2008**, *9*, 585–594. [CrossRef] [PubMed]
47. Bergmann, S.; Schumann, J.; Scherlach, K.; Lange, C.; Brakhage, A.A.; Hertweck, C. Genomics-driven discovery of PKS-NRPS hybrid metabolites from *Aspergillus nidulans*. *Nat. Chem. Biol.* **2007**, *3*, 213–217. [CrossRef] [PubMed]
48. Gui, C.; Li, Q.; Mo, X.; Qin, X.; Ma, J.; Ju, J. Discovery of a New Family of Dieckmann Cyclases Essential to Tetramic Acid and Pyridone-Based Natural Products Biosynthesis. *Org. Lett.* **2015**, *17*, 628–631. [CrossRef] [PubMed]
49. Greule, A.; Stok, J.E.; De Voss, J.J.; Cryle, M.J. Unrivalled diversity: The many roles and reactions of bacterial cytochromes P450 in secondary metabolism. *Nat. Prod. Rep.* **2018**, *35*, 757–791. [CrossRef]
50. Lee, D.; Kang, K.S.; Lee, H.J.; Kim, K.H. Chemical characterization of a renoprotective metabolite from termite-associated *Streptomyces* sp. RB1 against cisplatin-induced cytotoxicity. *Int. J. Mol. Sci.* **2018**, *19*, 174. [CrossRef]

51. Lee, D.; Lee, S.; Shim, S.H.; Lee, H.J.; Choi, Y.; Jang, T.S.; Kim, K.H.; Kang, K.S. Protective effect of lanostane triterpenoids from the sclerotia of *Poria cocos* Wolf against cisplatin-induced apoptosis in LLC-PK1 cells. *Bioorg. Med. Chem. Lett.* **2017**, *27*, 2881–2885. [CrossRef]
52. Lee, S.R.; Lee, D.; Lee, H.J.; Noh, H.J.; Jung, K.; Kang, K.S.; Kim, K.H. Renoprotective chemical constituents from an edible mushroom, *Pleurotus cornucopiae* in cisplatin-induced nephrotoxicity. *Bioorg. Chem.* **2017**, *71*, 67–73. [CrossRef]
53. Volarevic, V.; Djokovic, B.; Jankovic, M.G.; Harrell, C.R.; Fellabaum, C.; Djonov, V.; Arsenijevic, N. Molecular mechanisms of cisplatin-induced nephrotoxicity: A balance on the knife edge between renoprotection and tumor toxicity. *J. Biomed. Sci.* **2019**, *26*, 25. [CrossRef]
54. Oh, G.S.; Kim, H.J.; Shen, A.; Lee, S.B.; Khadka, D.; Pandit, A.; So, H.S. Cisplatin-induced kidney dysfunction and perspectives on improving treatment strategies. *Electrolyte Blood Press* **2014**, *12*, 55–65. [CrossRef] [PubMed]
55. Yao, X.; Panichpisal, K.; Kurtzman, N.; Nugent, K. Cisplatin nephrotoxicity: A review. *Am. J. Med. Sci.* **2007**, *334*, 115–124. [CrossRef] [PubMed]
56. Ojha, S.; Venkataraman, B.; Kurdi, A.; Mahgoub, E.; Sadek, B.; Rajesh, M. Plant-derived agents for counteracting cisplatin-induced nephrotoxicity. *Oxid. Med. Cell Longev.* **2016**, *2016*, 4320374. [CrossRef] [PubMed]
57. Zhang, Y.; Tao, X.; Yin, L.; Xu, L.; Xu, Y.; Qi, Y.; Han, X.; Song, S.; Zhao, Y.; Lin, Y.; et al. Protective effects of dioscin against cisplatin-induced nephrotoxicity via the microRNA-34a/sirtuin 1 signalling pathway. *Br. J. Pharmacol.* **2017**, *174*, 2512–2527. [CrossRef] [PubMed]
58. Bruhn, T.; Schaumlöffel, A.; Hemberger, Y.; Pescitelli, G. SpecDis, Version 1.70.1, Berlin, Germany. 2017. Available online: https://specdis-software.jimdo.com (accessed on 7 October 2019).

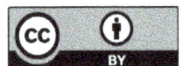

© 2019 by the authors. Licensee MDPI, Basel, Switzerland. This article is an open access article distributed under the terms and conditions of the Creative Commons Attribution (CC BY) license (http://creativecommons.org/licenses/by/4.0/).

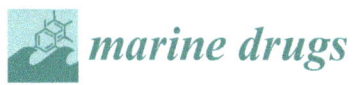

Article

Short Chain Fatty Acid Biosynthesis in Microalgae *Synechococcus* sp. PCC 7942

Yi Gong [1,2,3] and Xiaoling Miao [1,2,3,*]

[1] State Key Laboratory of Microbial Metabolism, School of Life Sciences & Biotechnology, Shanghai Jiao Tong University, 800 Dongchuan Road, Shanghai 200240, China; gongvsyi@126.com
[2] Joint International Research Laboratory of Metabolic & Developmental Sciences, Shanghai Jiao Tong University, Shanghai 200240, China
[3] Biomass Energy Research Center, Shanghai Jiao Tong University, Shanghai 200240, China
* Correspondence: miaoxiaoling@sjtu.edu.cn; Tel.: +86-21-34207028

Received: 19 April 2019; Accepted: 25 April 2019; Published: 28 April 2019

Abstract: Short chain fatty acids (SCFAs) are valued as a functional material in cosmetics. Cyanobacteria can accumulate SCFAs under some conditions, the related mechanism is unclear. Two potential genes Synpcc7942_0537 (*fabB/F*) and Synpcc7942_1455 (*fabH*) in *Synechococcus* sp. PCC 7942 have homology with *fabB/F* and *fabH* encoding β-ketoacyl ACP synthases (I/II/III) in plants. Therefore, effects of culture time and cerulenin on SCFAs accumulation, expression levels and functions of these two potential genes were studied. The results showed *Synechococcus* sp. PCC 7942 accumulated high SCFAs (C12 + C14) in early growth stage (day 4) and at 7.5g/L cerulenin concentration, reaching to 2.44% and 2.84% of the total fatty acids respectively, where *fabB/F* expression was down-regulated. Fatty acid composition analysis showed C14 increased by 65.19% and 130% respectively, when *fabB/F* and *fabH* were antisense expressed. C14 increased by 10.79% (*fab(B/F)*$^-$) and 6.47% (*fabH*$^-$) under mutation conditions, while C8 increased by six times in *fab(B/F)*$^-$ mutant strain. These results suggested *fabB/F* is involved in fatty acid elongation (C <18) and the elongation of *cis*-16:1 to *cis*-18:1 fatty acid in *Synechococcus* sp. PCC 7942, while *fabH* was involved in elongation of fatty acid synthesis, which were further confirmed in complementary experiments of *E. coli*. The research could provide the scientific basis for the breeding of SCFA-rich microalgae species.

Keywords: microalgae; *Synechococcus* sp. PCC 7942; short chain fatty acids; β-ketoacyl ACP Synthase

---

1. Introduction

Short chain fatty acids (SCFAs) are usually defined as the carbon number of fatty acids between 6 and 14 [1]. Due to corresponding glycerides with extraordinary characteristics such as low viscosity, high extensibility, low freezing point, low surface tension, high transparency and oxidation stability, SCFAs have very broad application in cosmeceuticals, nutraceuticals, nutritional supplements, chemical industry, etc. [2]. Currently, main sources of SCFAs are tropical plants, such as coconut and palm trees [3,4]. However, people have to turn their attention to the potential oleaginous microorganisms because of the high cost of vegetable oils and the limitation of climate and land resources [5]. It is widely reported that bacteria, mold, yeast and microalgae are important oleaginous microorganisms [5], of which microalgae has received much attention for its unique advantages such as fast growth rate, high oil content, high photosynthetic efficiency, low land requirements and environmental protection [6].

There are abundant algae in the ocean, the unique ecological environment of which causes the special bioactive metabolites accumulation in the algae. These metabolites have a series of biological effects, such as moisturizing [7], bacteriostasis [8], anti-inflammatory [9], antivirus [10], inhibiting the growth of tumor cells [11], and resisting ultraviolet radiation [12]. It was found that a kind of ancient cyanobacteria has antioxidant, immune and other biological activities [13]. In recent years, safety problems are often exposed in the cosmetics industry, when algae bioactive substances could be used as raw materials for new cosmeceuticals due to their low toxicity and high safety. Therefore, algae would be increasingly valued as a functional material in the field of cosmetics. At present, research on algae focuses on the active substances such as minerals, bioactive peptides, natural pigments, enzymes, polysaccharides and unsaturated fatty acids, etc. [14], while little research are about short carbon chain fatty acids. It was found that short carbon chain fatty acids were widely used in cosmetics, where they could replace white oil, lanolin and squalane. Compared with squalane, short carbon chain fatty acids are more easily absorbed by the skin and can be rapidly oxidized and metabolized. In addition, short carbon chain fatty acids have emulsifying stability and antioxidant properties, which can make cosmetics more uniform and delicate, improve product quality and storage period. In suntan lotion, short carbon chain fatty acids are non-greasy and uncomfortable feeling. In lipsticks, the short carbon chain fatty acids can eliminate the unique smell of lanolin, making the matrix tissue delicate, the pigment dispersion uniform and improving the surface gloss and spread ability [15].

Microalgae, as a high-quality oleaginous aquatic microorganism, are primarily used for biodiesel, polyunsaturated fatty acids and pigments, but rarely for SCFAs. The content of SCFAs in microalgae was not high under normal growth conditions [16–21]. Some microalgae can accumulate SCFAs when cultivated in stressed conditions [22], but the related mechanism of this is unclear. Studies on the synthesis mechanisms of SCFAs are mostly conducted in plants and bacteria [4], and mainly focused on the key enzymes such as thioesterases (TEs) and β-ketoacyl ACP (Acyl Carrier Protein) synthases (KAS). TEs are mainly present in plants and some eukaryotic microalgae, associated with the termination of the fatty acid synthesis cycle by catalyzing ACPs to remove from acyl-ACPs, producing free fatty acids [23,24]. Past efforts to increase medium chain fatty acid (MCFA) production in microalgae by genetic modifications of chain-length specific TEs have met with limited success, because of high specifics and substrate preferences of TEs. β-ketoacyl ACP synthases are associated with the carbon chain elongation of fatty acids, which are classified as KAS I, KAS II and KAS III, encoded by *fabB*, *fabF* and *fabH*, respectively [25,26]. It is reported that KAS III could catalyze the combination of acetyl-CoA with malonyl-CoA to generate 4:0-ACP, KAS I could catalyze 4:0-ACP to generate 16:0-ACP and KAS II could catalyze 16:0-ACP to generate 18:0-ACP as well as control the ratio of 16:0-ACP/18:0-ACP [27]. Verwoert et al. [28] overexpressed the *KAS III* gene from *E. coli* in rapeseed, causing changes in fatty acid composition, which decreased the content of C18:1 and increased the content of C18:2 and C18:3. Dehesh et al. [29] overexpressed the *KAS III* gene from spinach in three kinds of plants (Tobacco, *Arabidopsis thaliana*, Rape), leading to C16:0 fatty acid accumulation. Research on cyanobacteria *Synechococcus* sp. PCC 7002 revealed that KAS III initialized the synthesis of fatty acids circle, causing the condensation of malonyl ACP and acetyl CoA to form acetyl–acetyl ACP, which was thought of the only rate-limiting step in fatty acid synthesis of cyanobacteria [30]. The result is different from that of *E. coli*, where KAS III was not rate-limiting.

Although the fatty acids composition of microalgae varied with species and strains [31], but some cyanobacteria had strong ability to synthesize short carbon chain fatty acids. In the past, filamentous cyanobacteria *Trichodesmium erythraeum* has been found to produce 27% to 50% C10 fatty acids [32]. Later, Karatay et al. [33] reported *Synechococcus* sp. could accumulate about 23.8% of caprylic acid (C10:0) and myristic acid (C14:0) under nitrogen deficiency condition. Therefore, cyanobacteria may be an ideal species for the production of short carbon fatty acids. In addition, cyanobacteria, as prokaryotes, are more suitable for gene manipulation than eukaryotic microalgae, and some of which have completed whole genome sequencing. The sequencing information could also provide guidance for our research. Thus, *Synechococcus* sp. PCC 7942, whose genome have been sequenced, was used in the present study to explore the effects of cerulenin and culture time on the synthesis of SCFAs, the functions and expression regulation of genes related to the SCFAs synthesis were further investigated. The results may provide scientific guidance for the future development of short chain fatty acids resources in microalgae by means of metabolic engineering and molecular biology.

2. Results and Discussion

2.1. Fatty Acid Compositions of Synechococcus sp. PCC7942 under Different Conditions

Microalgae synthesize and store different types of lipids in a single cell [32]. In contrast to the conventional fatty acids (FAs) composition of microalgae that contain long chain fatty acids (LCFAs) from C16 to C18, SCFAs (from C8 to C14) are generally classified to be unusual. Generally, the content of SCFAs in microalgae is relatively low under normal growth conditions. In order to better understand the synthesis mechanism of SCFAs in microalgae from a physiological perspective preliminarily, the fatty acid profiles of *Synechococcus* sp. PCC 7942 under different culture time periods was investigated.

Table 1 shows the dynamic variations of fatty acids during the whole culture process. As shown in Table 1, the main fatty acid was C16 under different culture time periods, accounting for about 70%–80% of the total fatty acids, while little contents of LCFAs from C20 to C22 were detected. At the early growth stage (2 days–6 days), high content of SCFAs (C14 + C12) were observed, reaching highest content (2.44%) at day 4, among which C14:1 was 1.70% and C14:0 was 0.74% (Table 1). After day 8, contents of C14:0 and C14:1 did not change significantly, which were in the range of 0.3%–0.6% and 0.5%–0.9%, respectively, while C12 fatty acid could not be detected. These results suggested that the accumulation of SCFAs mainly occurred in the early growth stage (2 days–6 days), with C14 and C12 as the main composition. To our knowledge, this was the first report of SCFAs accumulation in the early growth stage in cyanobacteria.

Table 1. Fatty acid profile of *Synechococcus* sp. PCC 7942 under different culture time.

Fatty Acid (%)	Time (day)									
	2	4	6	8	10	12	14	16	18	20
12:0	0.02 ± 0.01	ND	0.02 ± 0.00	ND	ND	ND	ND	ND	ND	ND
14:0	0.63 ± 0.03	0.74 ± 0.15	0.56 ± 0.06	0.45 ± 0.03	0.62 ± 0.03	0.27 ± 0.03	0.33 ± 0.01	0.42 ± 0.03	0.34 ± 0.03	0.36 ± 0.03
14:1	0.98 ± 0.02	1.70 ± 0.19	1.17 ± 0.19	0.87 ± 0.10	0.90 ± 0.06	0.48 ± 0.03	0.55 ± 0.04	0.67 ± 0.06	0.57 ± 0.03	0.60 ± 0.06
16:0	42.14 ± 3.96	39.98 ± 2.67	45.42 ± 2.64	41.71 ± 2.22	38.65 ± 2.68	47.93 ± 2.00	45.41 ± 2.11	46.56 ± 2.04	46.63 ± 3.08	46.20 ± 2.05
16:1	34.72 ± 2.04	38.20 ± 1.89	36.80 ± 1.74	31.03 ± 1.25	31.32 ± 0.71	26.96 ± 1.71	31.94 ± 1.87	29.89 ± 0.89	29.60 ± 1.60	30.48 ± 1.89
16:2	ND	ND	ND	ND	ND	ND	ND	ND	0.13 ± 0.03	0.13 ± 0.02
17:0	0.13 ± 0.03	0.22 ± 0.03	0.09 ± 0.03	0.12 ± 0.03	0.11 ± 0.02	0.18 ± 0.04	0.11 ± 0.03	0.10 ± 0.00	0.13 ± 0.01	0.11 ± 0.00
17:1	0.22 ± 0.01	0.41 ± 0.01	0.14 ± 0.03	0.24 ± 0.05	0.27 ± 0.02	0.30 ± 0.00	0.33 ± 0.00	0.34 ± 0.03	0.32 ± 0.01	0.33 ± 0.03
18:0	1.70 ± 0.34	3.00 ± 0.21	0.24 ± 0.05	2.49 ± 0.24	3.11 ± 0.25	2.57 ± 0.25	1.89 ± 0.37	1.08 ± 0.11	1.85 ± 0.11	1.61 ± 0.03
18:1	2.51 ± 0.33	3.89 ± 0.29	1.80 ± 0.08	3.79 ± 0.11	4.48 ± 0.31	7.14 ± 0.75	6.42 ± 0.57	4.90 ± 0.36	6.15 ± 0.36	5.82 ± 0.23
18:2	0.31 ± 0.047	0.24 ± 0.09	3.16 ± 0.32	0.34 ± 0.04	0.39 ± 0.03	0.35 ± 0.02	0.68 ± 0.03	0.21 ± 0.03	0.41 ± 0.02	0.43 ± 0.03
20:0	0.04 ± 0.00	0.03 ± 0.00	0.04 ± 0.00	0.08 ± 0.03	0.12 ± 0.01	0.05 ± 0.01	ND	ND	0.06 ± 0.01	0.13 ± 0.02
22:0	0.04 ± 0.01	0.04 ± 0.01	0.05 ± 0.01	ND	0.19 ± 0.01	ND	ND	ND	0.26 ± 0.02	0.27 ± 0.04
22:1	0.05 ± 0.00	0.04 ± 0.00	0.04 ± 0.00	ND	0.11 ± 0.01	0.10 ± 0.00	0.07 ± 0.00	ND	ND	0.06 ± 0.00

The fatty acid synthesis system of plants and bacteria belonged to the type II, where the KASs were related to the fatty acid carbon chain elongation and generally divided into KAS I (FabB), KAS II (FabF) and KAS III (FabH) [25,26]. It was reported that fatty acid synthase inhibitors have effects on the fatty acids carbon chain elongation in bacteria [34,35], among which cerulenin mainly played its role on KAS I and KAS II. In order to further understand the SCFAs synthesis in *Synechococcus* sp. PCC 7942, effects of different cerulenin concentrations on SCFAs accumulation were studied.

As shown in Table 2, the content of SCFAs (C12 + C14) accumulated as high as 2.84% of the total fatty acids under cerulenin concentration of 7.5 g/L, among which the content of C14 fatty acids increased from 1.58% (0 g/L) to 2.75% (7.5 g/L), increasing by 74.05% ($p < 0.05$), and C12 fatty acids increased from 0.04% to 0.09%, increasing by 125% ($p < 0.05$). At this time, C16 fatty acids decreased from 63.49% to 57.35%, decreasing by 9.67%, C18 fatty acids decreased from 18.44% to 13.7%, decreasing by 25.7%, respectively. Israel et al. [36] found that after 40 min of adding cerulenin into the medium with *E. coli*, 90% of oil synthesis and 25% of RNA and DNA synthesis were inhibited, but the protein synthesis was not affected. In addition, a previous study [37,38] on antibacterial drug targets showed that cerulenin has specific inhibition on KAS I and KAS II, which are responsible for the carbon chain elongation of C4–C16 fatty acids in bacteria. As shown in Table 2, the contents of longer chain fatty acids (C18 + C16) decreased and the contents of SCFAs (C12 + C14) increased, with the increase of cerulenin concentration. These results suggested that KAS I/II in *Synechococcus* sp. PCC 7942 might be inhibited, which resulted in the increase of SCFAs (C12 + C14).

Table 2. Effects of different cerulenin concentrations on fatty acid profile in *Synechococcus* sp. PCC 7942 after 16 days cultivation.

Fatty Acid (%)	Cerulenin Concentration (g/L)				
	0	1	2.5	5	7.5
12:0	0.04 ± 0.00	0.05 ± 0.00	0.04 ± 0.01	0.07 ± 0.00	0.09 ± 0.01
14:0	0.71 ± 0.08	0.98 ± 0.09	0.77 ± 0.04	0.84 ± 0.09	1.25 ± 0.31
14:1	0.87 ± 0.15	1.1 ± 0.26	0.82 ± 0.08	1.35 ± 0.17	1.5 ± 0.31
15:0	0.07 ± 0.02	0.07 ± 0.01	ND	ND	ND
16:0	31.47 ± 2.48	41.74 ± 1.85	34.76 ± 1.68	35.43 ± 1.53	31.84 ± 2.46
16:1	31.75 ± 2.39	32.97 ± 2.56	25.66 ± 2.90	26.57 ± 3.38	25.43 ± 2.45
16:2	0.27 ± 0.03	0.07 ± 0.02	ND	0.06 ± 0.01	0.08 ± 0.01
17:0	0.49 ± 0.03	0.16 ± 0.04	0.16 ± 0.02	0.21 ± 0.02	0.47 ± 0.01
17:1	0.81 ± 0.12	0.43 ± 0.02	0.52 ± 0.06	0.51 ± 0.04	0.76 ± 0.11
18:0	1.79 ± 0.10	2.14 ± 0.42	3.33 ± 0.33	2.7 ± 0.15	3.57 ± 0.26
18:1	15.84 ± 0.98	8.02 ± 0.14	14.05 ± 1.47	12.13 ± 1.49	5.69 ± 0.04
18:2	0.81 ± 0.08	1.15 ± 0.11	0.69 ± 0.03	0.9 ± 0.10	4.44 ± 0.27
20:0	0.04 ± 0.03	0.05 ± 0.00	ND	ND	ND

Based on the above results, it is assumed that the low expression levels of the related genes *fabB/F* (KAS I/II) in *Synechococcus* sp. PCC 7942 might inhibit the carbon chain elongation of fatty acids, leading to the sufficient accumulation of SCFAs at this stage. Therefore, the related genes expression levels under the above conditions were further investigated.

2.2. Genes Expression under Different Conditions in Synechococcus sp. PCC7942

Bioinformatic analysis showed that Synpcc7942_0537 and Synpcc7942_1455 in *Synechococcus* sp. PCC 7942 might have homology with *fabB/F* and *fabH* of plants and bacteria.

As mentioned above, the influences of culture time period and cerulenin concentration on the fatty acid compositions of microalgae were significant. In order to understand the relationship between genes expression level and fatty acids (FAs) carbon chain elongation, the influences of cerulenin concentration and culture time on transcriptional levels of the relative genes (*fabB/F* and *fabH*) were explored.

As shown in Figure 1a, the expression level of *fabB/F* was relatively low in the early growth stage (2 days–6 days), and reached the highest expression level at day 8, then decreased in the later period of culture time (10 days–16 days). The overall trend of expression level of *fabB/F* increased first and then decreased, which was consistent with the variations of fatty acid composition (Table 1), that is to say, the SCFAs mainly accumulated in early growth stage. The result indicated that *fabB/F* played an important role on the synthesis of SCFAs. On the other side, during the whole cultivation phase, the expression level of *fabH* was not high enough, and showed a trend of gradual decrease, only with relatively high expression level in the early growth stage (2 days–6 days) (Figure 1b). Inhibition of the expression of *fabB/F* will hinder the transformation of SCFAs (C12, C14) to relatively longer chain fatty acids (C16, C18), leading to SCFAs accumulation, which also verified the previous hypothesis that *fabB/F* is a key gene promoting the synthesis of SCFAs (C12, C14) to longer chain fatty acids (C16, C18).

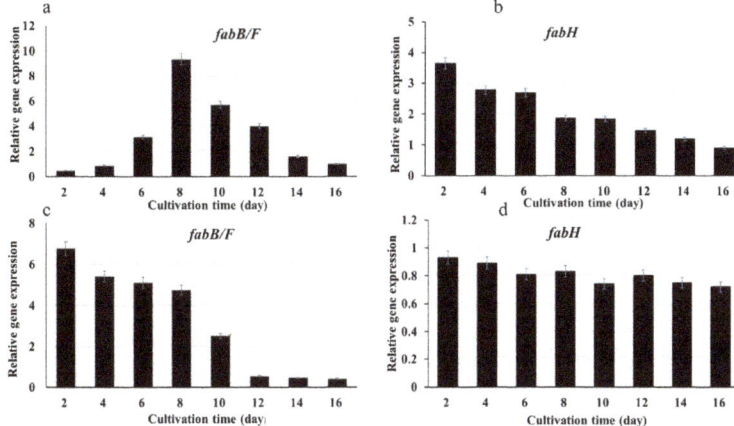

Figure 1. Dynamic change of expression levels of two related genes in *Synechococcus* sp. PCC 7942 under different conditions. (**a**) Expressions of Synpccw7942_0537 (*fabB/F*) under different culture time periods; (**b**) Expressions of Synpccw7942_1455 (*fabH*) under different culture time periods; (**c**) Expressions of Synpccw7942_0537 (*fabB/F*) under cerulenin concentration of 7.5 g/L; (**d**) Expressions of Synpccw7942_1455 (*fabH*) under cerulenin concentration of 7.5 g/L. The expression levels of genes Synpccw7942_0537 (*fabB/F*) and Synpccw7942_1455 (*fabH*) at 16 day (**a**,**b**) and cerulenin concentration of 0 g/L (**c**,**d**) were set to 1.

As shown in Figure 1c, under cerulenin concentration of 7.5 g/L, the expression level of *fabB/F* was relatively high at the early growth stage (2 days–8 days), then decreased significantly with the extension of culture time and reached the lowest expression level in the late growth stage (12 days–16 days). These results suggested that cerulenin could change the expression levels of *fabB/F* in *Synechococcus* sp. PCC 7942. Ter Beek et al. [39] also found that cerulenin could change the expression levels of fab (fatty acid biosynthesis) genes in fatty acid synthesis of *Bacillus subtilis*. The dynamic trend of *fabB/F* expression at 7.5 g/L of cerulenin was consistent with variation of SCFAs composition, compared with that in the absence of cerulenin or at low concentration of cerulenin (Table 2). The expression level of *fabH* gene did not change significantly during the whole cultivation period under 7.5 g/L cerulenin concentration (Figure 1d), which indicated that cerulenin also has specific inhibition on KAS I and KAS II in *Synechococcus* sp. PCC 7942. However, high cerulenin concentration could cause the inhibition of the growth of *Synechococcus* sp. PCC 7942. When the cerulenin concentrations were between 0 g/L and 7.5 g/L, the OD_{730} value of the same culture time period decreased with the increase of the concentration of cerulenin. At 7.5 g/L cerulenin concentration, the OD_{730} value was the lowest, which was about one third of that at 0 g/L (Figure S1, Supplementary Materials). Therefore, although there was no significant change during the whole cultivation period, the *fabH* expression level at 7.5 g/L cerulenin was much lower (Figure 1d) compared with that in the absence of cerulenin (Figure 1b). This is probably caused by the growth inhibition at 7.5 g/L cerulenin concentration (Figure S1). So, the above dynamic expressions of two related genes in *Synechococcus* sp. PCC 7942 may be the result of both growth and gene inhibition.

2.3. Fatty Acid Compositions in fabB/F and fabH Sense/Antisense Expression Strains

It is reported that deletion of some important enzymes in the fatty acid synthesis pathway may lead to cell death [40]. Therefore, sense and antisense expression strains of *fabB/F* and *fabH* were constructed first to investigate the functions of the two genes in the process of fatty acids synthesis. Chen et al. [41] reported that inhibiting the expression of phosphoenol pyruvate carboxylase (PEPC) gene in rapeseed by antisense RNA led the oil content of transgenic rapeseed to 6.4%–18%, which was higher than that of the control group. Song et al. [42] successfully antisense expressed the encoding gene (*pcc*) of PEPC in *Synechococcus* sp. PCC 7002, resulting in an oil content increase. It can be seen that antisense expression is very feasible in improving the oil content of microalgae.

As shown in Table 3, the SCFAs contents were not significantly changed in *Synechococcus* sp. PCC 7942 harboring sense plasmids pRL-Sense-*fabB/F* (Synpccw7942_0537) and pRL-Sense-*fabH* (Synpccw7942_1455) (The sense and antisense plasmids were all derived from pRL 489). Research in plants showed *fabB/F* was responsible for the longer chain fatty acids elongation, while *fabH* was related to the initiation of fatty acids synthesis and extending C2 to C4 [27]. The present study suggested that acyl-ACPs for longer chain fatty acids synthesis may enter the next step of fatty acid synthesis, which could not result in a massive accumulation of SCFAs (Table 3). It was also found that overexpression of KAS IV in a MCFA-producing strain of *Dunaliella tertiolecta* could allow MCFA accumulation [43], which lies in the control of a KAS enzyme to generate MCFA acyl-ACP substrates. We believed that enlargement of the MCFA acyl-ACP substrate pool by overexpressing KAS IV and concentration of MCFA acyl-ACP substrate pool caused by KAS enzyme all could lead to MCFAs accumulation [24]. Although the overexpression of *KAS III* gene in *E. coli* could change the fatty acid profile of *E. coli*, when C14:0 increased and C18:1 decreased [26], which were different from our results of *Synechococcus* sp. PCC 7942 with pRL-Sense-*fabH* (Table 3), indicating that the Synpccw7942_1455 (*KAS III*) gene had species difference. Furthermore, eukaryotic microalgae (*Dunaliella tertiolecta*) and bacteria/cyanobacteria are innately different, given that eukaryotic microalgae are capable to store free FAs in the form of SCFAs.

Table 3. Fatty acid profile of sense and antisense expression of Synpccw7942_0537 (*fabB/F*) and Synpccw7942_1455 (*fabH*) in *Synechococcus* sp. PCC 7942 after 16 days cultivation.

Fatty Acid (%)	Wild Type [a]	Sense-*fabB/F* [b]	Sense-*fabH* [c]	Antisense-*fabB/F* [d]	Antisense-*fabH* [e]
C12:0	0.04 ± 0.01	0.06 ± 0.01	0.05 ± 0.00	0.06 ± 0.00	0.05 ± 0.01
C14:0	0.71 ± 0.08	0.71 ± 0.06	0.65 ± 0.04	1.09 ± 0.16	1.35 ± 0.35
C14:1	0.87 ± 0.07	0.75 ± 0.07	0.66 ± 0.03	1.52 ± 0.12	2.28 ± 0.46
C15:0	0.07 ± 0.00	0.29 ± 0.03	0.44 ± 0.02	0.10 ± 0.00	0.06 ± 0.01
C16:0	31.47 ± 0.63	32.04 ± 1.38	38.06 ± 0.55	34.99 ± 0.72	36.09 ± 2.31
C16:1	31.75 ± 2.40	33.16 ± 0.53	34.26 ± 1.68	37.2 ± 1.35	39.4 ± 1.19
C16:2	0.27 ± 0.02	0.16 ± 0.03	0.05 ± 0.01	0.13 ± 0.02	0.07 ± 0.02
C17:0	0.49 ± 0.02	0.32 ± 0.05	0.39 ± 0.06	0.10 ± 0.01	0.24 ± 0.03
C17:1	0.81 ± 0.01	0.56 ± 0.02	0.49 ± 0.02	0.77 ± 0.01	0.39 ± 0.03
C18:0	1.79 ± 0.21	6.83 ± 0.74	8.3 ± 0.36	0.72 ± 0.11	0.82 ± 0.03
C18:1	15.84 ± 2.00	8.05 ± 0.10	8.49 ± 0.32	1.25 ± 0.05	4.52 ± 0.65
C18:2	0.81 ± 0.08	3.33 ± 0.20	0.33 ± 0.03	0.18 ± 0.07	0.13 ± 0.03
C20:0	0.04 ± 0.01	0.06 ± 0.00	ND	0.72 ± 0.03	ND

[a] Wild type strain of *Synechococcus* sp. PCC 7942; [b] *Synechococcus* sp. 7942 harboring pRL-Sense-*fabB/F* (Synpccw7942_0537); [c] *Synechococcus* sp. 7942 harboring pRL-Sense-*fabH* (Synpccw7942_1455); [d] *Synechococcus* sp. 7942 harboring pRL-Antisense-*fabB/F* (Synpccw7942_0537); [e] *Synechococcus* sp. 7942 harboring pRL-Antisense-*fabH* (Synpccw7942_1455).

The content of C18 of *Synechococcus* sp. PCC 7942 containing pRL-Antisense-*fabB/F* decreased from 18.44% of wild-type to 2.15% of antisense expression strain (Table 3), with a decrease of 88.34%. Meanwhile, the content of C14 in *Synechococcus* sp. PCC7942 containing pRL-Anti-*fabB/F* increased from 1.58% of the wild type to 2.61% of antisense expression strain (Table 3), with an increase of 65.19% ($p < 0.05$). This is because that the antisense gene fragment could inhibit the expression level of *fabB/F*. The expression levels of *fabB/F* in antisense expression of *fabB/F* strains were down-regulated ($p < 0.05$) as compared with that in the wild type strain during the whole growth period (Figure S2, Supplementary Materials). In addition, as shown in Table 3, C16:2 in *fabB/F* antisense expression strain decreased from 0.27% to 0.13%, C18:2 decreased from 0.81% to 0.18%, C17 (17:0 and 17:1) fatty acids decreased from 1.3% to 0.87%. By referring to the studies of other microorganisms [3], *fabB/F* might be related to the extension of longer chain fatty acids. Further analysis showed that C16:1 of the antisense expression strain increased from 31.75% to 37.20% and C18:1 decreased from 15.84% to 1.25%

(Table 3), which was consistent with the function of *fabF* for extending *cis*-16:1 into *cis*-18:1 mentioned in a previous report [44]. In *E. coli*, both KAS I (*fabB*) and KAS II (*fabF*) have the ability for longer chain elongation of saturated fatty acids. KAS I is one of the key enzymes involved in the de novo synthesis of unsaturated fatty acids, while KAS II only extends the *cis*-hexadecenoyl to *cis*-octadecanoyl and does not participate in *de novo* synthesis of unsaturated acyl [45]. Combined with the studies above, we speculated that *fabB/F* was involved in the synthesis of unsaturated fatty acids. Leonard et al. [46] have found that the gene with KAS II activity in *Cuphea wrightii* could regulate FA chain length regulation, and was co-expressed with specific thioesterases, leading the content of C10:0 and C12:0 accumulation. Besides, Pidkowich et al. [47] proved that KAS II had the function of extention 16:0-ACP to 18:0-ACP in plant. Our results suggested that Synpccw7942_0537 (*fabB/F*) also performed the function of *fabF* and *fabB* in microalgae.

The antisense expression *fabH* also caused the change of fatty acid composition. As Table 3 shows, the content of C18 of *Synechococcus* sp. PCC 7942 containing pRL-Antisese-*fabH* decreased from 18.44% of the wild-type strain to 5.47% of antisense expression strains, with a decrease of 70.34%. At the same time, the content of C14 increased from 1.58% of the wild type to 3.63% of the antisense expression strain (Table 3), with an increase of 130% ($p < 0.05$). In addition, C16:2, C17:0, C17:1 and C18:2 content of *fabH* antisense expression strain all decreased, when C16:2 decreased from 0.27% to 0.07%, C18:2 decreased from 0.81% to 0.13%, C17 (17:0 and 17:1) fatty acids decreased from 1.3% to 0.63%. It is generally believed that *fabH* was related to the initiation of fatty acid elongation and a rate-limiting step of fatty acid synthesis [30]. González-mellado et al. [48] found that KAS III in sunflower had a new substrate specificity, which could participate in the synthesis of C6 to C10 fatty acids. Our present results showed that the C18 fatty acid decreased with the increase of C14 fatty acid when the gene *fabH* was inhibited, suggesting that the Synpccw7942_1455 (*fabH*) in *Synechococcus* sp. PCC 7942 may only participate in the carbon chain extension (C < 18) (not the first condensation step in the fatty acid synthesis circle) and had acyl-ACP carbon chain substrate specificity. While antisense expression *fabB/F* and *fabH* are able to redirect FA synthesis from long to short chain lengths, the increases in yield are still not as high as those achieved in plants and some bacteria. It is thought that high content of SCFAs could be poisonous for microalgae growth. Therefore, SCFAs accumulation is not only governed by KAS, but also by the tolerance of SCFAs concentration in microalgae cells.

2.4. Fatty Acid Compositions of fabB/F and fabH Deletion Mutants

The functions of Synpccw7942_0537 (*fabB/F*) and Synpccw7942_1455 (*fabH*) were further explored by gene deletion mutants. Table 4 showed that C16 was the main fatty acid component in the *fab(B/F)*$^-$ mutant strain, accounting for about 60%–70% of the total fatty acid. The content of C8 increased by six times and C14 increased by 10.79%, while the content of C18 decreased by 9.87% (Table 4). In addition, the content of C15:0 fatty acid in the *fab(B/F)*$^-$ mutant strain was 0.48% of the total fatty acids, which was not detected in the wild type (Table 4). These results suggested that the mutation of *fabB/F* gene might block fatty acid elongation. It was reported that the homologous protein of FabB could not found in some bacteria, but the homologous protein of FabF (FabY) had the dual functions of KAS I and KAS II, but this is not common [40]. The above results suggested that *fabB/F* in *Synechococcus* sp. PCC 7942 might have the function of fatty acid carbon chain elongation (C < 18), which were consistent with the functions of *fabB* and *fabF* in *E. coli*, where they carried out the elongation steps in fatty acid synthesis. The *fabB/F* in *Synechococcus* sp. PCC 7942 was also involved in the *de novo* synthesis of the unsaturated fatty acids of the microalgae and forming *cis*-11-octadecenoyl ACP by extending palmitoyl-ACP.

Table 4. Fatty acid profile of Synpccw7942_0537 (*fabB/F*) and Synpccw7942_1455 (*fabH*) deletion mutants of *Synechococcus* sp. PCC 7942 after 16 days cultivation.

Fatty Acid (%)	Wild Type [a]	fab(B/F)⁻	fabH⁻
C8:0	0.01 ± 0.00	0.06 ± 0.02	0.02 ± 0.00
C14:0	0.54 ± 0.04	0.63 ± 0.02	0.67 ± 0.07
C14:1	0.85 ± 0.02	0.91 ± 0.02	0.81 ± 0.00
C15:0	ND	0.48 ± 0.05	0.41 ± 0.03
C16:0	34.30 ± 0.25	36.21 ± 0.40	33.16 ± 0.04
C16:1	32.43 ± 0.63	30.93 ± 0.32	34.86 ± 0.70
C16:2	0.51 ± 0.01	0.64 ± 0.04	0.06 ± 0.00
C17:0	0.26 ± 0.06	0.69 ± 0.03	0.38 ± 0.05
C17:1	0.78 ± 0.14	0.74 ± 0.04	0.52 ± 0.05
C18:0	1.85 ± 0.03	1.93 ± 0.03	6.23 ± 0.58
C18:1	15.69 ± 0.90	13.71 ± 0.39	8.17 ± 0.35
C18:2	0.69 ± 0.05	0.79 ± 0.03	2.51 ± 0.54
C20:0	0.05 ± 0.00	0.02 ± 0.01	0.04 ± 0.00

[a] Wild type strain of *Synechococcus* sp. PCC 7942.

Table 4 also showed that the content of C18 decreased from 18.23% in the wild type to 16.91% in *fabH*⁻ mutant, with a decrease of 7.24%. Meanwhile, the content of C14 increased from 1.39% of the wild type to 1.48% of the mutant, with an increase of 6.47%, and 0.41% content of C15 was obtained (Table 4). These results indicated that the longer chain fatty acids decreased and shorter chain fatty acids increased when *fabH* was mutated. Previous studies showed that *fabH* was a rate-limiting step and also the first condensation step in the fatty acid synthesis circle in plants and bacteria [29,49]. The present results suggested that Synpccw7942_1455 (*fabH*) might only participate in the fatty acid carbon chain elongation (C < 18).

Nonetheless, the increment of SCFAs in mutants we observed was modest, far from our expectation. It was also reported that some enzyme had the activity of KAS III, with the domain similar to FabH, but whose molecular weight is larger than FabH, initializing fatty acid synthesis in *Pseudomonas aeruginosa* [46]. Therefore, it is assumed that *fab(B/F)*⁻ and *fabH*⁻ mutants were considered as strains deficient in *fabB/F* and *fabH* gene expression but not complete inactivation, or other proteins with similar activity executed corresponding functions (KAS III).

2.5. Complementation of E. coli

In order to further verify the functions of the related genes, we attempted to construct mutant strains of KAS I/II/III of *E. coli* and compared the fatty acid compositions of mutants with that of their complementation.

As shown in Table 5, the content of C12, C14 and C16 in *fab(B/F/H)*⁻ mutants of *E. coli* BL21 all increased as compared with that of the wild type. These results were consistent with the results that KAS III could catalyze acetyl-CoA with malonyl-CoA to generate 4:0-ACP, KAS I could catalyze 4:0-ACP to generate 16:0-ACP and KAS II could catalyze 16:0-ACP to generate 18:0-ACP as well as regulate the ratio of 16:0-ACP/18:0-ACP [24]. Mutation of the genes might lead to changes in fatty acids.

Table 5. Fatty acid profile of wild type, mutation and complementary mutation of *E. coli*.

Fatty Acid (%)	*E. coli* BL21	*fabB*⁻	*fabF*⁻	*fabH*⁻	Com-*fabB* [a]	Com-*fabF* [b]	Com-*fabH* [c]
C12:0	0.23 ± 0.02	0.3 ± 0.00	0.72 ± 0.10	0.78 ± 0.13	0.31 ± 0.12	0.50 ± 0.10	0.23 ± 0.01
C13:0	1.33 ± 0.11	ND	ND	0.10 ± 0.00	1.19 ± 0.00	0.94 ± 0.23	1.87 ± 0.34
C14:0	2.88 ± 0.28	3.04 ± 0.23	3.69 ± 0.29	3.01 ± 0.46	2.88 ± 0.46	3.03 ± 0.33	3.87 ± 0.58
C14:1	ND	3.23 ± 0.20	0.21 ± 0.01	0.30 ± 0.00	ND	ND	ND
C15:0	8.25 ± 0.22	0.57 ± 0.03	1.02 ± 0.07	0.72 ± 0.15	6.32 ± 0.15	5.97 ± 0.55	12.45 ± 2.02
C16:0	33.98 ± 3.83	50.51 ± 2.75	48.59 ± 3.11	50.23 ± 3.64	33.82 ± 0.64	33.37 ± 2.50	34.76 ± 1.55
C16:1	2.78 ± 0.30	9.21 ± 0.22	9.94 ± 1.60	8.21 ± 0.94	2.60 ± 0.94	2.66 ± 0.35	3.08 ± 0.19
C17:0	5.02 ± 0.21	0.44 ± 0.04	0.60 ± 0.18	0.51 ± 0.07	3.56 ± 0.07	3.94 ± 0.42	7.57 ± 0.67
C17:1	2.69 ± 0.17	2.97 ± 0.31	2.46 ± 0.38	5.18 ± 0.56	3.71 ± 0.56	2.36 ± 0.34	1.99 ± 0.12
C18:0	2.30 ± 0.16	1.40 ± 0.15	2.93 ± 0.54	2.37 ± 0.40	2.62 ± 0.40	2.07 ± 0.23	2.20 ± 0.24
C18:1	20.57 ± 0.94	6.61 ± 0.51	7.12 ± 0.29	5.39 ± 0.68	20.51 ± 0.68	20.62 ± 2.83	5.55 ± 0.77
C18:2	0.17 ± 0.02	0.34 ± 0.02	0.52 ± 0.02	0.37 ± 0.03	0.16 ± 0.03	0.17 ± 0.03	8.36 ± 0.51
C19:0	1.11 ± 0.11	1.34 ± 0.05	1.22 ± 0.12	2.83 ± 0.29	5.20 ± 0.29	1.25 ± 0.15	0.96 ± 0.14
C20:0	0.03 ± 0.01	0.02 ± 0.00	0.04 ± 0.01	0.03 ± 0.00	0.04 ± 0.00	0.03 ± 0.00	0.03 ± 0.01
C20:1	1.59 ± 0.17	0.41 ± 0.04	0.73 ± 0.03	0.31 ± 0.03	1.76 ± 0.03	1.98 ± 0.17	1.03 ± 0.03
C21:0	0.01 ± 0.00	ND	0.02 ± 0.00	0.02 ± 0.01	0.01 ± 0.01	ND	ND
C22:0	0.12 ± 0.01	0.03 ± 0.00	0.14 ± 0.02	0.07 ± 0.01	0.11 ± 0.01	0.09 ± 0.02	0.16 ± 0.01
C22:1	0.05 ± 0.00	0.02 ± 0.01	ND	ND	0.08 ± 0.03	0.02 ± 0.00	ND
C23:0	0.10 ± 0.00	0.03 ± 0.01	0.05 ± 0.00	0.04 ± 0.01	0.06 ± 0.01	0.07 ± 0.00	0.17 ± 0.00
C24:0	0.09 ± 0.00	0.02 ± 0.00	0.05 ± 0.00	0.04 ± 0.01	0.06 ± 0.01	0.05 ± 0.00	0.15 ± 0.02

[a] *E. coli* BL21 *fabB* mutant complement with *fabB/F* of *Synechococcus* sp. PCC 7942. [b] *E. coli* BL21 *fabF* mutant complement with *fabB/F* of *Synechococcus* sp. PCC 7942. [c] *E. coli* BL21 *fabH* mutant complement with *fabH* of *Synechococcus* sp. PCC 7942.

Synpccw7942_0537 (*fabB/F*) and Synpccw7942_1455 (*fabH*) from *Synechococcus* sp. PCC 7942 were used for *E. coli* mutants (*fabB/F/H*)⁻ complementation. The results show that fatty acid compositions of mutants were basically restored to that of the wild type after complementation (Table 5). These suggested that the Synpccw7942_0537 (*fabB/F*) gene in *Synechococcus* sp. PCC 7942 has similar functions of *fabB* and *fabF* of *E. coli* and was related to the elongation of fatty acids. Synpccw7942_1455 (*fabH*) has similar function of *fabH*, which is also related to the elongation of fatty acid in *Synechococcus* sp. PCC 7942.

2.6. Fluorescence Localization of the Related Proteins

In order to describe the SCFAs synthesis pathway in microalgae, cellular localization of Synpccw7942_0537 (*fabB/F*) and Synpccw7942_1455 (*fabH*) by co-expressing green fluorescence protein gene and potential genes were carried out. Figure 2 shows that the fusion expressed proteins of eGFP-FabB/F and eGFP-FabH in *Synechococcus* sp. PCC 7942 were evenly dispersed on the cell membrane, indicating that the enzymes corresponding to *fabB/F* and *fabH* were located on the cell membrane. It is the first time to show the cell location of KASs.

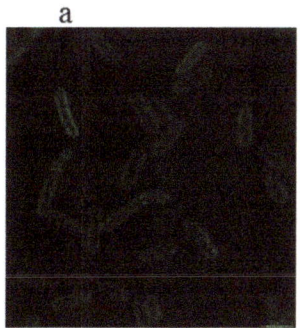 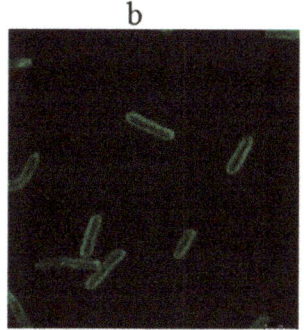

Figure 2. The fusion expressed proteins of FabB/F-eGFP (**a**) and FabH-eGFP (**b**) in *Synechococcus* sp. PCC 7942 observed under the confocal laser fluorescence microscope. (**a**) FabB/F labeled with eGFP in *Synechococcus* sp. PCC 7942 for fluorescence localization; (**b**) FabH labeled with eGFP in *Synechococcus* sp. PCC 7942 for fluorescence localization.

Based on the above studies, a possible pathway for the SCFAs synthesis in *Synechococcus* sp. PCC 7942 is proposed. As shown in Figure 3, CO_2 enters the microalgal cell and finally forms malonyl-ACP through de novo fatty acids synthesis, then goes into the fatty acid synthesis pathway, where KAS I/II (*fabB/F*) and KAS III (*fabH*) located on the cell membrane could catalyze condensation reactions to accumulate different chain length fatty acids less than 18 carbon atoms. Previous research found that fatty acids synthetic system started from acetyl-CoA carboxylase (ACCase), catalyzing the conversion of acyl-CoA to malonyl CoA, which was thought to be a limiting step [50]. KAS III had also been proved to be a limiting step in microalgae fatty acid biosynthesis. The above two limiting steps may affect the fixation of CO_2 in microalgae fatty acid biosynthesis. In the whole photosynthetic CO_2 fixation process, to increase the lipid productivity, ACCase and KAS III are the best options available for operation. Overexpression of *ACCase* and *KAS III* genes has succeeded to regulate the lipid synthesis [29,51,52].

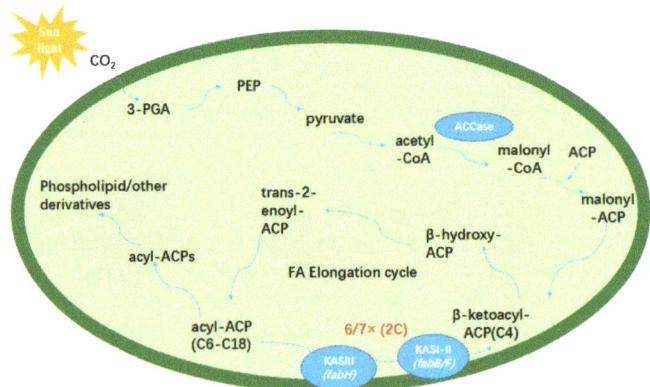

Figure 3. The proposed synthesis pathway of short carbon fatty acids (SCFAs) in *Synechococcus* sp. PCC 7942.

3. Materials and Methods

3.1. Microalgae Cultures

Synechococcus sp. PCC 7942 used in the study was provided by Prof. Dingji Shi (Shanghai Ocean University, Shanghai, China). Cells were preserved in the BG11 medium. The initial OD_{730} was 0.1, the initial pH was 7.8–8.0. The cultivation of *Synechococcus* sp. PCC 7942 was bubbled under $27 \pm 1\ °C$ and 140 mmol m^{-2} s^{-1} in 1 L Erlenmeyer flask with 500 mL working volume of BG11 medium. BG11 medium consists of (1 L) 1.5 g $NaNO_3$; 0.03 g K_2HPO_4; 0.075 g $MgSO_4·2H_2O$; 0.036 g $CaCl_2·2H_2O$; 0.006 g citric acid; 0.006 g ferric ammonium citrate; 0.001 g EDTA; 0.02 g Na_2CO_3 and 1 mL micronutrient solution. The microelement solution consists of (1 L) 2.86 g H_3BO_3; 1.81 g $MnCl_2·4H_2O$; 0.222 g $ZnSO_4·7H_2O$; 0.39 g $NaMoO_4·5H_2O$; 0.079 g $CuSO_4·5H_2O$ and 0.0494 g $Co(NO_3)_2·6H_2O$.

Cell growth in BG11 medium was set as the normal growth condition. Different cerulenin concentrations were set as follows: 0 g/L, 1 g/L, 2.5 g/L, 5 g/L and 7.5 g/L. Stock solution of cerulenin (100 mg/L, preserved in ethyl alcohol, $-20\ °C$) was added to BG11 medium with the final concentrations at 0 day.

3.2. Genomic DNA Extraction and PCR Analysis

Genomic DNA of *Synechococcus* sp. PCC 7942 was isolated as described previously by Kuo et al. [30]. Genomic DNA of *Synechococcus* sp. PCC 7942 transformant was prepared from exponential growth phase cultures using a procedure based on cetyltrimethylammonium bromide (CTAB) method. PCR analysis of transformants was carried out with genomic DNA as a template using primers as shown in Table S1 (Supplementary Materials). PCR amplification was performed for 30 cycles of 95 °C for 1 min, 56 °C for 30 s, and 72 °C for 30 s, followed by 72 °C for 10 min.

3.3. Sense and Antisense Expression Vector Construction

Bioinformatics showed that two enzymes in *Synechococcus* sp. PCC 7942 were annotated with β-ketoacyl ACP synthase activity. Alignments were proved that the sequence of Synpccw7942_0537 (Gene ID: 3774775) is similar to *fabB* and *fabF* in plants and bacteria, while the sequence of Synpccw7942_1455 (Gene ID: 3773627) is similar to *fabH* in plants and bacteria. In this experiment, we labeled them as *fabF/B* (Synpccw7942_0537) and *fabH* (Synpccw7942_1455), respectively.

The sequence Synpcc7942_0537 (*fabB/F*) and Synpcc7942_1455 (*fabH*) of *Synechococcus* sp. PCC 7942 were amplified by PCR from total DNA, using 7942-anti-fabB/F-F, 7942-anti-fabB/F-R and 7942-anti-fabH-F, 7942-anti-fabH-R (7942-sen-fabB/F-F, 7942-sen-fabB/F-R and 7942-sen-fabH-F, 7942-sen-fabH-R) primers (Table S1, Supplementary Materials) and then sub-cloned into pMD19-T vector (pMD19-T Vector Cloning Kit, TaKaRa Biotech Co., Dalian, China), resulting in pMD19T-anti*fabB/F* (pMD19T-sen*fabB/F*) and pMD19T-anti*fabH* (pMD19T-sen*fabH*) vectors. The amplified DNA fragments were digested with restriction enzymes XhoI and KpnI, and ligated into the corresponding sites of pRL489 vector to generate the antisense expression vectors (a) pRL-sen*fabB/F*, pRL-sen*fabH* and antisense expression vectors (b) pRL-antisen*fabB/F*, pRL-antisen*fabH*, using kanamycin as a selectable marker. These constructs were used for the natural transformation, then selected transformants by gradient antibiotics screening. Plasmids were propagated and purified using a standard procedure.

3.4. Deletion Mutant Construction

The plasmid pUC118 was constructed for gene deletion mutants of Synpcc7942_0537 (*fabB/F*) and Synpcc7942_1455 (*fabH*). DNA fragments upstream and downstream of Synpcc7942_0537 (*fabB/F*) and Synpcc7942_1455 (*fabH*) were amplified from *Synechococcus* sp. PCC 7942 genomic DNA using the primers in Table S1 (Supplementary Materials). Chloromycetin gene was amplified from pET28a. These upstream and downstream DNA fragments and chloromycetin gene were amplified by using overlap PCR to form *fabB/F*-cat and *fabH*-cat fragments, and inserted into pUC118, replacing the corresponding regions. The resulting plasmids (pUC118) contains homologous regions for gene deletion mutants of Synpcc7942_0537 (*fabB/F*) and Synpcc7942_1455 (*fabH*), and chloromycetin antibiotic resistance was used for selection. The deletion mutants were further confirmed by DNA sequence analysis (Figure S3, Supplementary Materials).

3.5. Fusion Expression Vector of Green Fluorescence Protein Construction

The plasmid pRL489 was used for fusion expression vectors of green fluorescence protein gene and Synpcc7942_0537 (*fabB/F*) and Synpcc7942_1455 (*fabH*). DNA sequences of Synpcc7942_0537 (*fabB/F*) and Synpcc7942_1455 (*fabH*) were amplified from *Synechococcus* sp. PCC 7942 genomic DNA using the primers in Table S1 (Supplementary Materials). Enhanced green fluorescent protein gene (*egfp*) fragment was from plasmid preserved in our laboratory. Synpcc7942_0537 (*fabB/F*) and Synpcc7942_1455 (*fabH*) and *egfp* gene were amplified by using overlap PCR to form egfp-fabB/F and egfp-fabH, and inserted into the pRL489, resulting pRL-egfp-*fabB/F* and pRL-egfp-*fabH*. Kanamycin antibiotic resistance was used for selection.

3.6. Liquid Culture and Screening of Transgenic Microalgae

Monoalgal colonies screened under antibiotic were cultured in BG11 medium containing kanamycin sulfate. Initially, transgenic microalgae was cultured in BG11 medium containing 25 g/L of kanamycin, and then the concentration of kanamycin (50 g/L, 100 g/L, 150 g/L, 200 g/L, 250 g/L, and 300 g/L) was gradually increased. When the concentration of antibiotic was increased to 300 g/L, wild type strains completely died under the pressure of antibiotic.

3.7. RNA Extraction and cDNA Synthesis

Total RNA extraction was treated with Trizol reagent (Sangon Biotech, Shanghai, China). Microalgal cells were harvested at different times (2 day intervals) by centrifugation. Approximately, microalgal cells (0.1 g) were ground in liquid nitrogen to powder before adding 1 mL Trizol reagent. After centrifugation at 12,000 r.p.m. for 10 min at 48 °C, 200 mL chloroform was added and mixed thoroughly. The sample was centrifuged at 12,000 r.p.m. for 15 min, then 450 mL of the uppermost layer was transferred into a fresh tube. Isopropanol (450 mL) was added to precipitated RNA and then centrifuged at 12,000 r.p.m. for 15 min, washed with 1 mL ethanol (75%, *v/v*) twice, dissolved in 30 mL diethyl pyrocarbonate treated distilled water. M-MLV (Moloney Murine Leukemia Virus) reverse transcriptase (TaKaRa Biotech Co., Dalian, China) was used to synthesize the cDNA. Two fatty acid synthetase genes (*fabF/B* and *fabH*) were investigated in this study. Genome annotation identified putative components of fatty acid biosynthetic pathway including *fabF/B* and *fabH*. Primers were designed according to the highly conserved regions obtained from the alignment of public database and the deduced amino acid sequences. The primers used in the experiment were shown in Table S1 (Supplementary Materials). After amplification, the PCR products were purified and cloned into pMD-19T vector for sequencing.

3.8. Quantitative Real-Time PCR

Real-time PCR was carried out on CFX96 Touch Real-Time PCR Detection System (Bio-Rad, Hercules, CA, USA) using SYBR Premix Ex TaqTMII (TaKaRa Biotech Co., Dalian, China). The reference gene was used as an internal standard, amplified with the *rnpB-F/rnpB-R* primers (Table S1, Supplementary Materials). Real-time PCR was conducted following the procedure: 95 °C for 30 s before performing 40 cycles of 95 °C for 5 s and 60 °C for 45 s, and a melting step at 60 °C–95 °C. PCR efficiency of each gene was calculated by relative standard curve using sequential dilutions of the cDNA. The $2^{-\Delta\Delta CT}$ method [53] was applied for the target gene expression calculation.

3.9. Lipid Extraction and Fatty Acid Analysis

Microalgal cells were harvested by centrifugation after cultivation. The total lipids were extracted according to the following method. Lyophilized microalgae powder (0.2 g) was pulverized in a mortar and extracted using 5 mL solvent mixture of chloroform:methanol (2:1, *v/v*). After shaking for 10 min, the samples were centrifuged (5804R, Eppendorf, Germany) at 10,000 r.p.m. for 10 min. The procedure was repeated three times to make sure the lipids were extracted completely. The solvent phase was transferred by pipette and evaporated in a water bath at 60 °C.

The fatty acids component of the lipids was analyzed by GC-linked mass spectrometry (GC-MS). Fatty acid methyl esters were obtained by acidic transesterification of the lipids. After reaction at 90 °C for 2 h, 2.5 mL hexane and 1 mL water were added to the sample, then vibrated gently and centrifuged. One milliliter of the organic upper phase was injected into an Auto System XL GC/Turbo Mass MS (Perkin Elmer, Germany) using a DB-5MS (5% phenyl)-methylpolysiloxane nonpolar column (30 m × 0.25 mm × 0.25 mm). At the beginning, the column temperature was kept at 60 °C for 4 min, then increased to 220 °C, and finally reached to 280 °C with a temperature gradient of 10 °C min, maintained for 10 min.

4. Conclusions

This study demonstrated that SCFAs synthesis of *Synechococcus* sp. PCC 7942 relied on β-ketoacyl ACP synthase (KAS), where Synpccw7942_0537 (*fabB/F*) had the function of short chain fatty acids elongation (C < 18) and elongation of C16:1 to C18:1, and Synpccw7942_1455 (*fabH*) could participate the SCFAs elongation (C < 18). Moreover, cerulenin, which could inhibit the expression level of Synpccw7942_0537 (*fabB/F*) and Synpccw7942_1455 (*fabH*), led to SFCAs accumulation. Based on these results, the SCFAs biosynthesis pathway in microalgae was proposed.

Supplementary Materials: The following are available online at http://www.mdpi.com/1660-3397/17/5/255/s1, Table S1: Primers used in this experiment; Figure S1: Effects of different cerulenin concentrations on the growth of *Synechococcus* sp. PCC 7942; Figure S2: The expression levels of *fabB/F* and *fabH* in *Synechococcus* sp. PCC 7942 with sense and antisense expression of Synpccw7942_0537 (*fabB/F*) and Synpccw7942_1455 (*fabH*). The expression levels of Synpccw7942_0537 (*fabB/F*) and Synpccw7942_1455 (*fabH*) in wild type strain were set to 1; Figure S3: DNA sequence analysis of the deletion mutants. (a) Alignment of construction of *fabB/F*-cat deletion mutation; (b) DNA fragment of *fabB/F*-cat; (c) alignment of construction of *fabH*-cat -cat deletion mutation; (d) DNA fragment of *fabH*-cat.

Author Contributions: Y.G. and X.M.: conceptualization; Y.G. and X.M.: methodology; Y.G.: software; Y.G. and X.M.: validation; Y.G.: formal analysis; Y.G.: investigation; Y.G. and X.M.: resources; Y.G.: data curation; Y.G.: writing—original draft preparation; Y.G. and X.M.: writing—review and editing; Y.G.: visualization; X.M.: supervision; X.M.: project administration; X.M.: funding acquisition.

Funding: This research was financially supported by the National Natural Science Foundation of China (No. 41476122). It was also supported by the National High Technology Research and Development Program (863 Program) of China (No. 2013AA065805).

Conflicts of Interest: The authors declare no conflict of interest.

References

1. Traul, K.A.; Driedger, A.; Ingle, D.L.; Nakhasi, D. Review of the toxicologic properties of medium-chain triglycerides. *Food Chem. Toxicol.* **2000**, *38*, 79–98. [CrossRef]
2. Cournarie, F.; Savelli, M.P.; Rosilio, V.; Bretez, F.; Vauthier, C.; Grossiord, J.L.; Seiller, M. Insulin-loaded W/O/W multiple emulsions: Comparison of the performances of systems prepared with medium-chain-triglycerides and fish oil. *Eur. J. Pharm. Biopharm.* **2004**, *58*, 477–482. [CrossRef] [PubMed]
3. Dehesh, K. How can we genetically engineer oilseed crops to produce high levels of medium-chain fatty acids? *Eur. J. Lipid Sci. Technol.* **2015**, *103*, 688–697. [CrossRef]
4. Xia, H.; Wang, X.; Li, M.; Xiao, H. Improving fatty acid composition and increasing triacylglycerol content in plants by gene engineering. *Chin. J. Biotech.* **2010**, *26*, 735–743.
5. Shi, T.T. *Screening of Oil-producing Strains*; Shandong Polytechnic University: Jinan, China, 2012.
6. Schenk, P.M.; Thomas-Hall, S.R.; Stephens, E.; Marx, U.C.; Mussgnug, J.H.; Posten, C.; Kruse, O.; Hankamer, B. Second Generation Biofiiels; High-Efficiency Microalgae for Biodiesel Production. *Bioenerg. Res.* **2008**, *1*, 20–43. [CrossRef]
7. Xu, L.; Li, Z.; Zhou, H.L.; Ding, Y.T.; Liu, L. Study of hygroscopic and moisturizing performance of oligosaccharides obtained from enzymolysis of algin. *China Surfactant Deterg. Cosmet.* **2011**, *41*, 42–45.
8. Lü, H.; Gao, Y.; Shan, H.; Lin, Y. Preparation and antibacterial activity studies of degraded polysaccharide selenide from *Enteromorpha prolifera*. *Carbohydr. Polym.* **2014**, *107*, 98–102. [CrossRef]
9. Abad, M.J.; Bedoya, L.M.; Bermejo, P. Natural marine anti-inflammatory products. *Mini Rev. Med. Chem.* **2008**, *8*, 740–754. [CrossRef] [PubMed]
10. Yang, C.; Chung, D.; Shin, I.S.; Lee, H.; Kim, J.; Lee, Y.; You, S. Effects of molecular weight and hydrolysis conditions on anticancer activity of fucoidans from sporophyll of *Undaria pinnatifida*. *Int. J. Biol. Macromol.* **2008**, *43*, 433–437. [CrossRef]
11. Shao, P.; Chen, X.; Sun, P. Chemical characterization, antioxidant and antitumor activity of sulfated polysaccharide from *Sargassum horneri*. *Carbohydr. Polym.* **2014**, *105*, 260–269. [CrossRef]
12. Adams, N.L.; Shick, J.M. Mycosporine-like amino acids provide protection against ultraviolet radiation in eggs of the green sea urchin *Strongylocentrotus droebachiensis*. *Photochem. Photobiol.* **1996**, *64*, 149–158. [CrossRef]
13. Zhang, Q.; Li, N.; Zhou, G.; Lu, X.; Xu, Z.; Li, Z. In vivo antioxidant activity of polysaccharide fraction from *Porphyra haitanesis* (Rhodophyta) in aging mice. *Pharmacol. Res.* **2003**, *48*, 151–155. [CrossRef]
14. Abidov, M.; Ramazanov, Z.; Seifulla, R.; Grachev, S. The effects of Xanthigen in the weight management of obese premenopausal women with non-alcoholic fatty liver disease and normal liver fat. *Diabetes Obes. Metab.* **2010**, *12*, 72–81. [CrossRef] [PubMed]
15. Chang, Z.C. Application of Bioengineering in Olechemical Industry (III)—Application of Medium Chain Length Fatty Acid Esters in Medical. *Nutr. Cosmet. China Oils Fats* **1999**, *6*, 50–52. [CrossRef]
16. Kim, I.H.; Kim, H.; Lee, K.T.; Chung, S.H.; Ko, S.N. Lipase-catalyzed acidolysis of perilla oil with caprylic acid to produce structured lipids. *J. Am. Oil Chem. Soc.* **2002**, *79*, 363–367. [CrossRef]

17. Murga, M.L.; Cabrera, G.M.; De Valdez, G.F.; Disalvo, A.; Seldes, A.M. Influence of growth temperature on cryotolerance and lipid composition of *Lactobacillus acidophilus*. *J. Appl. Microbiol.* **2000**, *88*, 342–348. [CrossRef]
18. Yumoto, I.; Yamazaki, K.; Hishinuma, M.; Nodasaka, Y.; Inoue, N.; Kawasaki, K. Identification of facultatively alkaliphilic *Bacillus* sp. strain YN-2000 and its fatty acid composition and cell-surface aspects depending on culture pH. *Extremophiles* **2000**, *4*, 285–290. [CrossRef]
19. Hartig, C.; Loffhagen, N.; Babel, W. Glucose stimulates a decrease of the fatty acid saturation degree in *Acinetobacter calcoaceticus*. *Arch. Microbiol.* **1999**, *171*, 166–172. [CrossRef]
20. Huang, J.Z.; Aki, T.; Hachida, K.; Yokochi, T.; Kawamoto, S.; Shigeta, S.; Ono, K.; Suzuki, O. Profile of Polyunsaturated Fatty Acids Produced by *Thraustochytrium* sp. KK17-3. *J. Am. Oil Chem. Soc.* **2001**, *78*, 605–610. [CrossRef]
21. Joestensen, J.P.; Landfald, B. Influence of growth conditions on fatty acid composition of a polyunsaturated-fatty-acid-producing Vibrio species. *Arch. Microbiol.* **1996**, *165*, 306–310. [CrossRef]
22. Han, J.C. *Research on the Collection and Lipid Systhesis Pathway of Oil-Producing Microalgae*; Ocean University of China: Qingdao, China, 2012.
23. Jones, A.; Davies, H.M.; Voelker, T.A. Palmitoyl-acyl carrier protein (ACP) thioesterase and the evolutionary origin of plant acyl-ACP thioesterases. *Plant Cell* **1995**, *7*, 359–371. [CrossRef]
24. Dehesh, K.; Jones, A.; Knutzon, D.S.; Voelker, T.A. Production of high levels of 8:0 and 10:0 fatty acids in transgenic canola by overexpression of *ChFatB2*, a thioesterase cDNA from *Cuphea hookeriana*. *Plant J.* **1996**, *2*, 167–172. [CrossRef]
25. Thelen, J.J.; Ohlrogge, J.B. Metabolic engineering of fatty acid biosynthesis in plants. *Metab. Eng.* **2002**, *4*, 12–21. [CrossRef]
26. Lu, S.F. Biosynthesis and Gene Engineering of Plant Fatty Acids. *Chin. Bull. Bot.* **2000**, *17*, 481–491.
27. Li, X.W. *Cloning and Analysis of Genes of Fatty Acid Biosynthesis-related Enzymes (KASI, FatB) and Genetic Transformation of ahFAD2B in Arachis hypogaea L.*; Shandong Agricultural University: Taian, China, 2011.
28. Verwoert, I.I.; van der Linder, K.H.; Walsh, M.C. Modification of *Brassica napus* seed oil by expression of the *Escherichia coli fabH* gene, encoding β-ketoacyl-acyl carrier protein synthase III. *Plant Mol. Biol.* **1995**, *27*, 875–886. [CrossRef]
29. Dehesh, K.; Tai, H.; Edwards, P.; Byrne, J.; Jaworski, J.G. Overexpression of β-ketoacyl-acyl-carrier protein synthase IIIs in plants reduces the rate of lipid synthesis. *Plant Physiol.* **2001**, *125*, 1103–1114. [CrossRef]
30. Kuo, J.; Khosla, C. The initiation keto synthase (*FabH*) is the sole rate-limiting enzyme of the fatty acid synthase of *Synechococcus* sp. PCC 7002. *Metab. Eng.* **2014**, *22*, 53–59. [CrossRef]
31. Renaud, S.M.; Thinh, L.V.; Lambrinidis, G.; Parry, D.L. Effect of temperature on growth, chemical composition and fatty acid composition of tropical Australian microalgae grown in batch cultures. *Aquaculture* **2002**, *211*, 195–214. [CrossRef]
32. Parker, P.L.; van Baalen, C.; Maurer, L. Fatty acids in eleven species of blue-green algae: Geochemical significance. *Science* **1967**, *155*, 707–708. [CrossRef] [PubMed]
33. Karatay, S.E.; Dönmez, G. Microbial oil production from thermophile cyanobacteria for biodiesel production. *Appl. Energ.* **2011**, *88*, 3632–3635. [CrossRef]
34. Arnvig, M.K.; McGuire, J.N.; von Wettstein-Knowles, P. Acyl carrier protein (ACP) inhibition and other differences between β-ketoacyl synthase (KAS) I and II. *Biochem. Soc. Trans.* **2000**, *28*, 607–610. [CrossRef]
35. Jin, L.M.; Liu, P.; Tian, W.J. Bacterial fatty acid biosynthesis enzymes-drug targets for antibacterial agent screen. *J. Shenyang Pharm. Univ.* **2006**, *23*, 814–818.
36. Israel, G.; James, R.; Konrad, B. Inhibition of Lipid Synthesis in *Escherichia coli* Cells by the Antibiotic cerulenin. *Antimicrob. Agents Chemother.* **1973**, *5*, 549–554.
37. Lin, P.H. *Preliminary Modeling Screening for Fatty Acid Synthase FabB/F Inhibitor*; Jiangxi Agricultural University: Nanchang, China, 2012.
38. Blatti, J.L.; Beld, J.; Behnke, C.A.; Mendez, M.; Mayfield, S.P.; Burkart, M.D. Manipulating fatty acid biosynthesis in microalgae for biofuel through protein-protein interactions. *PLoS ONE* **2012**, *7*, e42949. [CrossRef]
39. Ter Beek, A.; Keijser, B.J.; Boorsma, A.; Zakrzewska, A.; Orij, R.; Smits, G.J.; Brul, S. Transcriptome analysis of sorbic acid-stressed *Bacillus subtilis* reveals a nutrient limitation response and indicates plasma membrane remodeling. *J. Bacteriol.* **2008**, *190*, 1751–1761. [CrossRef] [PubMed]

40. Yu, Y.H.; Ma, J.R.; Miao, X.Y.; Wang, H.H. Biological Function Research of β-ketoacyl ACP Synthase III. *Prog. Biochem. Biophys.* **2016**, *43*, 1004–1012.
41. Chen, J.Q.; Lang, C.X.; Hu, Z.H. Antisense PEP Gene Regulates to Ratio of Protein and Lipid Content in *Brassica Napus* Seeds. *J. Agric. Biotechnol.* **1999**, *7*, 316–320.
42. Song, D.; Hou, L.; Shi, D. Exploitation and utilization of rich lipids-microalgae, as new lipids feedstock for biodiesel production—A review. *Chin. J. Biotechnol.* **2008**, *24*, 341–348. [CrossRef]
43. Lin, H.X.; Lee, Y.K. Genetic engineering of medium-chain-length fatty acid synthesis in *Dunaliella tertiolecta* for improved biodiesel production. *J. Appl. Phycol.* **2017**, *29*, 2811–2819. [CrossRef] [PubMed]
44. Ma, J.C.; Deng, L.T.; Tong, W.H.; Zhu, L.; Wang, H.H. Identification and Function Reasearch of Five β-Ketoacyl-ACP Synthase Homologues. *Prog. Biochem. Biophys.* **1997**, *41*, 887–895.
45. Qian, W.Z. *Preparation of Monoclonal Antibody against Protein FabB and Analysis of the Difference and Distribution of FabB in Different Bactieria Species*; Yangzhou University: Yangzhou, China, 2013.
46. Leonard, J.; Knapp, S.J.; Slabaugh, M.B. A Cuphea β-ketoacyl ACP synthase shifts the synthesis of fatty acids towards shorter chains in Arabidopsis seeds expressing Cuphea FatB thioesterases. *Plant J.* **1998**, *13*, 621–628. [CrossRef] [PubMed]
47. Pidkowich, M.S.; Nguyen, H.T.; Heilmann, I.; Ischebeck, T.; Shanklin, J. Modulating seed beta-ketoacyl-acyl carrier protein synthase II level converts the composition of a temperate seed oil to that of a palm-like tropical oil. *Proc. Natl. Acad. Sci. USA* **2007**, *104*, 4742–4747. [CrossRef]
48. González-Mellado, D.; von Wettstein-Knowles, P.; Garcés, R.; Martínez-Force, E. The role of β-ketoacyl-acyl carrier protein synthase III in the condensation steps of fatty acid biosynthesis in sunflower. *Planta* **2010**, *231*, 1277–1289. [CrossRef] [PubMed]
49. Brück, F.M.; Brummel, M.; Schuch, R.; Spener, F. In-vitro evidence for feed-back regulation of beta-ketoacyl-acyl carrier protein synthase III in medium-chain fatty acid biosynthesis. *Planta* **1996**, *198*, 271–278. [CrossRef]
50. Post-Beittenmiller, D.; JaworskiJ, G.; Ohlrogge, J.B. In vivo pools of free and acylated acyl carrier proteins in spinach. Evidence for Sites of regulation of fatty acid biosynthesis. *J. Biol. Chem.* **1991**, *266*, 1858–1865. [PubMed]
51. Roessler, P.G. Changes in the activities of various lipid and carbohydrate biosynthetic enzymes in the diatom *Cyclotella cryptica* in response to silicon deficiency. *Arch. Biochem. Biophys.* **1988**, *267*, 521–528. [CrossRef]
52. Courchesne, N.M.; Parisien, A.; Wang, B.; Lan, C.Q. Enhancement of lipid production using biochemical, genetic and transcription factor engineering approaches. *J. Biotechnol.* **2009**, *141*, 31–41. [CrossRef]
53. Perrineau, M.M.; Zelzion, E.; Gross, J.; Price, D.C.; Boyd, J.; Bhattacharya, D. Evolution of salt tolerance in a laboratory reared population of *Chlamydomonas reinhardtii*. *Environ. Microbiol.* **2014**, *16*, 1755–1766. [CrossRef] [PubMed]

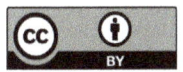

© 2019 by the authors. Licensee MDPI, Basel, Switzerland. This article is an open access article distributed under the terms and conditions of the Creative Commons Attribution (CC BY) license (http://creativecommons.org/licenses/by/4.0/).

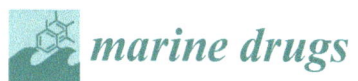

Article

Octominin: A Novel Synthetic Anticandidal Peptide Derived from Defense Protein of *Octopus minor*

Chamilani Nikapitiya [1], S.H.S. Dananjaya [1], H.P.S.U. Chandrarathna [1], Mahanama De Zoysa [1,*] and Ilson Whang [2,*]

1. College of Veterinary Medicine, Chungnam National University, Yuseong-gu, Daejeon 34134, Korea; chamilani14@gmail.com (C.N.); shsdananjaya@gmail.com (S.H.S.D.); surathsanda@gmail.com (H.P.S.U.C.)
2. National Marine Biodiversity Institute of Korea (MABIK), 75, Jangsan-ro 101beon-gil, Janghang-eup, Seochun-gun, Chungchungnam-do 33662, Korea
* Correspondence: mahanama@cnu.ac.kr (M.D.Z.); ilsonwhang@mabik.re.kr (I.W.)

Received: 30 October 2019; Accepted: 8 January 2020; Published: 15 January 2020

Abstract: The rapid emergence of multidrug-resistant pathogens makes an urgent need for discovering novel antimicrobial agents as alternatives to conventional antibiotics. Towards this end, we designed and synthesized a synthetic peptide of 23 amino acids (AAs) (^{1}GWLIRGAIHAGKAIHGLIHRRRH^{23}) from a defense protein 3 cDNA sequence of *Octopus minor*. The sequence of the peptide, which was named Octominin, had characteristic features of known antimicrobial peptides (AMPs) such as a positive charge (+5), high hydrophobic residue ratio (43%), and 1.86 kcal/mol of Boman index. Octominin was predicted to have an alpha-helix secondary structure. The synthesized Octominin was 2625.2 Da with 92.5% purity. The peptide showed a minimum inhibitory concentration (MIC) and minimum fungicidal concentration (MFC) of 50 and 200 µg/mL, respectively, against *Candida albicans*. Field emission scanning electron microscopy observation confirmed that Octominin caused ultrastructural cell wall deformities in *C. albicans*. In addition, propidium iodide penetrated the Octominin-treated *C. albicans* cells, further demonstrating loss of cell membrane integrity that caused cell death at both MIC and MFC. Octominin treatment increased the production of intracellular reactive oxygen species and decreased cell viability in a concentration dependent manner. Cytotoxicity assays revealed no significant influence of Octominin on the viability of human embryonic kidney 293T cell line, with over 95% live cells in the Octominin-treated group observed up to 100 µg/mL. Moreover, we confirmed the antifungal action of Octominin in vivo using a zebrafish experimental infection model. Overall, our results demonstrate the Octominin is a lead compound for further studies, which exerts its effects by inducing cell wall damage, causing loss of cell membrane integrity, and elevating oxidative stress.

Keywords: anticandidal activity; antimicrobial peptides; *Candida albicans*; Octominin; *Octopus minor*

1. Introduction

Candida albicans is one of the most dominant fungal species of the human microbiota and asymptomatically colonizes in the gastrointestinal and genitourinary tract in healthy people [1]. However, *C. albicans* is an opportunistic pathogen that can cause infections under certain pathological and physiological conditions such as in diabetes, pregnancy, under steroidal chemotherapy, and prolonged broad spectrum antibiotic administration, as well as in patients with acquired immunodeficiency syndrome [2]. Multidrug resistance is considered to be the major cause for failures in candidiasis treatment [3], and several pathogenic strains of *C. albicans* show multidrug resistance against currently used antifungal drugs such as fluconazole, itraconazole, nystatin, caspofungin, ketoconazole, flucytosine, and amphotericin B [4,5]. *C. albicans* shows a diversity of resistance mechanisms such as a decrease in drug accumulation or drug affinity of its targets and changes in drug metabolism [6].

Hence, it is important to identify and develop novel and less toxic anticandidal agents with high therapeutic efficacy to effectively control infections with drug-resistant strains of *C. albicans*.

Antimicrobial peptides (AMPs) are short peptides that typically consist of less than 50 amino acids (AAs) residues and exhibit antimicrobial activity [7]. To date, over 1200 AMPs have been identified or predicted from bacteria, fungi, plants, invertebrates, nonmammalian vertebrates, and mammals [8,9]. The genes encoding AMPs are highly evolutionarily conserved components of the host defense system against pathogenic microorganisms, and can thus be considered as "natural antibiotics" [10]. AMPs can also be described as "host defense peptides" owing to their additional immunomodulatory functions such as antitumor [11], antiendotoxin [12], cytokine and growth factor [6], immunomodulatory [9], and wound healing functions [13]. The antimicrobial activity of AMPs has been reported against a wide range of pathogens, including bacteria [14], yeast [15], fungi [16], viruses [17], and parasites [18]. Based on the secondary structure, AMPs can be classified into four major groups: α helical, β sheet, loop, and extended peptide [19]. A common characteristic of AMPs is their amphipathic nature with net positive charge due to the presence of multiple residues such as arginine (R), histidine (H) and lysine (K) and hydrophobic residues such as alanine (A), leucine (L), isoleucine (I), tyrosine (Y), and tryptophan (W) [20]. The ability of AMPs to kill microbial pathogens primarily depends on their interaction and binding capacity with the cell membrane or cell wall, which vary according to the net positive charge and ratio of hydrophobic AAs. This amphipathicity of AMPs is an important feature for interacting with cell membranes or their mimics to induce antimicrobial functions, and binding of AMPs to the cell membrane generally changes the membrane permeability and causes nonenzymatic disruption [6], resulting in the efflux of intracellular materials to exert rapid bactericidal/fungicidal activity [21].

Although various sources are available for isolating natural AMPs with different degrees of functional activities, it is difficult to obtain sufficiently large quantities of the peptides with the purity required for application in research or for therapeutic purposes. Therefore, the production of synthetic AMPs is becoming an increasingly popular strategy, which can lead to the development of novel therapeutic agents with a wide range of bioactivities [22]. Furthermore, intensifying the effort for the identification and development of novel AMPs is essential to help suppress the rapid spread and continued selection of multidrug-resistant pathogens.

Toward this end, the objective of this study was to screen for AMPs in the transcriptome of *Octopus minor*, and synthesize the peptide to investigate its antifungal effect. A novel AMP was screened and modified based on the defense protein 3 cDNA sequence of *Octopus minor*, which was named Octominin. To evaluate its anticandidal function and mode of action, *C. albicans* was used as a pathogenic model organism, and various parameters of Octominin in the presence of *C. albicans* were determined, including the minimum inhibitory concentration (MIC), minimum fungicidal concentration (MFC), and MFC/MIC ratios, along with the influence of the synthesized protein on the fungal cell, including change of cell membrane structure, cell viability, reactive oxygen species (ROS) production, propidium iodide (PI) uptake. Moreover, to establish the potential of Octominin for development in therapeutic application, we assessed its cytotoxicity in the human embryonic kidney HEK293T cell line. Based on the overall results and possible mode of action, we suggest that Octominin is a potential lead molecule with fungicidal activity that can be developed for commercial use.

2. Results

2.1. Designing, Synthesis, and Characteristics of Octominin

Upon screening of the transcriptome database of *O. minor* for selection of AMPs, defense protein 3 cDNA sequence was considered as one of the candidates. Based on the antimicrobial peptide prediction program [23], and subsequent modification of the sequence fragment, Octominin showed characteristics of known AMPs, including a total net charge of +5, high number of positively charged residues (17% R, 17% H), and hydrophobic residues (17% I, 8% L, 13% A, 4% W) with the total hydrophobic ratio of

43% and protein binding potential (Boman index) of 1.86 kcal/mol. Moreover, the predicted grand average hydropathy value (GRAVY) was −0.2696 and the predicted molecular weight of the peptide was 2626.1 Da. Negatively charged AAs such as aspartate (D) and glutamate (E) were absent in the Octominin sequence, and a total of eight hydrophobic residues were identified on the same surface of the peptide. The predicted secondary and tertiary (three-dimensional) structures of Octominin are shown in Figure 1, including an alpha-helix secondary structure. The molecular weight of synthesized Octominin was 2652.2 Da with 92.5% purity (Supplementary Figure S1).

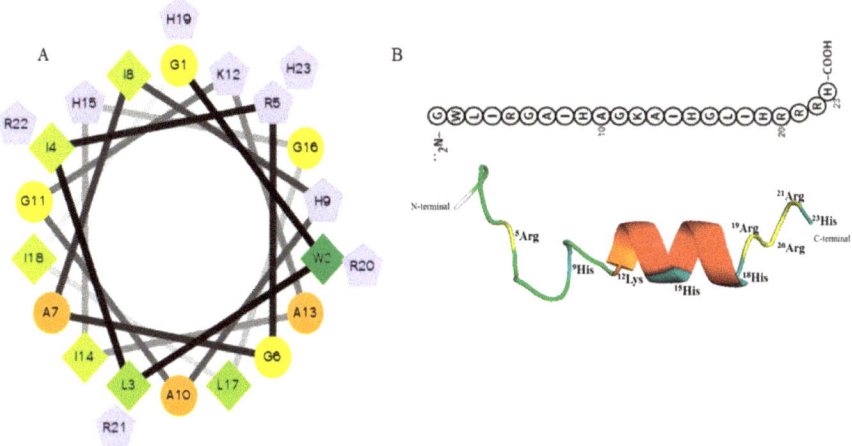

Figure 1. Predicted helical secondary and three-dimensional structures of Octominin. (**A**) Helical wheel of Octominin shows the AAs arrangement and the residue numbers which are counted from the amino (N) terminal of the peptide. The hydrophilic and hydrophobic residues are represented by circles and diamonds, respectively. The potentially charged (positively charged) residues are marked as pentagons in light blue. The most hydrophobic residue is green, and the amount of green is decreasing proportionally to the hydrophobicity, with zero hydrophobicity coded as yellow. (**B**) Three-dimensional structure and AA sequence of Octominin with positively charged residues.

2.2. MIC, MFC, and Growth Inhibition Profile of C. albicans Exposed to Octominin

We determined the MIC and MFC of Octominin to evaluate its ability for inhibiting the growth of *C. albicans* as a candidate anticandidal agent. Octominin demonstrated a clear anticandidal effect with a MIC and MFC of 50 and 200 µg/mL, respectively, representing a MFC/MIC ratio of 4.0. Moreover, the time–kill kinetic analysis revealed clear growth inhibition of *C. albicans* above the MIC level (Figure 2), which was similar to the growth inhibitory effect observed using the known antifungal agent nystatin (10 µg/mL) as a positive control. In addition, Octominin showed partial growth inhibition against *C. albicans* at a lower concentration (25 µg/mL) compared to that of the control.

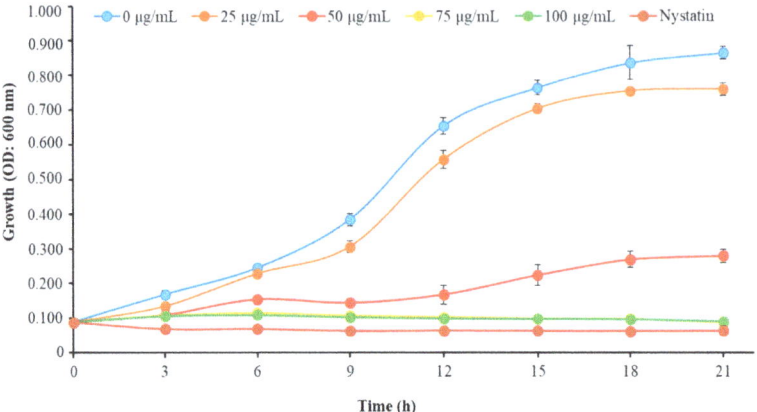

Figure 2. Time–kill kinetics of Octominin against *C. albicans*. *C. albicans* growth was assessed after Octominin treatment (0, 25, 50, 75, and 100 μg/mL) at 3 h intervals by measuring the optical density (OD) at 600 nm. The bars indicate the mean ± standard deviation ($n = 3$).

2.3. Effects of Octominin on Morphological Changes of C. albicans

To investigate the mode of action of Octominin, ultra-structural analysis of *C. albicans* was conducted using field-emission scanning electron microscopy (FE-SEM) after Octominin treatment. The SEM images clearly indicated membrane structural changes of *C. albicans* cells after treatment with Octominin at the MIC and MFC (Figure 3). As expected, untreated *C. albicans* cells displayed a smooth and undamaged cell surface (Figure 3A), whereas, swelling and severe cell wall alterations, including a rough membrane and irregular shape, were observed in the *C. albicans* treated with 50 (Figure 3B) and 200 μg/mL (Figure 3C) Octominin. Moreover, Octominin induced more severe morphological and structural changes at the MFC level than at the MIC level.

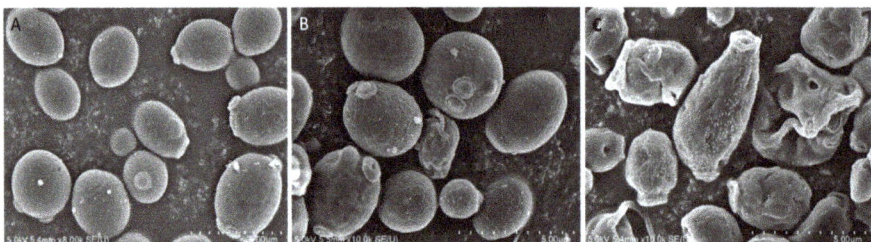

Figure 3. Effect of Octominin on morphological and structural changes of *C. albicans* assessed by field-emission scanning electron microscopy (FE-SEM). (**A**) Untreated *C. albicans*; (**B**) treated with 50 μg/mL (minimum inhibitory concentration; MIC;) Octominin; (**C**) treated with 200 μg/mL (minimum fungicidal concentration; MFC) Octominin.

2.4. Effects of Octominin on the Viability of C. albicans

The cell viability of *C. albicans* was determined by a 3-(4,5-dimethylthiazol-2-yl)-2,5-diphenyltetrazolium bromide (MTT) assay after treatment with different concentrations of Octominin (0–100 µg/mL). The cell viability was significantly decreased ($P < 0.05$) when *C. albicans* was treated with Octominin in a concentration dependent manner (Figure 4). The control group showed the highest cell viability, and the lowest cell viability of 9.25% was detected with treatment of Octominin at 100 µg/mL.

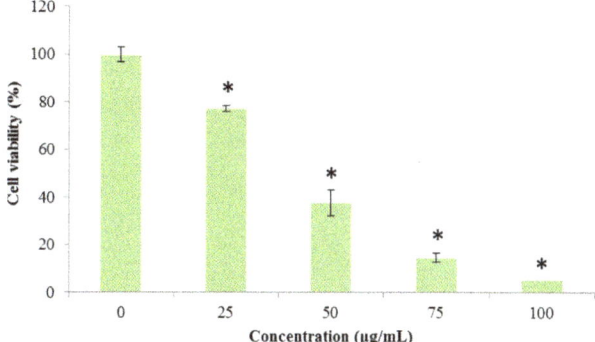

Figure 4. Effect of Octominin on the viability of *C. albicans*. Cell viability was assessed by the 3-(4,5-dimethylthiazol-2-yl)-2,5-diphenyltetrazolium bromide (MTT) assay after treatment with different concentrations of Octominin (0–100 µg/mL) until 24 h. * $P < 0.05$ compared to the control (untreated) group. The error bars indicate the mean ± standard deviation ($n = 3$).

2.5. Effect of Octominin on the Membrane Permeability of C. albicans

The PI uptake assay was performed to evaluate the effect of Octominin on the membrane permeability of *C. albicans* and its potential association with cell death. PI is an indicator stain that can penetrate dead or damaged cells and subsequently bind with the nucleus, emitting red fluorescence under a confocal laser scanning microscope (CLSM). The results of PI analysis showed that Octominin induced clear membrane damage to the *C. albicans* cells in a concentration-dependent manner (Figure 5). No PI-stained cells were detected in the untreated control group (Figure 5B,C). Both PI-stained and nonstained cells could be observed after treatment of *C. albicans* with the MIC of Octominin (Figure 5E,F), whereas all cells showed the red fluorescence signal after treatment with Octominin at the MFC, indicating the highest degree of membrane permeability (Figure 5H,I).

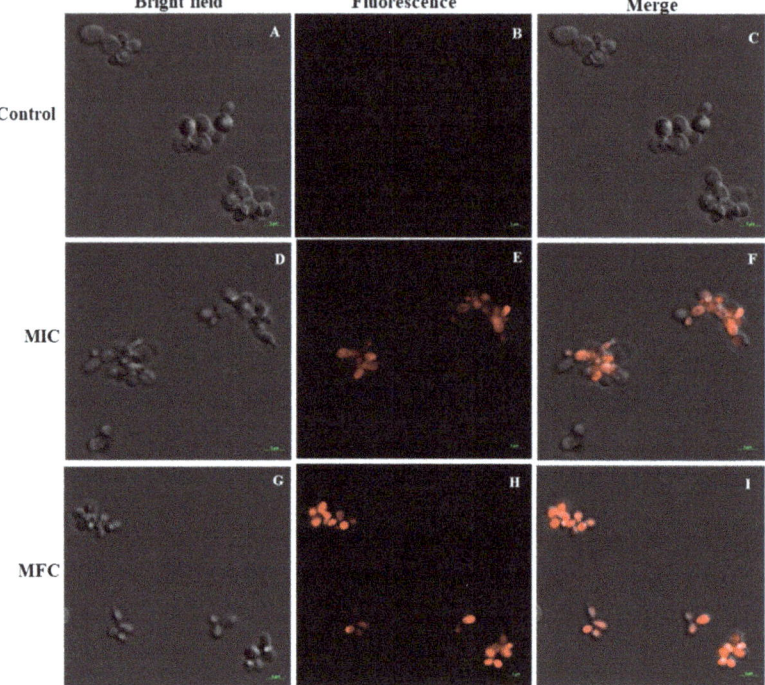

Figure 5. Effect of Octominin on membrane permeability in *C. albicans*. Confocal laser-scanning microscope (CLSM) merged and fluorescence images representing the cell membrane permeability by propidium iodide (PI) staining in *C. albicans* cells treated with Octominin at 30 °C for 6 h. (**A–C**) Untreated control; (**D–F**) treatment with Octominin at the MIC (50 µg/mL); (**G–I**) treatment with Octominin at the MFC (200 µg/mL).

2.6. Effects of Octominin on ROS Production in C. albicans

To investigate the mechanism of action of Octominin, we examined the change in the level of endogenous ROS production in *C. albicans* after Octominin treatment, which was assessed by staining of the fluorescent probe 5-(and-6)-carboxy-2,7-dihydrodichlorofluorescein diacetate (carboxy-H2DCF-DA). The ROS level was increased in a concentration dependent manner when *C. albicans* was treated with Octominin (Figure 6). Furthermore, *C. albicans* treated with 50 µg/mL (MIC) and 200 µg/mL (MFC) of Octominin showed higher levels of ROS compared to those of untreated cells, indicating that Octominin induced high oxidative stress in the cells.

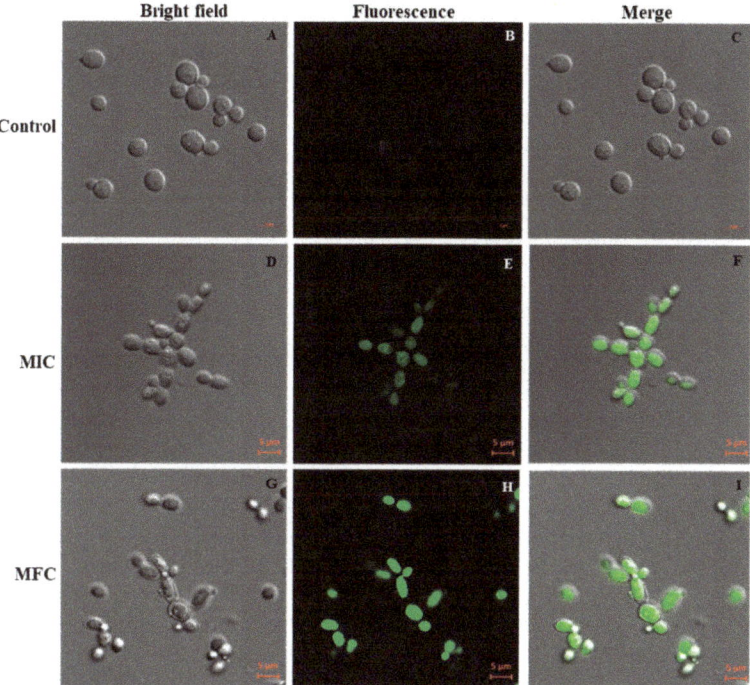

Figure 6. Effect of Octominin on reactive oxygen species (ROS) production of *C. albicans*. CLSM merged and fluorescence images representing ROS production in *C. albicans* with Octominin treatment at the MIC and MFC. (**A–C**) Untreated control; (**D–F**) treatment with Octominin at the MIC (50 μg/mL); (**G–I**) treatment with Octominin at the MFC (200 μg/mL).

2.7. Cytotoxicity of Octominin to Mammalian Cells

To further explore the potential safety of Octominin in therapeutic application, its cytotoxicity was tested using human embryonic kidney 293 (HEK293) cells with the EZ-Cytox enhanced cell viability assay kit. No morphological changes of the cells were observed when treated with Octominin up to 100 μg/mL (Figure 7B–D). There was no significant difference in cell viability between the Octominin-treated samples and untreated control ($P < 0.05$), with over 95% of the HEK293 cells remaining viable under all Octominin-treated concentrations up to 100 μg/mL (Figure 7E). Overall, these results confirmed that 100 μg/mL, which inhibits the growth of *C. albicans* by its anticandidal effects, was not toxic to human cells, demonstrating its potential for use in vivo treatments after clinical trials.

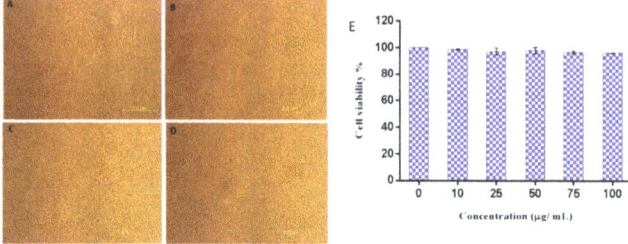

Figure 7. Cytotoxic effect of Octominin on HEK293 cells. (**A–D**) Representative images of Octominin-treated HEK293 cells at 48 h post treatment. (**A**) Untreated (control), (**B**) 10 µg/mL Octominin, (**C**) 75 µg/mL Octominin, (**D**) 100 µg/mL of Octominin. (**E**) Cell viability percentage of HEK293 cells treated with Octominin at different concentrations (0, 10, 25, 50, 75, and 100 µg/mL). Data are expressed as the mean ± standard error ($n = 3$).

2.8. Efficacy of Octominin Treatment on C. albicans Infection in a Zebrafish Model

C. albicans cells were injected to the dorsal muscle of adult zebrafish to study the effectiveness of Octominin treatment under in vivo conditions. The cumulative mortality at 72 h post treatment was 84% and 25% in the control and Octominin-treated (100 µg/fish per day) groups, respectively. Moreover, superficial fungal growth and a wound around the infected site were clearly observed in control (water-treated) fish (Figure 8A–C) at 24, 48, and 72 h post infection (hpi) compared to Octominin-treated fish (Figure 8D–F). In addition, the histopathological data confirmed the treatment effect against *C. albicans*, demonstrating less leukocyte infiltration around the infected site of Octominin-treated fish (Figure 8I) than the infected and untreated fish (Figure 8H) at 72 hpi.

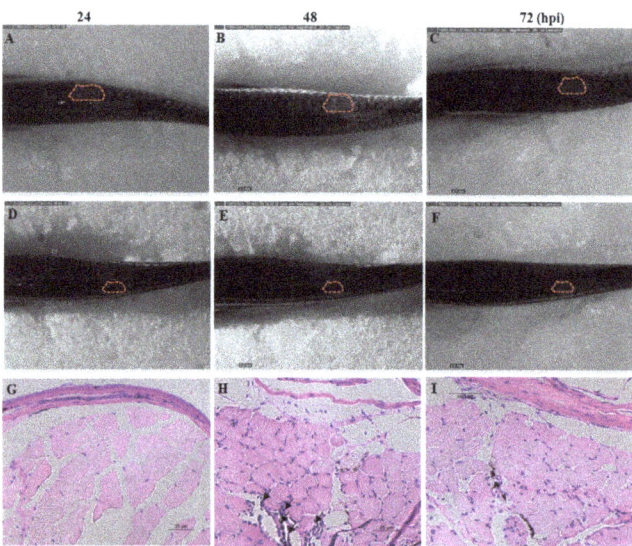

Figure 8. Anticandidal effect of Octominin in *C. albicans*-infected zebrafish. *C. albicans* growth and wound area at 24, 48, and 72 h post treatment of Octominin compared with the control (water-treated) fish. (**A–C**) *C. albicans* infected nontreated control. (**D–F**) *C. albicans*-infected Octominin treated fish. Effect of Octominin treatment in zebrafish muscle tissue upon *C. albicans* infection evaluated by periodic acid-Schiff-hematoxylin (PAS-H)-stained sections under microscope (400×). Muscle tissues of uninfected (**G**), infected and untreated treated (**H**), and infected and Octominin-treated (**I**) zebrafish. Black arrowhead shows the leukocyte infiltration in the muscle tissue of zebrafish.

3. Discussion

Discovery of novel AMPs is important to identify potential drug candidates for treating infections with multidrug-resistant pathogens such as *C. albicans*. Several AMPs with diversified antimicrobial functions have been identified from many species of the phylum Mollusk including abalone [14]. We previously reviewed the AMPs in marine mollusks and their potential biomedical applications [24]; thus, the present study represents a further extension of our AMPs research in different mollusk species of the class Cephalopoda. Through screening of the transcriptome database of *O. minor*, we discovered a defense protein 3 cDNA sequence, and a fragment of its AAs sequence was selected and modified, and named Octominin for development of a novel AMP. Octominin shares 92% and 88% identity with two related AMPs namely Chrysophsin-2 and Chrysophsin-1, respectively [25]. We further confirmed that Octominin inhibits the growth of *C. albicans* with a MIC and MFC of 50 and 200 μg/mL, respectively. A chemically synthesized porcine peptide PMAP-23 was reported to have marked antifungal activity (MIC 2–5 μM) against *C. albicans* [26]. In addition, Nikawa et al. [27] synthesized three new cationic peptides with an α-helical structure and amphipathic properties and their abilities to inhibit *C. albicans* were compared to those of known antifungals. The authors suggested that the α-helicity of the peptides has a limited contribution to the killing effect; however, the *p*-value was positively correlated with greater antifungal activity. Although the MIC of Octominin is relatively high, *C. albicans* growth was still delayed by about 3 h (in time–kill kinetics) as same to the 100 μg/mL. Moreover, 50 and 100 μg/mL of Octominin treatment resulted 35% and 5% cell viability at 24 h, respectively. This indicates that the viable cell number decreases rapidly under Octominin treatment, suggesting the efficient killing of the *C. albicans* cells. Therefore, the anticandidal activity of Octominin could be associated with its amphipathic nature, total hydrophobicity (43%), and net positive charge (+5).

Several peptides have been reported to cause ultrastructural damage to the cell wall of *C. albicans*. For example, a short peptide bovine lactoferrin (FKARRWQWRM) showed efficient inhibitory activity against *Candida* by damaging the cell wall via direct interaction with the cell surface, followed by induction of the autolytic response [28]. Moreover, the chemically synthesized HP (2-20) peptide derived from the N-terminus *Helicobacter pylori* ribosomal protein L1 showed free diffusion of PI suggesting that the *C. albicans* cell membrane was damaged [29]. Similarly, PMAP-23 exerts its antifungal activity by creating pores in the cell membrane rather than to the cell wall [26]. Another synthetic hybrid peptide, HP(2-9)-magainin 2(1-12), showed strong antifungal activity via damage to the fungal cell membrane, resulting in K^+ release from the cells [18]. The FE-SEM images of Octominin-treated cells clearly demonstrated its ability to damage the cell wall and the membrane based on the high number of malformed cells. Moreover, free diffusion of PI into the cytoplasm of *C. albicans* suggested that Octominin might have strong damaging effects on the *C. albicans* cell wall and/or cytoplasmic membrane.

Furthermore, we demonstrated that at least part of the mode of action of Octominin in *C. albicans* cells was associated with the accumulation of ROS based on oxidation of the fluorescent dye DCFH-DA (an indicator of ROS). The formation of ROS such as superoxide anion (O_2^-), hydroxyl radical (^-OH), hydrogen peroxide (H_2O_2), and singlet oxygen ($^1O_2$) can lead to oxidative stress in cells, consequently inducing damage to the macromolecules such as DNA, RNA, and proteins. A state of oxidative stress could activate degradation of the structural components, i.e., cellular membranes, and inactivate their basic functions by increasing the permeability, ultimately resulting in exposure of the cellular contents to the extracellular environment [30]. Indeed, the formation of ROS has been suggested as a critical step in the fungicidal mechanism of several AMPs [31]. However, Veerman et al. [32] suggested that ROS production did not play a role in the killing effect of the human salivary peptide histatin 5 in *C. albicans*. Moreover, histatins bind to a receptor on the fungal cell membrane and enter the cytoplasm, subsequently the mitochondrion, suggesting a role in oxidative stress [33]. Thus, the precise mode of action of some of the antifungal peptides against *C. albicans* remains controversial or unclear.

Based on its physico-chemical properties (alpha-helical, amphipathic, hydrophobic, and cationic), FE-SEM images, PI uptake, and ROS accumulation, we suggest that Octominin has multifactorial effects on *C. albicans*, resulting in structural disruption of the cell wall and the membrane to ultimately kill the fungal cells. We propose that Octominin may directly interact with the cell wall and then the phospholipid bilayer of the fungal cell membrane, leading to alterations of lipid organization in the membrane or the formation of ion-permeable channels (i.e., pores) in the membranes allowing for diffusion of the cell contents. Further, Octominin might directly interact with the cell membrane of *C. albicans* to disrupt its function and enhance its permeability. Octominin could then reach intracellular targets, the nucleus and DNA, leading to apoptosis. However, the exact mechanism by which Octominin exerts its fungicidal activity will need to be explored and identified in future studies.

One of the crucial problems associated with the development of an antifungal therapeutic drug is the cytotoxicity of the peptide that limits its safety and application. Here, we conformed that Octominin does not influence the viability of mammalian cells. Further, the overall results of in vivo experiments with a zebrafish infection model suggested that Octominin could effectively reduce the *C. albicans* infection; however, complete recovery was not observed, which may have been due to loss of some Octominin in the water after the treatment. Nevertheless, this result suggests that Octominin has good potential for triggering the host defense against *C. albicans*, supporting its functional novelty. Moreover, Octominin can be used safely as an anticandidal agent against *C. albicans* with maximum efficacy. However, its safety and mechanism of action need to be elucidated more detail in future studies.

In summary, although the properties of Octominin are somewhat inconsistent with those of previously reported anticandidal peptides, the basic characteristics as an AMP were confirmed. The net positive (+5) charge of the novel peptide Octominin leads to its affinity towards the lipid plasma membrane and specificity for *Candida*, and favors the interaction towards the anionic components in the *C. albicans* plasma membrane. Octominin showed a potent anticandidal activity without mammalian cell toxicity, demonstrating its potential for development as a novel anticandidal therapeutic agent. Despite expanding knowledge of antifungal peptides in recent years, this study demonstrates the untapped potential for discovering novel effective antifungal compounds, which can help to overcome current challenges of the treatment of drug resistant infections.

4. Materials and Methods

4.1. Design and Synthesis of the Screened AMP in O. minor

We screened the immune functional gene sequences from our *O. minor* transcriptome database for selection of candidate AMPs. The defense protein 3 cDNA sequence was selected and submitted to the National Center for Biotechnology Information (NCBI) (https://www.ncbi.nlm.nih.gov/) database under the accession number MN876862. The *N*-terminal region of the defense protein 3 AA sequence was selected as a template for designing the Octominin peptide using the prediction tool of the antimicrobial peptide database (APD) (http://aps.unmc.edu/AP), [23] according to the criteria of hydrophobicity, net charge, total hydrophobic ratio, and protein binding potential. We modified the selected sequence by increasing the number of hydrophobic (2 to 4 I, 1 to 2 L, 1 to 3 A, and 0 to 1 W) and positively charged residues (3 to 4 R and 0 to 4 H) to obtain the characteristic features of an AMP, resulting in the novel 23-AA Octominin peptide (^{1}GWLIRGAIHAGKAIHGLIHRRRH^{23}). The peptide was synthesized by a solid-phase peptide synthesis technique (AnyGen Co., Gwangju, Korea) and purified by reverse phase high performance liquid chromatography using a SHIMADZU C18 analytical column (Shimadzu HPLC LabSolution, Kyoto, Japan).

4.2. Culture of C. albicans

We used the *C. albicans* strain KCTC 27242 from the Korean Collection for Type Culture. A single colony picked up from a potato dextrose agar (PDA) plate was cultured in potato dextrose broth (PDB) under aerobic conditions at 30 °C for 24 h in a shaking incubator at 180 rpm. The *C. albicans* culture was centrifuged at 3500 rpm for 10 min to harvest the cells and washed twice with phosphate buffered saline (PBS, pH 7.4) followed by re-suspension in PBS (OD_{600} 0.1) to adjust the concentration of 10^6 colony forming units per milliliter (CFU/mL), which was measured using a hemocytometer [30].

4.3. Determination of MIC and MFC of Octominin for C. albicans

The MIC and MFC levels of Octominin on *C. albicans* were determined using the broth microdilution susceptibility test and subculture, respectively according to the guidelines of the Clinical and Laboratory Standards Institute (CLSI, 2008 M27-A3). Different concentrations (0–200 μg/mL) of Octominin were tested with 10 μg/mL nystatin (Sigma-Aldrich, Saint Louis, USA) as a standard antifungal drug (positive control) [33]. The MIC was determined as the minimal concentration required to inhibit the visual growth of *C. albicans*. The MFC was determined by sub-culturing 10 μL of the medium collected from the wells showing no microscopic growth after 48 h on PDA medium plates, representing the lowest concentration that yielded no colonies after 24 h growth on agar. The calculated MFC/MIC ratio was used to determine whether the AMPs Octominin had more fungistatic (MFC/MIC ≥ 4) or fungicidal (MFC/MIC < 4) activity according to previously reported criteria [34]. For the time kill kinetic analysis, *C. albicans* (10^6 CFU/mL) was incubated with Octominin at various concentrations (0–100 μg/mL) in PDB at 30 °C, and the inhibitory effects were investigated after incubation at different time intervals (0, 3, 6, 9, 12, 15, 18, and 21 h) by measuring the absorbance at 600 nm using a microplate reader (Bio-Rad, Saint Louis, USA). The time–kill analysis experiment was performed in triplicate.

4.4. Determination of the Effect of Octominin on C. albicans Cell Viability

The effects of Octominin on the viability of *C. albicans* were tested by MTT assay as described by Dananjaya et al. [30]. In brief, *C. albicans* was cultured in PDB (1×10^6 CFU/mL) and treated with the different concentrations of Octominin at 30 °C for 24 h in a shaking incubator at 180 rpm. The culture was then centrifuged at 3500 rpm for 10 min and the cells were washed with PBS. For the cell viability assay, *C. albicans* cells were reacted with 20 μL of MTT reagent (Sigma Aldrich, Saint Louis, USA) for 30 min, and the samples were re-suspended with dimethyl sulfoxide (Sigma Aldrich, Saint Louis City, USA). The cell viability was calculated based on the OD at 570 nm using a microplate reader (Bio- Rad, Saint Louis, USA).

4.5. Analysis of Morphological Changes of C. albicans upon Octominin Treatment

To investigate the effect of Octominin on the cell morphology of *C. albicans*, FE-SEM analysis was conducted as described by Dananjaya et al. [30] with some modifications. *C. albicans* cells (10^6 CFU/mL) were treated with Octominin at the MIC (50 μg/mL) and MFC (200 μg/mL) for 6 h. As a control, *C. albicans* cells were left untreated and cultured for the same period. The cells were pelleted, washed with PBS, and prefixed with 2.5% glutaraldehyde for 30 min. The prefixed cells were then washed with PBS, and serially (30%, 50%, 70%, 80%, 90%, and 100%) dehydrated using ethanol. The fixed cells were dried and coated with platinum using an ion sputter (E-1030, Hitachi, Japan). Treated and control *C. albicans* cells were observed by FE-SEM (Sirion FEI, Eindhoven, The Netherlands).

4.6. Determination of the Effect of Octominin on the Membrane Permeability of C. albicans

To determine the effect of Octominin on membrane permeability, a PI uptake assay was conducted as described by Dananjaya et al. [30]. PI is a red-fluorescent nuclear and chromosome counterstain that indicates changes of cell membrane permeability, and is commonly used to detect the presence of dead cells. Octominin-treated (MIC; 50 μg/mL and MFC; 200 μg/mL levels) and control cell suspensions of *C. albicans* were centrifuged (5000 rpm for 2 min) and the pellets were resuspended in PBS. The cells were then incubated with 5 μg/mL of PI (Sigma Aldrich, Saint Louis, USA) at 30 °C for 15 min in the dark, and then the excess stain was washed with PBS. Finally, one drop of each suspension was placed on a cover slip, and fluorescence images were observed using a CLSM with a scan head integrated to the Axiovert 200 M inverted microscope (Carl Zeiss, Jena, Germany). The PI fluorescence emission was recorded at 585 nm.

4.7. Effect of Octominin on ROS Production in C. albicans

Accumulation of ROS in *C. albicans* was quantified using fluorescent probe carboxy-H2DCF-DA (Invitrogen, Carlsbad, USA). In brief, *C. albicans* culture (10^6 CFU/mL) was treated with Octominin (MIC; 50 µg/mL and MFC; 200 µg/mL) and incubated at 30 °C for 6 h. The cells were then harvested by centrifugation at 5000 rpm for 2 min. To detect ROS levels, the cells were stained with H_2DCF-DA (30 µg/mL) and incubated for 30 min at room temperature (24 ± 1 °C) followed by centrifugation at 5000 rpm for 2 min. The cells were washed with ×1 PBS and the dichloro-fluorescein (DCF) fluorescence was measured using CLSM (LSM5 Live Configuration Variotwo VRGB, Zeiss, Germany) at an excitation wavelength of 488 nm and an emission wavelength of 535 nm.

4.8. Analysis of Octominin Cytotoxicity on Mammalian Cells

To determine the cytotoxicity of Octominin, HEK293T cells (American Type Culture Collection ATCC-11268) were treated with Octominin, and the cell viability was assessed. In brief, HEK293T cells were seeded in Dulbecco's modified Eagle's medium (Invitrogen, Carlsbad, USA) with 1% antibiotic/antimycotic solution (Glibco, Carlsbad, USA) and 10% fetal bovine serum (Hyclone, Carlsbad, USA). The cells were then seeded in 96-well flat bottom microtiter plates at a density of 1.5×10^4 cells per well with 100 µL of medium, and incubated at 37 °C in a 5% CO_2 atmosphere. After 24 h of culture, the medium was aspirated out, and the cells were washed with PBS. Each well was treated with different Octominin concentrations (0–100 µg/mL). Untreated cells were used as a control. Ultimately, cell viability was determined at 48 h post treatment using EZ-Cytox Enhanced cell viability assay kit (DoGenBio Co., Seoul, Korea) following the manufacturer's protocol.

4.9. In Vivo Efficacy of Octominin upon C. albicans Infection in a Zebrafish Model

4.9.1. Zebrafish Husbandry

All zebrafish experiments were conducted in accordance with the institutional animal ethics guidelines and under supervision and approval of the committees of Chungnam National University (CNU-00866). Wild-type AB zebrafish were maintained under standard culturing conditions using an automated water recirculating system (14 h:10 h light:dark cycle at 28 ± 0.5 °C, conductivity of 500 + 50 µS/sm, feeding equivalent to 4% of their body weight per day) throughout the experimental period.

4.9.2. Determination of In Vivo Efficacy of Octominin upon *C. albicans* Infection

The effectiveness of Octominin as an antifungal agent was tested using a zebrafish model of *C. albicans* infection according to the method described by Kulatunga et al. [35]. In brief, a total of 18 zebrafish (average weight: 0.35 ± 0.05 g) were divided into three groups: (1) Uninfected control with water treatment (Control), (2) *C. albicans* infected and water treated (Water treated), and (3) *C. albicans*-infected and Octominin-treated (Octominin-treated). The fish were anesthetized using system water containing 160 µg/mL of buffered tricaine (Ethyl 3-aminobenzoate methanesulfonate). *C. albicans* (4 µL) was injected intramuscularly into the dorsal muscle of the water-treated and Octominin-treated zebrafish groups at a dose of 1×10^6 cells/fish using Hamilton®syring (10 µL). Fish in the control group were injected with 4 µL of autoclaved distilled water. Twenty microliters of Octominin (100 µg/fish) was treated to the fish as a topical application by placing it at the site of fungal injection. Treatment was administered after the infection (0 h) and then every 24 hpi up to 72 hpi. After the treatment, fish were kept outside for 3 min to allow for Octominin absorption to the infection site and then released back to the aquarium tanks. The water-treated group received the same treatment but with the same volume of water. All fish were kept in individual tanks during the experiment period. To confirm the antifungal effect of Octominin, photographs of both the water- and Octominin-treated fish were acquired for comparing the infected/healed area at 24, 48, and 72 hpi. For histological examinations, fish were euthanized with an over dose of tricaine, and then the muscle tissues at the infection site were collected and preserved in 10% neutral buffered formalin for 24 h. Formalin fixed muscle tissues were processed

(Leica® TP1020 Semi-enclosed Benchtop Tissue Processor, Nussloch, Germany), embedded (Leica EG1150 Tissue Embedding Center, Nussloch, Germany), and sectioned into 4 µm thickness (Leica RM2125 microtome, Nussloch, Germany). The tissue samples were stained by standard PAS staining. Briefly, the sections were deparaffinized in xylene, and rehydrated in a series of ethanol using, distilled water. The sections were then treated with periodic acid (0.5 mg/mL), washed well in distilled water, and stained with Schiff's reagent. Stained sections were then washed well in fast running lukewarm tap water, the nuclei were stained with hematoxylin, and the sections were rinsed in tap water followed by differentiation in acid alcohol and bluing in Scott's tap water. Finally, the sections were dehydrated in a series of ethanol, cleared in xylene, and mounted with a xylene based medium. Sections were examined under a light microscope (Leica 3000 LED, Wetzlar, Germany) and the images were captured with a Leica DCF450-C camera (400×).

4.10. Statistical Analysis

All experimental data were analyzed using GraphPad Prism software version 5 (GraphPad Software Inc., La Jolla, USA). One way of analysis of variance and unpaired two-tailed t-test were performed to find the significant ($P < 0.05$) differences between controls and peptide treated samples and the data are presented as means ± standard deviations for replicates.

Supplementary Materials: The following are available online at http://www.mdpi.com/1660-3397/18/1/56/s1, Supplementary Figure S1.

Author Contributions: Conceptualization, funding acquisition, project administration, resources, supervision, writing—review and editing, I.W.; Conceptualization, methodology, project administration, supervision, Writing—review and editing, M.D.Z.; Formal analysis, investigation, writing—original draft, C.N.; Formal analysis, investigation, S.H.S.D.; Formal analysis, investigation, H.P.S.U.C. All authors have read and agree to the published version of the manuscript.

Acknowledgments: This work was supported by the Research Program of the National Marine Biodiversity Institute of Korea (MABIK2020M00600)) funded by the Ministry of Oceans and Fisheries and by the National Research Foundation of Korea (NRF) grant funded by the Korea government (MSIT) (2019R1A2C1087028).

Conflicts of Interest: The authors declare that they have no conflict of interest.

References

1. De Alteriis, E.; Maselli, V.; Falanga, A.; Galdiero, S.; Di Lella, F.M.; Gesuele, R.; Guida, M.; Galdiero, E. Efficiency of gold nanoparticles coated with the antimicrobial peptide indolicidin against biofilm formation and development of *Candida* spp. clinical isolates. *Infect. Drug Resist.* **2018**, *11*, 915–925. [CrossRef] [PubMed]
2. Manohar, V.; Ingram, C.; Gray, J.; Talpur, N.A.; Echard, B.W.; Bagchi, D.; Preuss, H.G. Antifungal activities of origanum oil against *Candida albicans*. *Mol. Cell Biochem.* **2001**, *228*, 111–117. [CrossRef] [PubMed]
3. Amigo-Benavent, M.; Wang, S.; Mateos, R.; Sarriá, B.; Bravo, L. Antiproliferative and cytotoxic effects of green coffee and yerba mate extracts, their main hydroxycinnamic acids, methylxanthine and metabolites in different human cell lines. *Food Chem. Toxicol.* **2017**, *106*, 125–138. [CrossRef]
4. Lee, W.; Lee, D.G. A novel mechanism of fluconazole: Fungicidal activity through dose-dependent apoptotic responses in *Candida albicans*. *Microbiology* **2018**, *164*, 194–204. [CrossRef]
5. Samaranayake, Y.H.; Cheung, B.P.K.; Wang, Y.; Yau, J.Y.Y.; Yeung, K.W.S.; Samaranayake, L.P. Fluconazole resistance in *Candida glabrata* is associated with modification of its virulence attributes. *J. Med. Microbiol.* **2012**, *62*, 303–318. [CrossRef]
6. Pfaller, M.A. Antifungal drug resistance: Mechanisms, epidemiology, and consequences for treatment. *Am. J. Med.* **2012**, *125*, 3–13. [CrossRef]
7. Zhang, L.; Gallo, R.L. Antimicrobial peptides. *Curr. Biol.* **2016**, *26*, R1–R21. [CrossRef]
8. Giuliani, A.; Pirri, G.; Nicoletto, S.F. Antimicrobial peptides: An overview of a promising class of therapeutics. *Cent. Eur. J. Biol.* **2007**, *2*, 1–33. [CrossRef]
9. Lai, Y.; Gallo, R.L. AMPed up immunity: How antimicrobial peptides have multiple roles in immune defense. *Trends Immunol.* **2009**, *30*, 131–141. [CrossRef] [PubMed]

10. López-Abarrategui, C.; Alba, A.; Silva, O.N.; Reyes-Acosta, O.; Vasconcelos, I.M.; Oliveira, J.T.; Migliolo, L.; Costa, M.P.; Costa, C.R.; Silva, M.R.; et al. Functional characterization of a synthetic hydrophilic antifungal peptide derived from the marine snail *Cenchritis muricatus*. *Biochimie* **2012**, *94*, 968–974. [CrossRef] [PubMed]
11. Silphaduang, U.; Noga, E.J. Peptide antibiotics in mast cells of fish. *Nature* **2001**, *414*, 268. [CrossRef] [PubMed]
12. Scott, M.G.; Yan, H.; Hancock, R.E. Biological properties of structurally related α-helical cationic antimicrobial peptides. *Infect. Immun.* **1999**, *67*, 2005–2009. [PubMed]
13. Gallo, R.L.; Ono, M.; Povsic, T.; Page, C.; Eriksson, E.; Klagsbrun, M.; Bernfield, M. Syndecans, cell surface heparan sulfate proteoglycans, are induced by a proline-rich antimicrobial peptide from wounds. *Proc. Natl. Acad. Sci. USA* **1994**, *91*, 11035–11039. [CrossRef] [PubMed]
14. De Zoysa, M.; Nikapitiya, C.; Whang, I.; Lee, J.S.; Lee, J. Abhisin: A potential antibacterial peptide derived from histone H2A of disk abalone. *Fish Shellfish Immun.* **2009**, *27*, 639–646. [CrossRef]
15. Ribeiro, S.F.; Carvalho, A.O.; Da Cunha, M.; Rodrigues, R.; Cruz, L.P.; Melo, V.M.; Vasconcelos, I.M.; Melo, E.J.; Gomes, V.M. Isolation and characterization of novel peptides from chilli pepper seeds: Antimicrobial activities against pathogenic yeasts. *Toxicon* **2007**, *50*, 600–611. [CrossRef]
16. Ye, X.Y.; Ng, T.B. Isolation of a new cyclophilin-like protein from chickpeas with mitogenic, antifungal and anti-HIV-1 reverse transcriptase activities. *Life Sci.* **2002**, *70*, 1129–1138. [CrossRef]
17. Chia, T.J.; Wu, Y.C.; Chen, J.Y.; Chi, S.C. Antimicrobial peptides (AMP) with antiviral activity against fish nodavirus. *Fish Shellfish Immunol.* **2010**, *28*, 434–439. [CrossRef]
18. Park, Y.; Jang, S.H.; Lee, D.G.; Hahm, K.S. Antinematodal effect of antimicrobial peptide, PMAP-23, isolated from porcine myeloid against *Caenorhabditis elegans*. *J. Pept. Sci.* **2004**, *10*, 304–311. [CrossRef]
19. Hancock, R.E.W.; Diamond, G. The role of cationic antimicrobial peptides in innate host defences. *Trends Microbiol.* **2000**, *8*, 402–410. [CrossRef]
20. Park, S.C.; Kim, J.Y.; Jeong, C.; Yoo, S.; Hahm, K.S.; Park, Y. A plausible mode of action of pseudin-2, an antimicrobial peptide from *Pseudis paradoxa*. *Biochim. Biophys. Acta.* **2011**, *1808*, 171–182. [CrossRef]
21. Yeaman, M.R.; Yount, N.Y. Mechanisms of antimicrobial peptide action and resistance. *Pharmacol. Rev.* **2003**, *55*, 27–55. [CrossRef] [PubMed]
22. Diehnelt, C.W. Peptide array based discovery of synthetic antimicrobial peptides. *Front. Microbiol.* **2013**, *4*, 402. [CrossRef] [PubMed]
23. Wang, Z.; Wang, G. APD: The antimicrobial peptide database. *Nucleic Acids Res.* **2004**, *32*, D590–D592. [CrossRef] [PubMed]
24. De Zoysa, M. Chapter 35: Antimicrobial Peptides in Marine Mollusks and their Potential Applications. In *Marine Proteins and Peptides: Biological Activities and Applications*, 1st ed.; Wiley-Blackwell: Chichester, UK, 2013; pp. 695–707.
25. Iijima, N.; Tanimoto, N.; Emoto, Y.; Morita, Y.; Uematsu, K.; Murakami, T.; Nakai, T. Purification and characterization of three isoforms of chrysophsin, a novel antimicrobial peptide in the gills of the red sea bream, *Chrysophrys major*. *Eur. J. Biochem.* **2003**, *270*, 675–686. [CrossRef] [PubMed]
26. Lee, D.G.; Kim, D.H.; Park, Y.; Kim, H.K.; Kim, H.N.; Shin, Y.K.; Choi, C.H.; Hahm, K.S. Fungicidal Effect of Antimicrobial Peptide, PMAP-23, Isolated from Porcine Myeloid against *Candida albicans*. *Biochem. Biophys. Res. Commun.* **2001**, *282*, 570–574. [CrossRef]
27. Nikawa, H.; Fukushima, H.; Makihira, S.; Hamada, T.; Samaranayake, L.P. Fungicidal effect of three new synthetic cationic peptides against *Candida albicans*. *Oral Dis.* **2004**, *10*, 221–228. [CrossRef]
28. Bellamy, W.; Wakabayashi, H.; Takase, M.; Kawase, K.; Shimamura, S.; Tomita, M. Killing of *Candida albicans* by lactoferricin B, a potent antimicrobial peptide derived from the N-terminal region of bovine lactoferrin. *Med. Microbiol. Immunol.* **1993**, *182*, 97–105. [CrossRef]
29. Lee, D.G.; Park, Y.; Kim, H.N.; Kim, H.K.; Kim, P.I.; Choi, B.H.; Hahm, K.S. Antifungal mechanism of an antimicrobial peptide, HP (2-20), derived from N-terminus of *Helicobacter pylori* ribosomal protein L1 against *Candida albicans*. *Biochim. Biophys. Research Commun.* **2002**, *291*, 1006–1013. [CrossRef]
30. Dananjaya, S.H.S.; Udayangani, R.M.C.; Oh, C.; Nikapitiya, C.; Lee, J.; De Zoysa, M. Green synthesis, physio-chemical characterization and anti-candidal function of a biocompatible chitosan gold nanocomposite as a promising antifungal therapeutic agent. *RSC Adv.* **2017**, *7*, 9182–9193. [CrossRef]

31. Maurya, I.K.; Pathak, S.; Sharma, M.; Sanwal, H.; Chaudhary, P.; Tupe, S.; Deshpande, M.; Chauhan, V.S.; Prasad, R. Antifungal activity of novel synthetic peptides by accumulation of reactive oxygen species (ROS) and disruption of cell wall against *Candida albicans*. *Peptides* **2011**, *32*, 1732–1740. [CrossRef]
32. Veerman, E.C.; Nazmi, K.; Van't Hof, W.; Bolscher, J.G.; Den Hertog, A.L.; Nieuw Amerongen, A.V. Reactive oxygen species play no role in the candidacidal activity of the salivary antimicrobial peptide histatin 5. *Biochem. J.* **2004**, *381*, 447–452. [CrossRef] [PubMed]
33. Kavanagh, K.; Dowd, S. Histatins: Antimicrobial peptides with therapeutic potential. *J. Pharm. Pharmacol.* **2004**, *56*, 285–289. [CrossRef] [PubMed]
34. Peixoto, L.R.; Rosalen, P.L.; Ferreira, G.L.; Freires, I.A.; de Carvalho, F.G.; Castellano, L.R.; de Castro, R.D. Antifungal activity, mode of action and anti-biofilm effects of *Laurus nobilis* Linnaeus essential oil against Candida spp. *Arch. Oral Biol.* **2017**, *73*, 179–185. [CrossRef] [PubMed]
35. Kulatunga, D.C.M.; Dananjaya, S.H.S.; Godahewa, G.I.; Lee, J.; De Zoysa, M. Chitosan silver nanocomposite (CAgNC) as an antifungal agent against *Candida albicans*. *Med. Mycol.* **2017**, *55*, 213–222. [CrossRef] [PubMed]

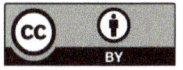

© 2020 by the authors. Licensee MDPI, Basel, Switzerland. This article is an open access article distributed under the terms and conditions of the Creative Commons Attribution (CC BY) license (http://creativecommons.org/licenses/by/4.0/).

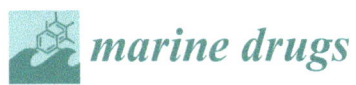

Review

Marine-Derived Natural Lead Compound Disulfide-Linked Dimer Psammaplin A: Biological Activity and Structural Modification

Qinxue Jing [1,†], Xu Hu [1,†], Yanzi Ma [1], Jiahui Mu [1], Weiwei Liu [2], Fanxing Xu [2], Zhanlin Li [1], Jiao Bai [1,*], Huiming Hua [1,*] and Dahong Li [1,*]

1. Key Laboratory of Structure-Based Drug Design & Discovery, Ministry of Education, School of Traditional Chinese Materia Medica, Shenyang Pharmaceutical University, Shenyang 110016, China
2. Wuya College of Innovation, Shenyang Pharmaceutical University, Shenyang 110016, China
* Correspondence: baijiao@hotmail.com (J.B.); huimhua@163.com (H.H.); lidahong0203@163.com (D.L.); Tel.: +86-24-23986465 (J.B., H.H. & D.L.)
† These authors contributed equally to this work.

Received: 21 May 2019; Accepted: 25 June 2019; Published: 27 June 2019

Abstract: Marine natural products are considered to be valuable resources that are furnished with diverse chemical structures and various bioactivities. To date, there are seven compounds derived from marine natural products which have been approved as therapeutic drugs by the U.S. Food and Drug Administration. Numerous bromotyrosine derivatives have been isolated as a type of marine natural products. Among them, psammaplin A, including the oxime groups and carbon–sulfur bonds, was the first identified symmetrical bromotyrosine-derived disulfide dimer. It has been found to have a broad bioactive spectrum, especially in terms of antimicrobial and antiproliferative activities. The highest potential indole-derived psammaplin A derivative, UVI5008, is used as an epigenetic modulator with multiple enzyme inhibitory activities. Inspired by these reasons, psammaplin A has gradually become a research focus for pharmacologists and chemists. To the best of our knowledge, there is no systematic review about the biological activity and structural modification of psammaplin A. In this review, the pharmacological effects, total synthesis, and synthesized derivatives of psammaplin A are summarized.

Keywords: psammaplin A; marine natural product; biological activity; structural modification

1. Introduction

Accumulating evidence indicates that natural products isolated from plants, animals, and microorganisms have played irreplaceable roles in the development of new drugs for human therapeutics [1–9]. It is noteworthy that marine natural products are considered to be extremely valuable resources of natural products and are furnished with diverse chemical structures and various bioactivities [10–12]. With the rapid development of technologies of scuba diving and marine prospection, great interest has been shown in unexplored marine natural products, which are considered to be potential sources for drug discovery [13–16]. To date, seven compounds derived from marine natural products, including cytarabine [17], vidarabine [18], ziconotide [19], omega-3 acid ethyl esters [20], eribulin mesylate [21], brentuximab vedotin [22], and *iota*-carrageenan [17], have been approved as therapeutic drugs by the U.S. Food and Drug Administration. The symmetrical disulfide dimer psammaplin A (**1**, Figure 1), belonging to open-chain α-oximinoamidesis, was originally isolated from *Psammaplysilla* (revised to *Pseudoceratina*) sp. and an unidentified sponge in 1987 [23–25], which represents the first isolated natural product containing oxime and disulfide moieties from marine sponge. Subsequently, biprasin, psammaplin C, psammaplin E, psammaplin F, psammaplin G, and psammaplin K (Figure 1) were also obtained [26–29]. Of these compounds, psammaplin A has attracted much attention because of its strong antimicrobial and cytostatic properties. Psammaplin A displays antibacterial activity mainly against *Staphylococcus aureus* (SA) and methicillin-resistant *Staphylococcus aureus* (MRSA) due to DNA gyrase inhibition and bacterial DNA synthesis arrest [30]. It was also reported that psammaplin A possesses antiproliferative activities against various cancer cell lines, including triple-negative breast (TNBC, MDA-MB-231), doxorubicin-resistant human breast (MCF-7/adr), colon (HCT15), ovarian (SK-OV-3), lung (A549, LM4175), bone (BoM1833), endometria, brain (BrM-2a), skin (SK-MEL-2), and central nervous system (XF498) cancer cell lines [29,31–34]. Additionally, the bactericidal and cytotoxic effects of psammaplin A were related to multiple enzyme inhibition, such as DNA gyrase [30], topoisomerase II [35], chitinase [36], farnesyl protein transferase [37], mycothiol-*S*-conjugate amidase [38], leucine aminopeptidase [37], DNA polymerase α-primase [39], aminopeptidase N [40], and especially potent inhibitory effects on histone deacetylases (HDAC) and DNA methyltransferase (DNMT) enzymes [28]. These enzymes exert extremely important roles in the epigenetic regulation of gene expression. Moreover, psammaplin A also exhibits potent enzyme inhibitory and antiproliferative activities under reduced conditions in cells, which indicates that psammaplin A could be used as a natural prodrug [41]. Although psammaplin A possesses a broad spectrum of bioactivities, its in-depth study has been hindered due to the limited amount of the compound that can be isolated from marine microorganism sources, as well its poor physiological stability. Inspired by this, many research groups have carried out its total synthesis and synthesis of derivatives. For example, the most potential indole-derived psammaplin A derivative, UVI5008 (Figure 1), was used as an epigenetic modulator with multiple enzyme inhibitory activities [42].

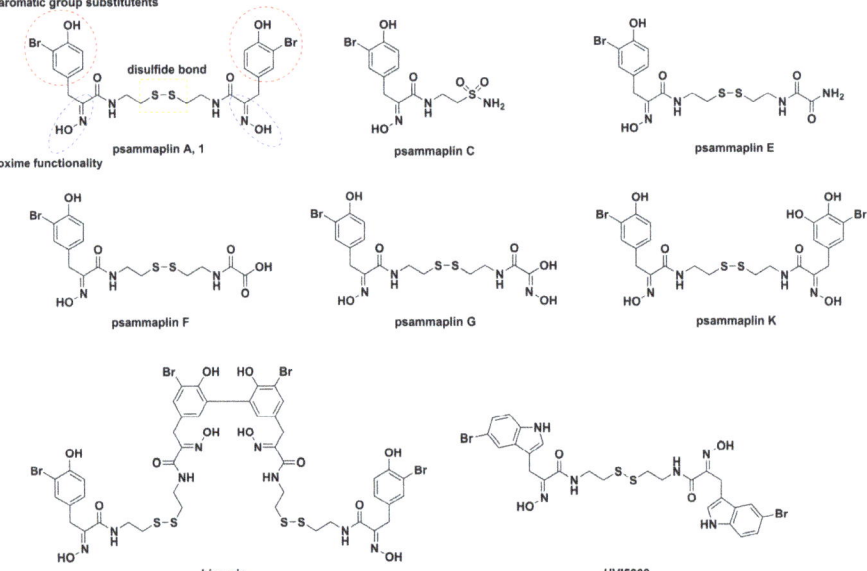

Figure 1. The chemical structure of psammaplin compounds, biprasin and UVI5008.

Over the last two decades, more than ten reviews have covered the field of marine natural products from various distinct viewpoints [43–57]. Hentschel et al. published an excellent paper on the synthesis of oximinotyrosine-derived marine natural products, including psammaplin A, covering the literature until 2009 [43]. Therefore, the synthetic methods of psammaplin A summarized in this review are those reported after 2009. In addition, structural modification work, structure–activity relationships, and further mechanistic studies of psammaplin A in the field of antibacterial activity and cytotoxicity have been studied by some research groups; these studies consistently confirm that the disulfide bond and the oxime moieties are indispensable for the bioactivities of psammaplin A. However, there is no systematic review of the biological activity and structural modification of psammaplin A. Thus, in this review, the pharmacological effects, total synthesis, and derivatives of psammaplin A are summarized.

2. Synthetic Chemistry

Although psammaplin A possesses a broad bioactive spectrum, its in-depth study has been hindered due to the limited amount of the compound that can be isolated from marine microorganism sources. Consequently, many research groups have carried out its total synthesis. To the best of our knowledge, Hentschel et al. have summarized the total synthesis of psammaplin A, covering the literature until 2009 [43]. Therefore, here, we update the total synthesis methods.

Psammaplin A (**1**, Figure 1) consists of a symmetrical disulfide with a cystamine linker functionalized on both sides by tyrosine-derived α-(hydroxyimino)acyl moieties [58]. Briefly, the conventional total synthesis method of psammaplin A is initiated from tyrosine or phenylpyruvic acid derivatives [59–62]. Then, the Lindel group optimized the synthetic method of psammaplin A through the Horner–Wadsworth–Emmons (HWE) route (Scheme 1) [63]. The intermediate **4** was synthesized by the HWE reaction of phosphonate **3** with aldehyde **2**, then oxime **5** was formed after desilylation of **4** under the condition of NEt$_3$·3HF. Debenzylation of **5** in the presence of H$_2$/Pd–C gave the hydroxyimino isomers; later, methyl ester saponification with lithium hydroxide obtained acid **6**. Finally, the esterification of **6** with two equivalents of cystamine dihydrochloride under the condition of NEt$_3$, DCC, and N-hydroxysuccinimide (NHS) in DMF generated the natural product psammaplin A.

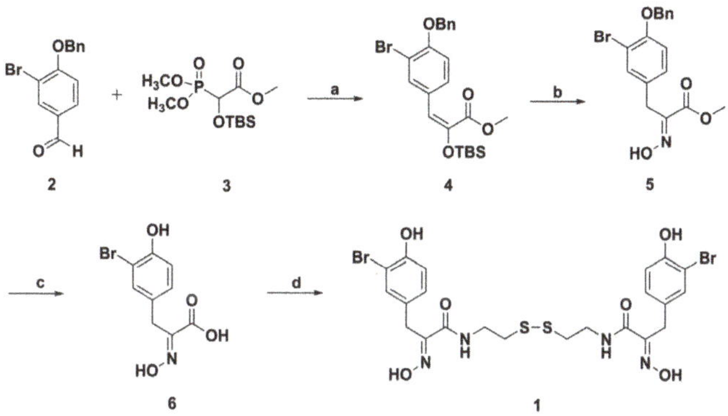

Scheme 1. Synthesis route of psammaplin A by the Lindel group. Reagents and conditions: (**a**) LDA, THF, −78 °C, 15 h; (**b**) NEt$_3$·3HF, MeOH, rt, 30 min; (**c**) (i) H$_2$, Pd/C, dioxane, rt, 41 h; (ii) LiOH·H$_2$O, THF/H$_2$O, rt, 40 h; (**d**) cystamine dihydrochloride, NHS, DCC, Et$_3$N, DMF, rt, 15 h.

The Harburn group reported another synthetic route starting from the benzaldehyde **2** (Scheme 2) [64]. Firstly, **2** was converted to benzylidene rhodanine **7** in excellent yield. Then, hydrolysis, acidification, and oximation of **7** afforded O-benzyl protected oximino acid **8**. The coupling of **8** with cystamine generated sponge metabolite **9** protected by the benzyl group. Finally, deprotection of **9** proceeded successfully in CH$_2$Cl$_2$ using TMSI to provide psammaplin A.

The Park group developed a new efficient and concise synthetic method for preparing psammaplin A (Scheme 3) [65,66]. Initially, the α,β-unsaturated ester **11** was obtained by Knoevenagel condensation of 4-hydroxybenzaldehyde (**10**) with ethyl acetoacetate using acetic acid and piperidine. Then the catalytic hydrogenation of **11** generated compound **12** through Pd/C and H$_2$ in methanol. The bromination of **12** with KBrO$_3$ and KBr in methanol under the condition of 0.5 M-HCl provided **13**. The treatment of n-butylnitrite with **13** in ethanol under the condition of sodium ethoxide at 0 °C yielded α-NO substituted **13** analogue. After α-nitrosation, the fragmentation initiated by addition of ethoxide anion to the acetyl group led to ethyl acetate release, followed by rearrangement to obtain the α-oxime ester **14**. The oxime hydroxyl group of **14** was protected with dihydropyran (DHP) under the condition of catalytic amount *p*-toluenesulfonic acid (PTSA) to obtain **15**. Then, **15** was hydrolyzed to the acid **16** with 1 N potassium hydroxide in ethanol. **16** and *N*-hydroxyphthalimide were coupled under the condition of EDC in 1,4-dioxane to synthesize **17**, followed by adding cystamine to afford the THP-protected psammaplin A. Finally, the THP-protected psammaplin A was deprotected in the presence of the solution of methanolic hydrochloride to get psammaplin A.

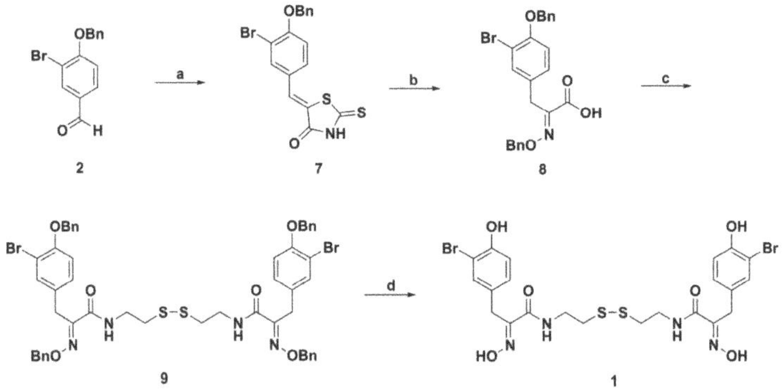

Scheme 2. Synthesis route of psammaplin A of the Harburn Group. Reagents and conditions: (**a**) Rhodanine, NH$_4$OAc, toluene, reflux; or Rhodanine, NaOAc, AcOH, reflux; (**b**) (i) NaOH, H$_2$O; (ii) HCl (10%), 0 °C; (iii) HCl·NH$_2$OBn, NaOAc, EtOH, 70 °C; (**c**) cystamine dihydrochloride, EDC, HOBt, Et$_3$N, CH$_2$Cl$_2$; (**d**) TMSI, CH$_2$Cl$_2$.

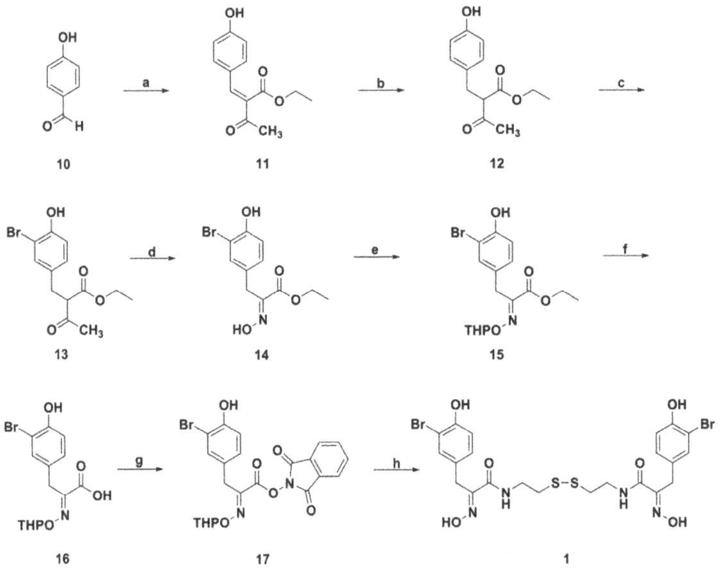

Scheme 3. Synthesis route of psammaplin A of the Park group. Reagents and conditions: (**a**) ethyl acetoacetate, piperidine, AcOH; (**b**) H$_2$, Pd/C, MeOH; (**c**) KBrO$_3$, KBr, 0.5 M-HCl, MeOH; (**d**) *n*-BuONO, AcOEt, NaOEt, EtOH, 0 °C; (**e**) DHP, PTSA, CH$_2$Cl$_2$; (**f**) 1 N-KOH, EtOH; (**g**) *N*-hydroxyphthalimide, EDC, 1,4-dioxane; (**h**) (i) cystamine, Et$_3$N, MeOH, 1,4-dioxane; (ii) 1 N HCl/Et$_2$O CH$_2$Cl$_2$/MeOH.

3. Pharmacological Activity

The pharmacological activities of psammaplin A and its derivatives include antibacterial, antiviral, anticancer, insecticidal, embryo development promotive, chemical defensive eryptosis inducing, and anticancer activities. These works can be classified as follows.

3.1. Antimicrobial Activity

Sortase enzymes, transpeptidases from Gram-positive bacteria, are responsible for anchoring surface protein virulence factors to the peptidoglycan cell wall layer. In Gram-positive SA, sortase isoform deletion results in significant reduction in infection potential and virulence. Psammaplin A showed potent inhibition of Sortase A and B, and adhesion of SA cells to fibronectin (Figure 2) [67].

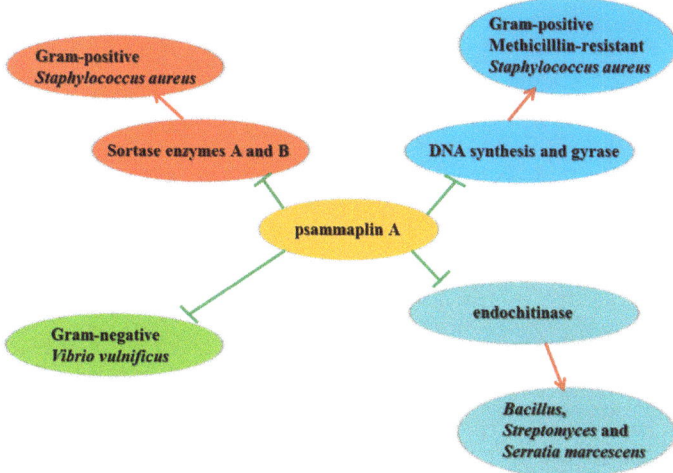

Figure 2. Schematic representation of the antimicrobial activity of psammaplin A.

The threat of multidrug-resistant bacterial strains against human health is increasing, and a large number of people die every year from the spread of resistant strains. Studies by Kim et al. showed that psammaplin A could inhibit Gram-positive bacteria, such as MRSA. Psammaplin A inhibited DNA synthesis with an IC_{50} value of 2.83 μg/mL, and DNA gyrase activity with an IC_{50} value of 100 μg/mL. [30]. Franci et al. screened a group of previously identified epigenetic regulators, and some could change the growth of Gram-positive bacteria. UVI5008 (Figure 1), a derivative of psammaplin A, was identified. The growth inhibition activity against MRSA was caused by cell wall modification [68].

Lee et al. measured the inhibition of Gram-negative *Vibrio vulnificus* (*V. vulnificus*)-induced cytotoxicity by 12 compounds from natural seafood in intestinal epithelial cells (INT-407). The results showed that psammaplin A significantly inhibited *V. vulnificus*-induced cytotoxicity, which indicated that psammaplin A could be developed for the prevention and treatment of *V. vulnificus* infection [69].

Tabudravu et al. tested the chitinase inhibition activity of psammaplin A in *Bacillus*, *Streptomyces*, and *Serratia marcescens*. The results showed that psammaplin A noncompetitively inhibited endochitinase activity with IC_{50} values of ranging from 50 to 100 μM [36].

3.2. Antiviral Activity

As a chronic infectious disease, hepatitis C can cause liver cancer; NS3 nucleoside triphosphatase (NTPase)/helicase plays an important role in hepatitis C virus (HCV) replication. Salam et al. screened inhibitors of NS3 helicase from marine organism extracts by a photo-induced electron transfer (PET) system. Psammaplin A showed the apparent Km value of 0.4 μM of NS3 ATPase activity which indicated no influence. The inhibitory effect of psammaplin A on viral replication was verified by experiments and it can be used as a potential antiviral agent [70]. Psammaplin A also shows anti-HIV activity. Richard et al. reported that psammaplin A could induce the expression of latent HIV-1 provirus in Jurkat full-length T cell lines (clones 8.4, 9.2, and 10.6). Psammaplin A synergistically enhanced the expression of HIV-1 when combined with the protein kinase C (PKC) activator prostratin, but not the histone deacetylase inhibitor (HDACi) panobinostat, indicating its latency to be a reversing agent (LRA) to induce proviral expression [71].

3.3. Embryo Development Promotive Activity

Reprogramming of donor somatic nuclei to an omnipotent embryonic state is a major obstacle to successful cloning, and treatment of cloned embryos with epigenetic modifiers such as HDACi can improve cloning efficiency. Acting as a novel HDACi, the effects of psammaplin A on the development and quality of cloned mouse embryos were investigated by Mallol et al. The experimental results confirmed that psammaplin A increased the cloning efficiency of mice more than valproic acid (VPA) [72].

For the development of somatic cell nuclear transfer (SCNT) embryos, the embryonic stem cell (ESC)-derived rates from the obtained blastocysts and intracytoplasmic sperm injection (ICSI) fertilized embryos were determined with or without treatment of psammaplin A. The results showed that psammaplin A-treated SCNT exerted increased nuclear transfer ESC derivation and blastocyst rates, and further increased embryo delay, which was not necessarily related to the epigenetic effects [73].

3.4. Insecticidal Activity

Chitinase is an interesting target that interferes with growth and develops alternative strategies for controlling pests. Psammaplin A is a chitinase inhibitor and acts as an effective active ingredient for the termite bait program. Husen et al. evaluated the impact of psammaplin A on *Reticulitermes flavipes* (*R. flavipes*) by using a no-choice feeding bioassay of eastern underground termites. The results indicated that chitinase inhibitor psammaplin A was toxic to *R. flavipes* and induced mortality in a non-concentration-dependent manner [74]. After that, Husen et al. further designed a trial to evaluate the palatability, feeding deterrence, consumption, and subsequent mortality. Psammaplin A was incorporated into filter paper diets and the treated filter papers were used as food source or bait for termite workers used in this study. In the no-selective feeding trial, the diet consumption of termites fed a 0.3% (2–5 weeks) and 0.15% (4–5 weeks) psammaplin A treatment diet was significantly reduced. In the double selection test, termites consumed almost the same amount of diet treated with psammaplin A as an untreated diet (except for diets treated with 0.3% psammaplin A). Additionally, in the no-select bioassay, termite mortality from diets treated with chitinase inhibitors was significantly higher than in untreated diets; at the same time, the biological activity of psammaplin A-treated diets in the double-select feeding arenas was reduced by more than 50%. These results indicate that chitinase inhibitors have new potential [75].

Psammaplin A can also be used as an aphid management tool. In a previous study, Saguez et al. reported the aphicidal effects of psammaplin A. Psammaplin A reduced fecundity, increased larval mortality, and reduced body size. An artificial diet was used to provide *M. persicae* with active (1, 10, 100 and 500 μg/mL) and inactive (500 μg/mL) bacterial (*Serratia marcescens*) chitinase. These compounds increased the nymphal viability at all active chitinase doses compared to the control diet, whereas inactive chitinase cannot [76]. Afterward, four chitinase inhibitors, cyclo-(histidine-valine), cyclo-(valine-tyrosine), psammaplin A, and allosamidin, were selected for feeding experiments with *M. persicae* (Sulzer), the peach-potato aphid. Artificial feed was used to supply 10, 50, and 100 μg/mL. The results showed that psammaplin A was the most toxic compound, increasing the mortality of all aphids at 50 and 100 μg/mL [77,78].

3.5. Active Chemical Defense

Active chemical defense, which rapidly transforms precursor molecules of defensive compounds after tissue damage, is widely found in terrestrial and marine plants, but is extremely rare in marine invertebrates. Thoms et al. observed that wound activation converted psammaplin A sulfate to psammaplin A in the tissue of the tropical sponge *Aplysinella rhax*. The same group, in a feeding test of the puffer fish *Canthigaster solandri*, showed that the antifeeding activity of psammaplin A was increased compared with the sulfate, which suggested that psammaplin A possessed defensive activity. A series of observations on their response to other sponge species indicated that marine organisms may have more active defenses [79].

3.6. Eryptosis Induction Acitivity

The cellular mechanisms that stimulate eryptosis include oxidative stress, cytosolic Ca^{2+} activity ($[Ca^{2+}]_i$), and increased ceramide; Abdulla Al Mamun Bhuyan et al. found that psammaplin A increased ceramide abundance and dichlorodihydrofluorescein diacetate (DCFDA) fluorescence and triggered cell shrinkage and phospholipid scrambling of the erythrocyte cell membrane, caused by induction of oxidative stress, increase of $[Ca^{2+}]_i$, and enhanced appearance of ceramide [80].

3.7. Anticancer Effects

The underlying anticancer properties of psammaplin A may depend on its efficacy in regulating enzymes that regulate apoptosis, differentiation, invasion, proliferation, angiogenesis, and DNA replication and transcription (Figure 3). Jiang et al. found that psammaplin A showed significant cytotoxic activity against the RAW264.7 cell line and could substantially inhibit SV40 DNA replication. The polymerase α-primase was one of the main targets [39]. Psammaplin A radiosensitization of glioblastoma U-373MG and lung cancer A549 cell lines might be due to the inhibition of DNA repair [81]. Godert et al. found that psammaplin A was a potent DNMT inhibitor in vitro, but it failed to alter the level of genomic DNA methylation in treated human colon carcinoma HCT116 cells [59]. Psammaplin A also inhibited cell growth of lung cancer NCI-H226 Bap1 null cells at a concentration between 1/10,000 μL and 1/1000 μL, while exhibiting minimal toxicity to human neuroblastomal SKN cells. When CPT was added, the performance strongly indicated that psammaplin A could exert a synergetic DNA damaging effect [82]. Kim et al. reported the tissue distribution and pharmacokinetics of psammaplin A as a DNMT and HDAC inhibitor in mice. The intravenous injection dose was 10 mg/kg and psammaplin A was rapidly eliminated, with the average half-life of 9.9 min and the systemic clearance (CLs) was 925.1 ± 570.1 mL/min. Psammaplin A was highly distributed in lung tissues, with lung-to-serum partition coefficients (Kp) of 49.9 to 60.2, while the concentrations in other tissues were either comparable to or less than serum concentrations [83].

Epigenetic dysregulation is one of the causes of cancer, and epigenetic factors are condidered as therapeutic targets. Nebbioso et al. pointed out that UVI5008 was an epigenetic modifier that inhibited HDAC, DNMT, and sirtuins, which efficiently induced selective death of cancer cells and exerted its activity in genetic mouse models of human breast cancer and several human tumor xenografts. Its anticancer activity involved the activation of reactive oxygen species and death receptors. UVI5008 showed strong anticancer properties with IC_{50} values from 0.2 to 3.1 μM. It also showed activity in vivo in HCT116- or MCF-7-xenografted mice (40 mg/kg) and ex vivo in acute myeloid leukemia (AML) blasts (5 μM) [84].

Massague et al. found that psammaplin-based HDAC inhibitors differentially induced hypoxia-inducible factor 1 (hif-1) activation, inhibited HDAC activity, and disrupted the growth of organic metastatic TNBC subclones. The results showed that psammaplins significantly inhibited the growth of bone (BoM1833) tumor spheres in the 3D culture system [31]. Peroxisome proliferator-activated receptors (PPARs) are ligand-activated transcription factors which have been shown to inhibit the growth of human breast tumor cells, induce apoptosis, and promote terminal differentiation. Psammaplin A can activate PPARγ and induces apoptosis in MCF-7 cells [85].

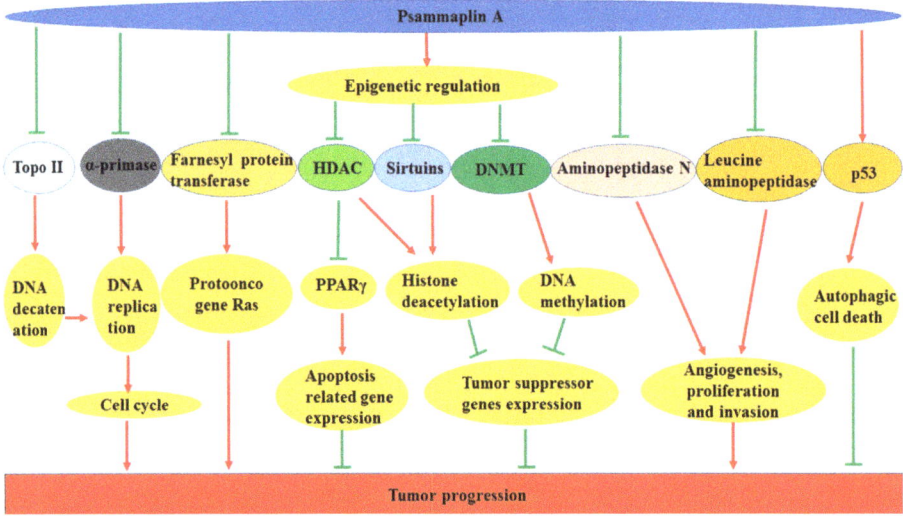

Figure 3. Schematic representation of the cytotoxic effects of psammaplin A.

Psammaplin A showed inhibitory activity in enzyme assays and antiproliferation assays with IC_{50} values of 0.003 and 1 µM, respectively. It selectively induced high acetylation of histones, resulting in upregulation of the well-known HDAC target gene gelsolin at the transcriptional level. Furthermore, the reduced psammaplin A showed stronger inhibitory activity than the unreduced one. It is noteworthy that glutathione-depleted cells were not sensitive to psammaplin A, which indicated that cellular reduction was responsible for HDAC inhibition [41]. Baud et al. also reported the cytotoxicity and enzyme inhibitory activity against recombinant HDAC1 by the active monomer (thiol) form of psammaplin A [86]. DNMT1 inhibitory activity was not found in another study [60].

In addition, psammaplin A inhibits aminopeptidase N (APN), which plays an important role in tumor progression and is involved in processes such as proliferation, adhesion, angiogenesis, and tumor invasion [40]. Psammaplin A also has the ability to inhibit mycothiol-*S*-conjugate amidase (MCA) [38], topoisomerase II [35], farnesyl protein transferase [37], and leucine aminopeptidase [37]. In addition, psammaplin C is a natural product of primary sulfonamide. Mujumdar et al. evaluated its inhibitory properties for the treatment-related carbonic anhydrase (CA) zinc metalloenzyme. At the same time, the analog psammaplin C showed unprecedented inhibition levels with a K_i of 0.79 nM of isoenzyme hCA XII. They also proposed the protein X-ray crystal structure of psammaplin C complexed with human CA and determined the binding posture with the hCA II, hCA IX, and hCA XII mimetic active sites [26]. Psammaplin C also reduced the efflux of temozolomide by P-glycoprotein and resensitizes the primary neurosphere to temozolomide. Salaroglio et al. revealed that the interaction of CA XII and Pgp could ultimately block the efflux function of Pgp to improve the prognosis of patients with glioblastoma [87].

Targeting the autophagic pathway plays a key role in chemotherapeutic approaches to treat human cancers and preventing tumor-derived chemoresistance; at the same time, some marine-derived compounds show this potency. Ratovitski et al. used psammaplin A to induce the expression of several autophagic signaling intermediates in human glioblastoma, squamous cell carcinoma, and colorectal cancer cells through transcriptional regulation by tumor protein p53 family members [34].

Psammaplin A also shows anticancer activity by inducing cell cycle arrest and apoptosis. Kim et al. reported that psammaplin A could significantly inhibit the proliferation of MCF-7/adr cells in a dose-dependent manner, and the cells arrested at the G_2/M phase [33]. Ahn et al. investigated the antitumor effect on Ishikawa endometrial human cancer cells. The results showed that psammaplin A could significantly inhibit Ishikawa cell proliferation in a dose-dependent manner. Psammaplin A significantly induced the expression of acetylated H3 and H4 histones, resulted in significant apoptosis associated with p53-independent p21WAF1 expression, and showed antiproliferative effects by selectively inducing genes involved cell cycle arrest [32].

4. Medicinal Chemistry

Inspired by the unique symmetrical structure of bromotyrosine-derived disulfide dimer scaffolds, a collection of derivatives was constructed and synthesized through structural modifications, aiming to explore potential therapeutic value and study the structure–activity relationships. With this consideration in mind, we reviewed the derivatives of psammaplin A (Figure 1) as follows, according to their different activities.

4.1. Antibacterial Derivatives

Some homodimeric and heterodimeric analogues of psammaplin A were refined by Nicolaou and coworkers utilizing combinatorial chemistry through a disulfide exchange strategy [61]. Combinatorial chemistry techniques have played an important role in the synthesis and structural activity optimization of bioactive natural products [88]. Among the synthetic homodimeric derivatives, compounds **18**, **19**, **20**, and **21** (Figure 4) showed significant antibacterial effects against MRSA. Moreover, the heterodimeric derivatives fell into three types (A–C) (Figure 5). Type A representative compound **22** consisted of two similar psammaplin-like structures. Type B representative compounds **23–26** were comprised of one psammaplin-like component conjugated to an alkyl or aryl group. Type C representative compounds **27** and **28** had no resemblance to the original psammaplin A structure. Among these heterodimeric derivatives, compounds **23–28**, with MIC values of 1.22, 2.43, 1.61, 3.90, 4.10, and 3.14 µg/mL, respectively, possessed higher antibacterial activity than psammaplin A (MIC 5.47 µg/mL). Especially, compound **23** showed similar activity to clinically used drugs vancomycin and ciprofloxacin, with MIC values of 0.83 and 0.89 µg/mL, respectively.

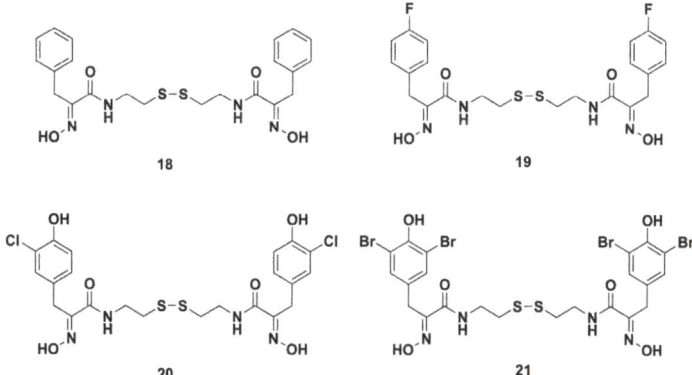

Figure 4. Chemical structures of the synthetic homodimeric derivatives **18-21**.

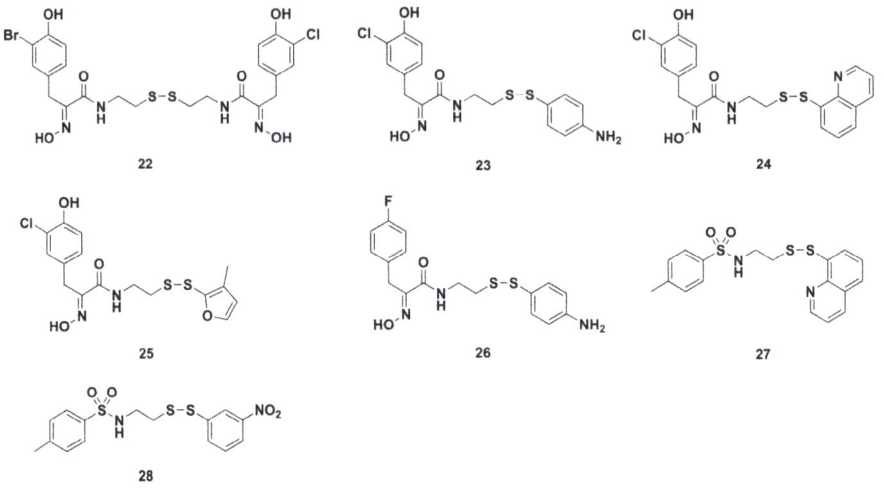

Figure 5. Chemical structures of three types of psammaplin A derivatives 22-28.

In the same year, in order to obtain better antimicrobial agents, Nicolaou and coworkers continued to optimize the heterodimeric lead compounds 23–26, mainly by studying the toxicity, potency, and nonspecific protein-binding effects through molecular design, structural modification, and mechanism of action [89]. Subsequently, a series of highly potent heterodimeric derivatives were afforded by parallel synthesis. Some representative compounds 29–33 (Figure 6) possessed 50-fold higher activities than their parent against both SA and MRSA. The average MIC values of compounds 30–33 were 0.09, 0.12, 0.29, and 0.12 µg/mL against SA, respectively, and 0.09, 0.11, 0.27, and 0.11 µg/mL against MRSA, respectively. In an in vitro toxicity assay, a therapeutic index (TI) ratio, as an estimate of the selectivity of the heterodimeric derivatives afforded the average IC_{50} value of a compound against fibroblast and lymphocyte cells, and was divided by the average MIC value against SA and MRSA strains, and the results showed that heterodimer 31, comprised of 3-bromo-phenyl alaine and 4'-fluorophenyl groups, had a good TI of 37.5, which indicated low toxicity and good selectivity. The mechanism study failed to confirm the reported inhibition of DNA gyrase [30] by psammaplin A and its derivatives. However, their studies also propose a nonspecific redox-based mechanism for these heterodimers.

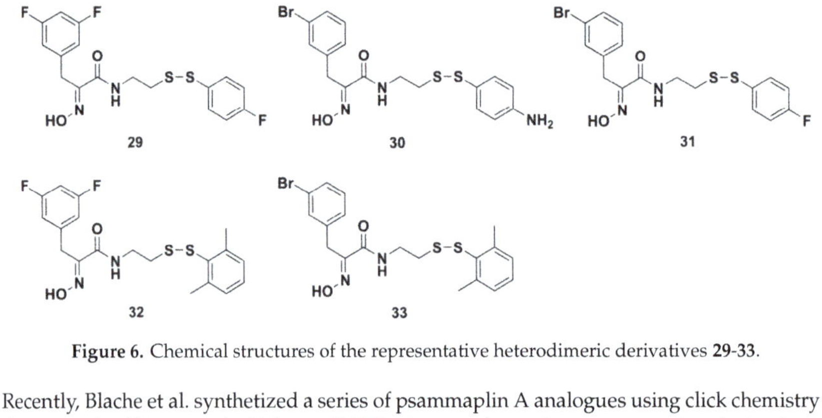

Figure 6. Chemical structures of the representative heterodimeric derivatives 29-33.

Recently, Blache et al. synthetized a series of psammaplin A analogues using click chemistry based on a framework of bis-triazole (Scheme 4) [90]. Among them, the representative derivatives of the dimethylaminoethyl chain 40 and the dimethylaminopropyl chain 41 possessed potent antibiofilm activity against three Gram-negative strains, including *Pseudoalteromonas lipolytica* (TC8), *Paracoccus* sp. Strain (4 M6), and *Pseudoalteromonas ulvae* (TC14), with EC_{50} close to tributyltin oxide and ampicillin. Furthermore, compounds **40** and **41** were not lethal to bacteria at low concentrations and showed weak bactericidal effects at high concentrations, which indicated they might be used as coantibiotics or nontoxic cobiocides.

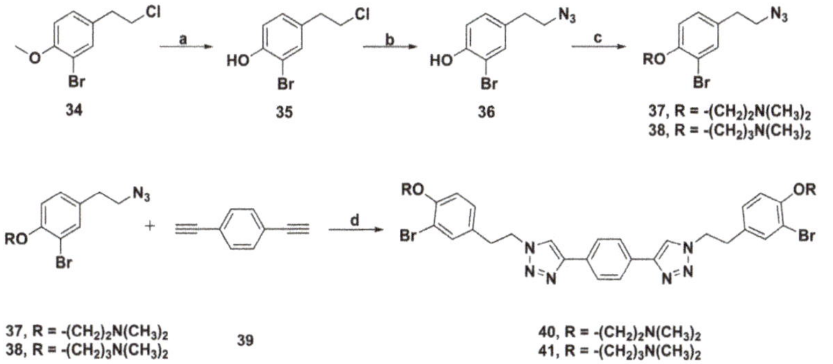

Scheme 4. Synthesis of psammaplin A bis-triazole derivatives **40** and **41**. Reagents and conditions: (a) BBr_3/CH_2Cl_2, 0 °C, rt, 4 h; (b) NaN_3/DMF, 5 h, 90 °C; (c) K_2CO_3, 18-crown-6, 2-dimethylaminoethyl chloride or 3-chloro-*N*,*N*-dimethylpropan-1-amine, acetone, reflux; (d) $CuSO_4$/sodium ascorbate, DMF/H_2O (2:1), 24 h, rt.

4.2. Anticancer Derivatives

A collection of more than 70 psammaplin A analogues were synthesized by Fuchter and coworkers [91]. The enzyme inhibitory activities against histone deacetylase 1 (HDAC 1) and HDAC 6 were evaluated. The derivatives **46**, **47**, **53**, and **54** (Scheme 5) showed more potent activity than psammaplin A and current inhibitors including trichostatin A and SAHA. Moreover, these compounds also displayed good selectivity for HDAC 1 over HDAC 6. In short, the structure–activity relationship indicated that the derivatives with the electron withdrawing group or the electron donating group in the benzene ring exhibited higher enzyme inhibitory activity than psammaplin A.

Subsequently, this group synthesized a library of psammaplin A derivatives (Figure 7) by modifying the disulfide bond, the aromatic group substituents, and the oxime functionality, aiming to study the enzymatic selectivity and mechanism of action against DNA methyltransferases and histone deacetylases [92]. The HDAC assays showed that the disulfide analogues **55**–**62** were less potent than their reduced products containing the free thiol. When the sulfur end group was protected, analogues **63**–**70** showed low to no inhibition of both HDAC 1 and HDAC 6. However, hydroxamic derivative **71** possessed highly potent activities against HDAC 1 (2 nM) and HDAC 6 (190 nM). Among the derivatives changed by the oxime functionality, the oxime-containing analogue **72** and hydrazone analogues **73** and **74** were 444–611 and 80–183-fold more potent, respectively, than the α-ketoamide-containing compounds **75** and **76** against HDAC 1. In the derivatives of aromatic group substituents, compound **77** exhibited the highest selectivity against HDAC 1. However, its potency was minor compared to the presence of the oxime and the free thiol. Unfortunately, psammaplin A and its derivatives were found to have weak inhibitory effects against DNA methyltransferases. On the other hand, the cytotoxicity studies showed that compound **72** had the smallest IC_{50} values of 0.16 and 0.61 µM against human lung carcinoma A549 and human breast carcinoma MCF-7, respectively. Amazingly, **73** was particularly selective against MCF-7 (IC_{50} 3.42 µM) with a ten-fold increase compared to the other cancer cell lines. Besides, hydroxamic acid **55** showed significant antiproliferative activity against A549 and MCF-7, which indicated that the cytotoxicity of derivatives might be related to HDAC inhibition. Western blot analysis showed that treatment with compound **71** could upregulate histone acetylation levels and not affect the tubulin acetylation levels. According to docking studies with HDAC 1, psammaplin A and its derivatives could bind to Zn^{2+}.

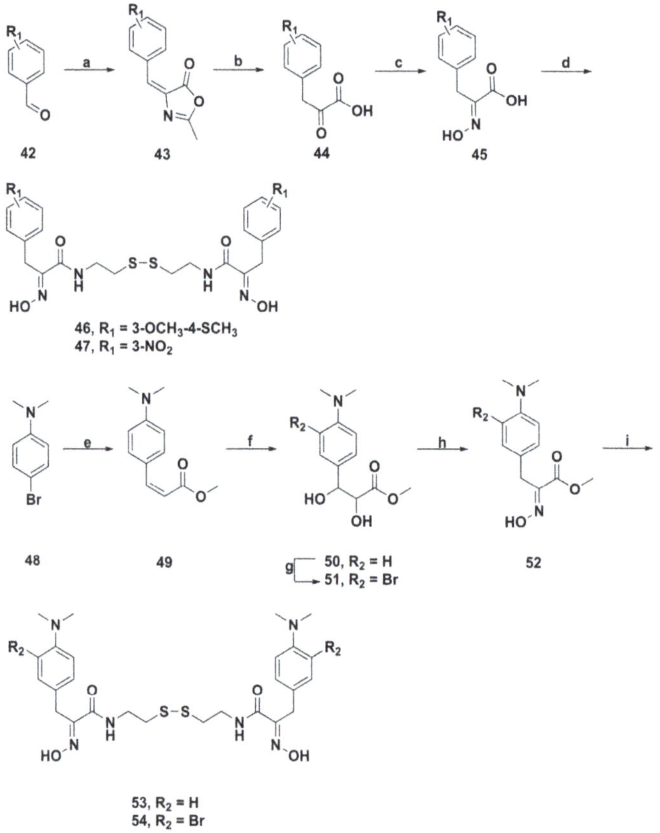

Scheme 5. Synthesis of psammaplin A analogues **46**, **47**, **53**, and **54**. Reagents and conditions: (a) NaOAc, N-Ac-Gly, Ac$_2$O; (b) HCl; (c) HONH$_2$·HCl, pyridine; (d) EDCI, N-hydroxy-succinamide dioxane; nucleophile, NEt$_3$, dioxane/MeOH; HCl, CH$_2$Cl$_2$/Et$_2$O/MeOH; (e) Pd(OAc)$_2$, P(o-Tol)$_3$, NEt$_3$, DMF; (f) osmium(VIII) oxide, NMO, MeCN/water; (g) NBS, DMF; (h) p-TsOH·H$_2$O, benzene; HONH$_2$·HCl, NaOAc, MeOH; (i) cystamine, AlMe$_3$, CH$_2$Cl$_2$.

In order to focus on the structure–activity relationship of the antiproliferative activities of psammaplin A derivatives, de Lera and coworkers synthesized five series of derivatives (Figure 8) by modifications in the halo-tyrosine aryl ring, the oxime bond, the connecting chain length, and the disulfide unit [60]. Subsequently, the HDAC inhibition tests showed that the derivatives **82** and **83** substituted on aryl rings possessed more potent inhibitory activity than psammaplin A. However, compounds **84–89** showed no apparent inhibitory effect, which suggested the oxime and disulfide bonds were indispensable for the HDAC inhibition activity. The cell-based assays on the U937 myeloid leukemia cells indicated that derivatives **85**, **82**, and **83** lacking the oxime could cause cell cycle arrest at G$_1$ phase, and the spirocycle derivative **86** lacking the free oxime and flexibility could induce apoptosis and arrest cell cycle at the G$_2$ phase. The homologues **78–81**, including three to six methylene units, and dimer **84**, containing an ethylene group replacing the disulfide bond, had weak apoptotic effects against the U937 cells. Mechanically, compounds **78–81**, **84**, **86**, **87**, and **89** could decrease the expression levels of p21WAF1 and tubulin acetylation. The derivative **82** could upregulate the levels of p21WAF1 even higher than SAHA. Moreover, **82** and **83** could increase the acetylated histone H3 levels.

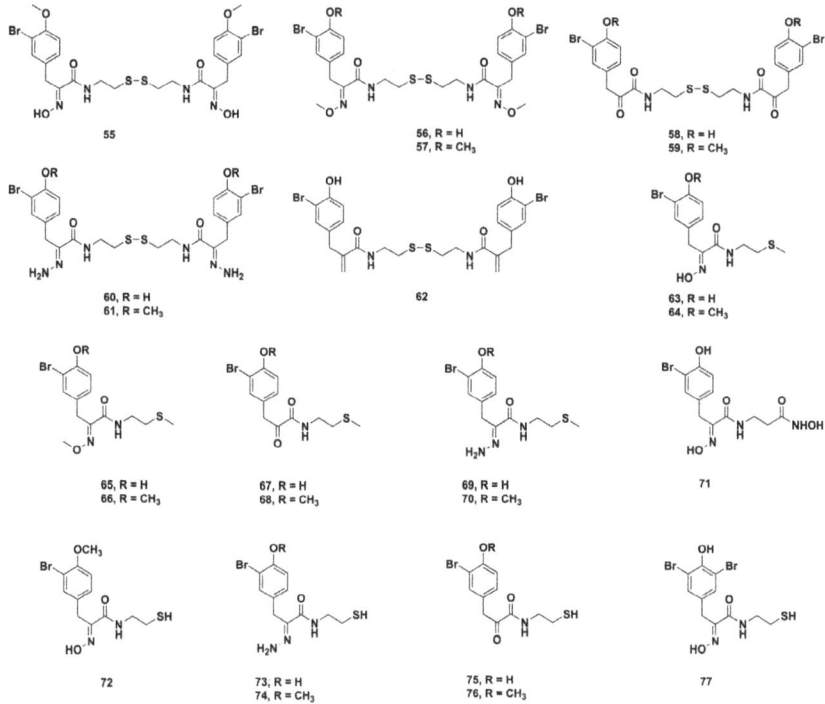

Figure 7. Chemical structures of the psammaplin A derivatives 55-77.

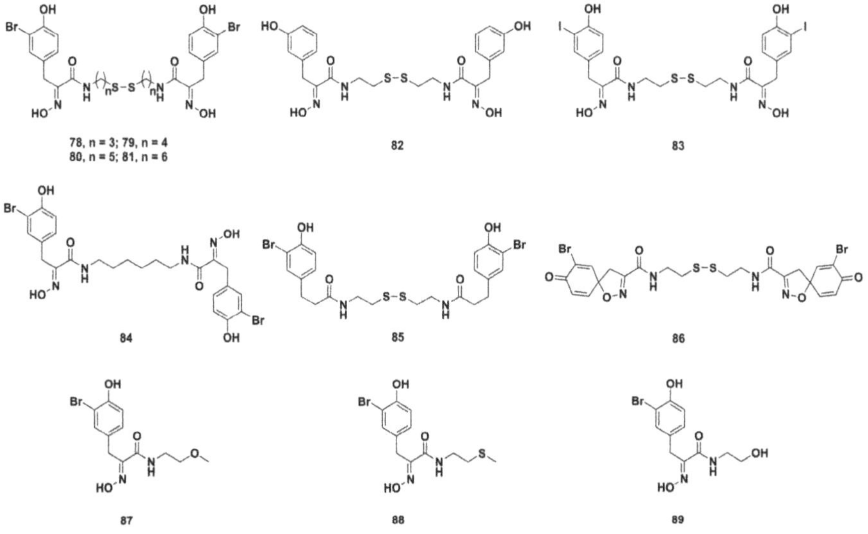

Figure 8. Chemical structures of the psammaplin A derivatives 78-89.

With continued research by de Lera and coworkers [42], a number of indole-based psammaplin A derivatives were designed and synthesized by replacing the *o*-bromophenol group with an indole ring to pursue more potent molecules for epigenetic disorder modulation, such as cancer. Especially, the induction ability of U937 acute myeloid leukemia (AML) cell apoptosis by compound **96** (Scheme 6) was stronger than that of the parent. Cell-based assays affirmed that the presence of disulfide bridge from **96** is essential for cell cycle arrest, differentiation, and induction of apoptosis. Besides, **96** could more efficiently induce α-tubulin acetylation as a sign of HDAC6 inhibition and increase the expression of histone H3 and p21 protein. Derivative **96** also induced cell cycle arrest and apoptosis in ex vivo AML patient blasts. In enzyme-based assays, **96** not only possessed the stronger inhibitory activities against HDAC and DNMT enzymes, but also inhibited the NAD$^+$-dependent SIRT deacetylase enzymes. In vivo pharmacokinetics study showed that **96**, as a prodrug, could immediately transform into the glutathione intermediate to exert multiple enzyme inhibitory activities [77]. More importantly, the maximum tolerated dose of **96** was higher than that of listed HDAC inhibitors, which merited further investigation for cancer therapy.

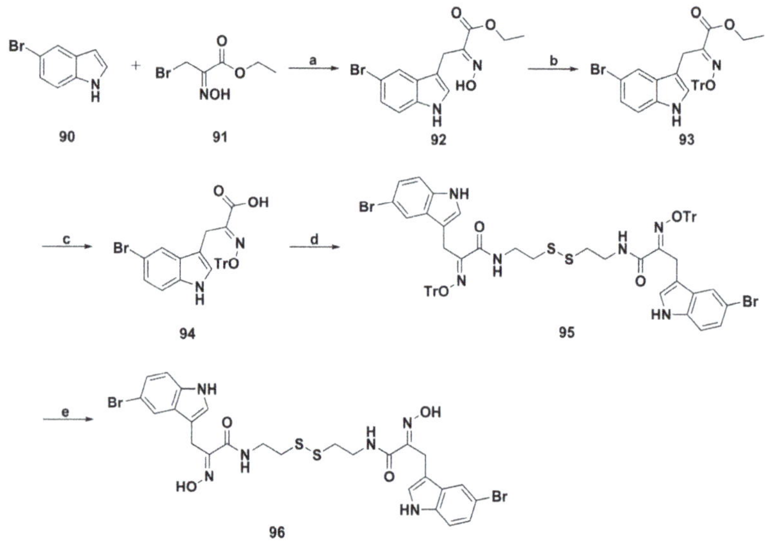

Scheme 6. Synthesis of indole-based psammaplin A derivative **96**. Reagents and conditions: (a) K$_2$CO$_3$, CH$_2$Cl$_2$, 25 °C, 20 h; (b) K$_2$CO$_3$, CH$_2$Cl$_2$, TrCl, 25 °C, 20 h; (c) LiOH·H$_2$O, THF/H$_2$O (1:1), 25 °C, 20 h; (d) cystamine, EDC, NHS, dioxane, 25 °C, 2 h; (e) 1 M HCl in Et$_2$O, CH$_2$Cl$_2$, 25 °C, 2 h.

Some psammaplin A fluorescent analogs were synthesized by Lindel and coworkers [63]. The cytotoxicity studies showed the fluorescent 4-coumarinacetyl-α-(hydroxyimino)acyl derivatives **97** and **98** (Figure 9) with IC$_{50}$ values of 0.93 and 1.10 µg/mL, respectively, were about two-fold stronger than that of psammaplin A (IC$_{50}$ 0.42 µg/mL) against the mouse fibroblast L-929 cells. Furthermore, bis- and mono (coumarinyl) derivatives **99** and **100** (Figure 9) lacking α-(hydroxyimino)acyl moieties were not cytotoxic. The HDAC inhibitory activities of the coumarin–psammaplin hybrid **97** (IC$_{50}$ 0.011 µM) was two-fold more potent than psammaplin A (IC$_{50}$ 0.028 µM) by a fluorometric HDAC assay. Afterwards, fluorescence microscopy revealed that compounds **97** and **98** lacking α-(hydroxyimino)acyl units were taken up into the cytoplasm, leading to fluorescence in the nuclear envelope, not in the nucleus, which indicated the disulfide bonds were reduced to the thiol before the disulfide penetrated the nucleus [93].

Soon afterwards, Lindel and coworkers synthesized the first photoreactive psammaplin A derivative **111** by adding 1-azi-2,2,2-trifluoroethyl moieties to benzene rings (Scheme 7) [94]. Photopsammaplin **111** showed antiproliferative activity in vitro with an average IC$_{50}$ value of 1.4 µM against 42 human cancer cell lines, which was especially sensitive to lung cancer (LXFA 526), melanoma (MEXF 276), mammary cancer (MAXF 401 and MCF-7), and bladder cancer (T-24), with IC_{50} values below 0.6 µM. Furthermore, the fluorometric HDAC assay showed **111** was also a potent HDAC inhibitor, with an IC_{50} value of 35 nM. With this information, photopsammaplin **111** might be considered as a good candidate of photoaffinity labeling, which played an important role in new targets identification of psammaplin A.

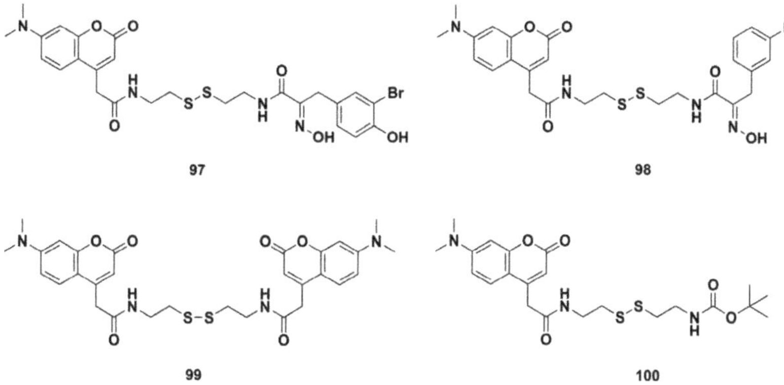

Figure 9. Chemical structures of the psammaplin A fluorescent derivatives **97-100**.

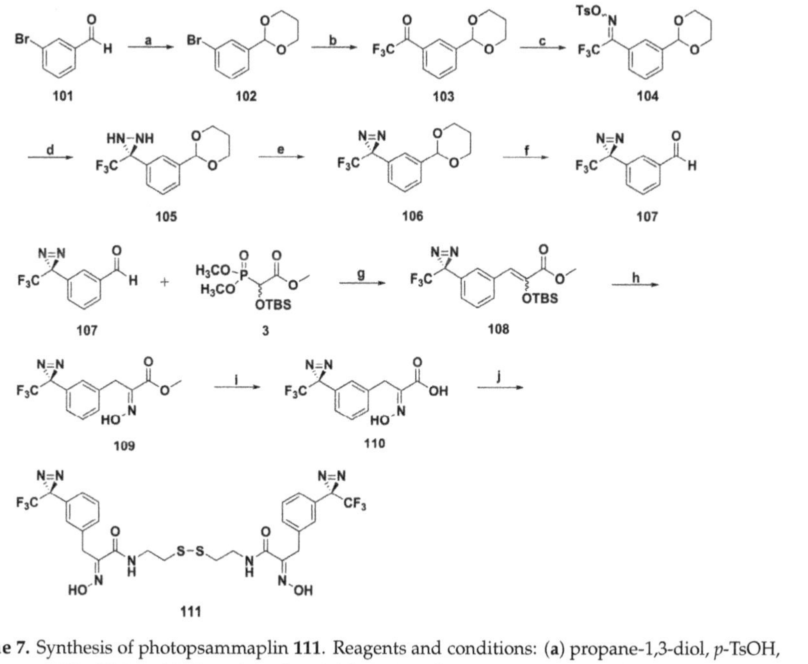

Scheme 7. Synthesis of photopsammaplin **111**. Reagents and conditions: (**a**) propane-1,3-diol, p-TsOH, toluene, rt, 2.5 h; (**b**) Mg, THF, rt, 2 h; then 0 °C, 2,2,2-trifluoro-1-(piperidin-1-yl)ethanone, 2 h, rt; (**c**) (i) $HONH_2 \cdot HCl$, pyridine, rt, 9 h; (ii) NEt_3, p-TsCl, 24 h, 0 °C to rt; (**d**) NH_3, 6 h, −78 °C to rt; (**e**) NEt_3, I_2, 15 min, 0 °C, then 3 h, rt, avoiding daylight; (**f**) 0.5 M H_2SO_4, acetone/H_2O, rt, 12 h, quant; (**g**) LDA, THF, −78 °C, 14 h; (**h**) (i) $NEt_3 \cdot 3HF$, MeOH, rt, 2 h; (ii) $HONH_2 \cdot HCl$, MeOH, rt, 17 h, quant; (**i**) $LiOH \cdot H_2O$, THF/H_2O, rt, 20 h, quant; (**j**) cystamine dihydrochloride, NHS, DCC, NEt_3, DMF, rt, 15 d.

Innovative synthesis of psammaplin analogues is proposed by Bertrand and coworkers through superacid, microwaves, and S-ene chemistry reactions as zinc-dependent HDAC inhibitors [95]. Among them, the thiol derivative **119** (Scheme 8) was five-fold more selective for HDAC 6 compared to HDAC 2. Moreover, in the bioluminescent resonance energy transfer tests, the HDAC inhibition activity of **119** confirmed the oxidative process importance in cancer cells in the environment of biomolecules being oxidized or reduced.

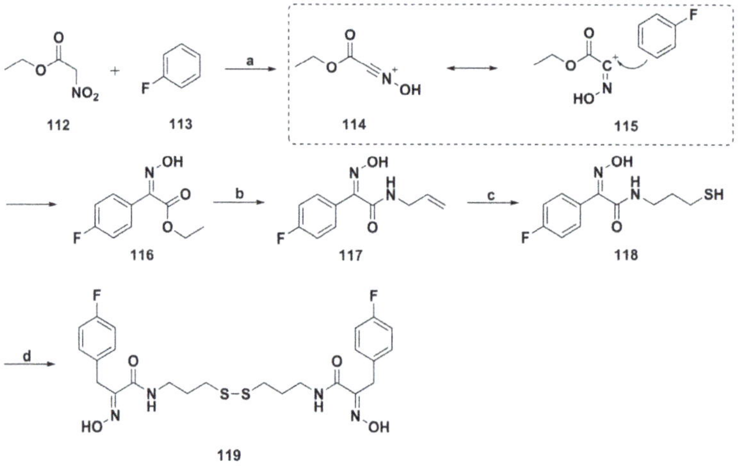

Scheme 8. Synthesis of psammaplin A analogue **119**. Reagents and conditions: (**a**) CF_3SO_3H; (**b**) amine, heating neat or microwave neat; (**c**) hν, R_2-SH; (**d**) air.

Twenty-eight derivatives of psammaplin A were prepared by Park and coworkers using a new concise approach [65]. Among them, compounds **120–124** (Figure 10) displayed comparable cytotoxicity to the parent compound. Especially, **120** possessed the highest antiproliferative activity against A549 cells with an IC_{50} value of 1.20 μM. Study of the structure–activity relationship revealed the disulfide bond and oxime group might be primary pharmacophores for high cytotoxicity. Furthermore, the fluorometric HDAC assay showed that **120** could inhibit the HDAC enzyme activity and enhance the expression of acetylated H3 in the A549 cells. The mechanism study showed **120** restrained the growth of A549 cells through the AKT and ERK signaling pathways. The in vivo study reconfirmed that **120** could inhibit tumor size outgrowth.

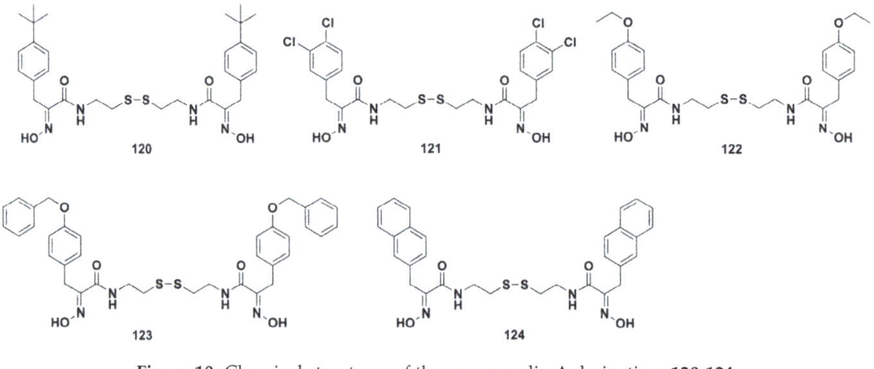

Figure 10. Chemical structures of the psammaplin A derivatives **120-124**.

A collection of novel psammaplin A derivatives were synthesized by Zhao and coworkers [96]. The derivatives **133** and **134** (Scheme 9) showed potent cytotoxicity against four cancer cell lines (PC-3, MCF-7, A549, and HL-60) and better HDAC inhibition than psammaplin A. Molecular docking simulation showed that the hydrogen atom of the oxime group could interact with the active site of Asp 99 of HDAC1 via hydrogen bonding, and the hydroxyl group which could interact with Glu 203 at the entrance to the active site tunnel was optimally attached on the *para*-position of the benzene ring.

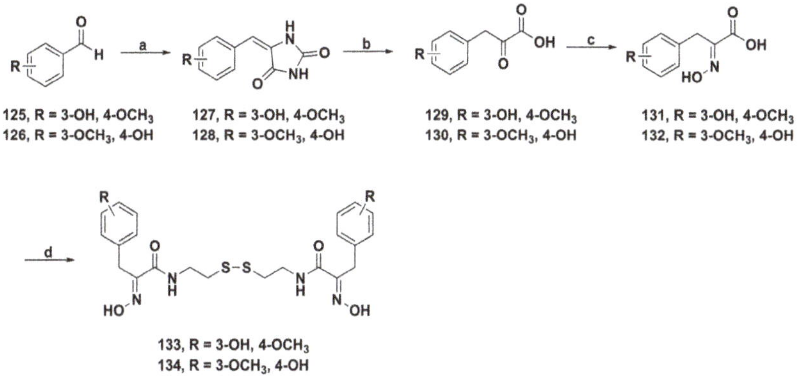

125, R = 3-OH, 4-OCH$_3$
126, R = 3-OCH$_3$, 4-OH

127, R = 3-OH, 4-OCH$_3$
128, R = 3-OCH$_3$, 4-OH

129, R = 3-OH, 4-OCH$_3$
130, R = 3-OCH$_3$, 4-OH

131, R = 3-OH, 4-OCH$_3$
132, R = 3-OCH$_3$, 4-OH

133, R = 3-OH, 4-OCH$_3$
134, R = 3-OCH$_3$, 4-OH

Scheme 9. Synthesis of psammaplin A analogues **133** and **134**. Reagents and conditions: (**a**) hydantoin, ethanolamine, EtOH, H$_2$O, reflux, 5 h; (**b**) NaOH, H$_2$O, reflux, 12 h; (**c**) NH$_2$OH·HCl, NaOH, NaHCO$_3$, H$_2$O, rt, overnight; (**d**) cystamine dihydrochloride, EDCI, HOBt, THF, rt, 24 h.

5. Conclusions

In summary, marine natural products, as extremely valuable resources, have become significant enablers of new drug development due to their extensive chemical variability and diverse bioactivities. Unfortunately, their in-depth study and application are restricted due to the low natural isolated yield from marine microorganisms and their poor physiological stability. Therefore, a great deal of interest has been shown in the total synthesis of marine natural products. The conventional total synthesis methods of psammaplin A were initiated from tyrosine or phenylpyruvic acid derivatives. Since 2009, improved synthesis methods have mainly used various substituted benzaldehydes as the starting materials, which made psammaplin A easier to obtain. Moreover, the pharmacological activities and structural modifications of the dimeric marine natural product psammaplin A were comprehensively summarized. Psammaplin A possesses a wide range of pharmacological activities, including antimicrobial, anticancer, antiviral, embryo development promotive, insecticidal, active chemical defense, and eryptosis-inducing activities. More importantly, it displays antibacterial and antiproliferative activities mainly through inhibiting multiple enzymes, including chitinase, HDAC, and others. To further improve its drug-like properties, a collection of psammaplin A derivatives were synthesized through structural modifications aimed to explore their potential therapeutic value and to study the structure–activity relationships. Among them, some antibacterial derivatives showed stronger antimicrobial activity against SA and MRSA via inhibiting DNA gyrase and bacterial DNA synthesis enzymes. Furthermore, the promising anticancer derivatives not only possessed stronger antiproliferative activities against various cancer cell lines, but also indicated higher HDAC 1 inhibitory activity. Finally, the structure–activity relationships revealed that the disulfide bond and the oxime moieties are indispensable pharmacophores for its bioactivities. Collectively, we hope this review will aid researchers in further studying psammaplin A.

Author Contributions: Q.J. and X.H. contributed equally to this work. Q.J. and X.H. conceived and wrote the review; Y.M. and J.M. edited the chemical structures; W.L., F.X. and Z.L. offered important advice to improve the review; J.B., H.H. and D.L. conceived the review and revised the paper.

Funding: This paper was financially supported by the Career Development Support Plan for Young and Middle-aged Teachers in Shenyang Pharmaceutical University.

Conflicts of Interest: The authors declare no conflict of interest.

References

1. Paterson, I.; Anderson, E.A. The renaissance of natural products as drug candidates. *Science* **2005**, *310*, 451. [CrossRef] [PubMed]
2. Cragg, G.M.; Grothaus, P.G.; Newman, D.J. Impact of natural products on developing new anti-cancer agents. *Chem. Rev.* **2009**, *109*, 3012–3043. [CrossRef] [PubMed]
3. Blunt, J.W.; Copp, B.R.; Keyzer, R.A.; Munro, M.H.; Prinsep, M.R. Marine natural products. *Nat. Prod. Rep.* **2016**, *33*, 382–431. [CrossRef] [PubMed]
4. Newman, D.J.; Cragg, G.M. Natural products as sources of new drugs from 1981 to 2014. *J. Nat. Prod.* **2016**, *79*, 629–661. [CrossRef] [PubMed]
5. Harvey, A.L.; Edrada-Ebel, R.; Quinn, R.J. The re-emergence of natural products for drug discovery in the genomics era. *Nat. Rev. Drug Discov.* **2015**, *14*, 111–129. [CrossRef]
6. Koehn, F.E.; Carter, G.T. The evolving role of natural products in drug discovery. *Nat. Rev. Drug Discov.* **2005**, *4*, 206–220. [CrossRef]
7. Sparks, T.C.; Hahn, D.R.; Garizi, N.V. Natural products, their derivatives, mimics and synthetic equivalents: Role in agrochemical discovery. *Pest. Manag. Sci.* **2017**, *73*, 700–715. [CrossRef]
8. Mishra, B.B.; Tiwari, V.K. Natural products: An evolving role in future drug discovery. *Eur. J. Med. Chem.* **2011**, *46*, 4769–4807. [CrossRef]
9. Tang, C.; Wu, B.; Wu, J.; Zhang, Z.; Yu, B. Novel strategies using total gastrodin and gastrodigenin, or total gastrodigenin for quality control of gastrodia elata. *Molecules* **2018**, *23*, 270. [CrossRef]
10. Soldatou, S.; Baker, B.J. Cold-water marine natural products, 2006 to 2016. *Nat. Prod. Rep.* **2017**, *34*, 585–626. [CrossRef]
11. Chen, J.; Wang, B.; Lu, Y.; Guo, Y.; Sun, J.; Wei, B.; Zhang, H.; Wang, H. Quorum sensing inhibitors from marine microorganisms and their synthetic derivatives. *Mar. Drugs* **2019**, *17*, 80. [CrossRef] [PubMed]
12. Choudhary, A.; Naughton, L.M.; Montánchez, I.; Dobson, A.D.W.; Rai, D.K. Current status and future prospects of marine natural products (MNPs) as antimicrobials. *Mar. Drugs* **2017**, *15*, 272. [CrossRef] [PubMed]
13. Molinski, T.F.; Dalisay, D.S.; Lievens, S.L.; Saludes, J.P. Drug development from marine natural products. *Nat. Rev. Drug Discov.* **2009**, *8*, 69–85. [CrossRef] [PubMed]
14. Pereira, F. Have marine natural product drug discovery efforts been productive and how can we improve their efficiency? *Expert Opin. Drug Discov.* **2019**, *15*, 1–6. [CrossRef] [PubMed]
15. Huang, C.; Zhang, Z.; Cui, W. Marine-derived natural compounds for the treatment of Parkinson's disease. *Mar. Drugs* **2019**, *157*, 221. [CrossRef] [PubMed]
16. Wu, Q.; Nay, B.; Yang, M.; Ni, Y.; Wang, H.; Yao, L.; Li, X. Marine sponges of the genus *Stelletta* as promising drug sources: Chemical and biological aspects. *Acta. Pharm. Sin. B* **2019**, *9*, 237–257. [CrossRef]
17. Mudit, M.; El Sayed, K.A. Cancer control potential of marine natural product scaffolds through inhibition of tumor cell migration and invasion. *Drug Discov. Today* **2016**, *21*, 1745–1760. [CrossRef]
18. Mayer, A.M.S.; Glaser, K.B.; Cuevas, C.; Jacobs, R.S.; Kem, W.; Little, R.D.; McIntosh, J.M.; Newman, D.J.; Potts, B.C.; Shuster, D.E. The odyssey of marine pharmaceuticals: A current pipeline perspective. *Trends Pharmacol. Sci.* **2010**, *31*, 255–265. [CrossRef]
19. Olivera, B.M.; Cruz, L.J.; de Santos, V.; LeCheminant, G.W.; Griffin, D.; Zeikus, R.; McIntosh, J.M.; Galyean, R.; Varga, J.; Gray, W.R. Neuronal calcium channel antagonists. Discrimination between calcium channel subtypes using omega-conotoxin from Conus magus venom. *Biochemistry* **1987**, *26*, 2086–2090. [CrossRef]
20. Heydari, B.; Abdullah, S.; Pottala, J.V.; Shah, R.; Abbasi, S.; Mandry, D.; Francis, S.A.; Lumish, H.; Ghoshhajra, B.B.; Hoffmann, U.; et al. Effect of omega-3 acid ethyl esters on left ventricular remodeling after acute myocardial infarction: The OMEGA-REMODEL randomized clinical trial. *Circulation* **2016**, *134*, 378–391. [CrossRef]
21. Newland, A.M.; Li, J.X.; Wasco, L.E.; Aziz, M.T.; Lowe, D.K. Brentuximab vedotin: A CD30-directed antibody-cytotoxic drug conjugate. *Pharmacotherapy* **2013**, *33*, 93–104. [CrossRef] [PubMed]

22. Jordan, M.A.; Kamath, K.; Manna, T.; Okouneva, T.; Miller, H.P.; Davis, C.; Littlefield, B.A.; Wilson, L. The primary antimitotic mechanism of action of the synthetic halichondrin e7389 is suppression of microtubule growth. *Mol. Cancer Ther.* **2005**, *4*, 1086–1095. [CrossRef] [PubMed]
23. Quiñoà, E.; Crews, P. Phenolic constituents of Psammaplysilla. *Tetrahedron Lett.* **1987**, *28*, 3229–3232. [CrossRef]
24. Rodriguez, A.D.; Akee, R.K.; Scheuer, P.J. Two bromotyrosine-cysteine derived metabolites from a sponge. *Tetrahedron Lett.* **1987**, *28*, 4989–4992. [CrossRef]
25. Arabshahi, L.; Schmitz, F.J. Brominated tyrosine metabolites from an unidentified sponge. *J. Org. Chem.* **1987**, *52*, 3584–3586. [CrossRef]
26. Mujumdar, P.; Teruya, K.; Tonissen, K.F.; Vullo, D.; Supuran, C.T.; Peat, T.S.; Poulsen, S.A. An unusual natural product primary sulfonamide: Synthesis, carbonic anhydrase inhibition, and protein X-ray structures of psammaplin C. *J. Med. Chem.* **2016**, *59*, 5462–5470. [CrossRef] [PubMed]
27. Yang, Q.; Liu, D.; Sun, D.; Yang, S.; Hu, G.; Wu, Z.; Zhao, L. Synthesis of the marine bromotyrosine psammaplin F and crystal structure of a psammaplin A analogue. *Molecules* **2010**, *15*, 8784–8795. [CrossRef] [PubMed]
28. Pina, I.C.; Gautschi, J.T.; Wang, G.Y.S.; Sanders, M.L.; Schmitz, F.J.; France, D.; Cornell-Kennon, S.; Sambucetti, L.C.; Remiszewski, S.W.; Perez, L.B.; et al. Psammaplins from the sponge *Pseudoceratina purpurea*: Inhibition of both histone deacetylase and DNA methyltransferase. *J. Org. Chem.* **2003**, *68*, 3866–3873. [CrossRef] [PubMed]
29. Park, Y.; Liu, Y.; Hong, J.; Lee, C.O.; Cho, H.; Kim, D.K.; Im, K.S.; Jung, J.H. New bromotyrosine derivatives from an association of two sponges, *Jaspis wondoensis* and *Poecillastra wondoensis*. *J. Nat. Prod.* **2003**, *66*, 1495–1498. [CrossRef]
30. Kim, D.; Lee, I.S.; Jung, J.H.; Yang, S.I. Psammaplin A, a natural bromotyrosine derivative from a sponge, possesses the antibacterial activity against methicillin-resistant *Staphylococcus aureus* and the DNA gyrase-inhibitory activity. *Arch. Pharm. Res.* **1999**, *22*, 25–29. [CrossRef]
31. Zhou, Y.D.; Li, J.; Du, L.; Mahdi, F.; Le, T.P.; Chen, W.L.; Swanson, S.M.; Watabe, K.; Nagle, D.G. Biochemical and anti-triple negative metastatic breast tumor cell properties of psammaplins. *Mar. Drugs* **2018**, *16*, 442. [CrossRef]
32. Ahn, M.Y.; Jung, J.H.; Na, Y.J.; Kim, H.S. A natural histone deacetylase inhibitor, psammaplin A, induces cell cycle arrest and apoptosis in human endometrial cancer cells. *Gynecol. Oncol.* **2008**, *108*, 27–33. [CrossRef] [PubMed]
33. Kim, T.H.; Kim, H.S.; Kang, Y.J.; Yoon, S.; Lee, J.; Choi, W.S.; Jung, J.H.; Kim, H.S. Psammaplin A induces sirtuin 1-dependent autophagic cell death in doxorubicin-resistant MCF-7/adr human breast cancer cells and xenografts. *Biochim. Biophys. Acta.* **2015**, *1850*, 401–410. [CrossRef] [PubMed]
34. Ratovitski, E.A. Tumor protein (TP)-p53 members as regulators of autophagy in tumor cells upon marine drug exposure. *Mar. Drugs* **2016**, *14*, 154. [CrossRef] [PubMed]
35. Kim, D.; Lee, I.S.; Jung, J.H.; Lee, C.O.; Choi, S.U. Psammaplin A, a natural phenolic compound, has inhibitory effect on human topoisomerase II and is cytotoxic to cancer cells. *Anticancer Res.* **1999**, *19*, 4085–4090. [PubMed]
36. Tabudravu, J.N.; Eijsink, V.G.H.; Gooday, G.W.; Jaspars, M.; Komander, D.; Legg, M.; Synstad, B.; van Aalten, D.M.F. Psammaplin A, a chitinase inhibitor isolated from the Fijian marine sponge *Aplysinella rhax*. *Bioorg. Med. Chem.* **2002**, *10*, 1123–1128. [CrossRef]
37. Shin, J.; Lee, H.S.; Seo, Y.; Rho, J.R.; Cho, K.W.; Paul, V.J. New bromotyrosine metabolites from the sponge *Aplysinella rhax*. *Tetrahedron* **2000**, *56*, 9071–9077. [CrossRef]
38. Nicholas, G.M.; Eckman, L.L.; Ray, S.; Hughes, R.O.; Pfefferkorn, J.A.; Barluenga, S.; Nicolaou, K.C.; Bewley, C.A. Bromotyrosine-derived natural and synthetic products as inhibitors of mycothiol-s-conjugate amidase. *Bioorg. Med. Chem. Lett.* **2002**, *12*, 2487–2490. [CrossRef]
39. Jiang, Y.; Ahn, E.Y.; Ryu, S.H.; Kim, D.K.; Park, J.S.; Yoon, H.J.; Yoo, S.; Lee, B.J.; Lee, D.S.; Jung, J.H. Cytotoxicity of psammaplin A from a two-sponge association may correlate with the inhibition of DNA replication. *BMC Cancer* **2004**, *4*, 70. [CrossRef]
40. Shim, J.S.; Lee, H.S.; Shin, J.; Kwon, H.J. Psammaplin A, a marine natural product, inhibits aminopeptidase N and suppresses angiogenesis in vitro. *Cancer Lett.* **2004**, *203*, 163–169. [CrossRef]

41. Kim, D.H.; Shin, J.; Kwon, H.J. Psammaplin A is a natural prodrug that inhibits class I histone deacetylase. *Exp. Mol. Med.* **2007**, *39*, 47–55. [CrossRef] [PubMed]
42. Pereira, R.; Benedetti, R.; Pérez-Rodríguez, S.; Nebbioso, A.; García-Rodríguez, J.; Carafa, V.; Stuhldreier, M.; Conte, M.; Rodríguez-Barrios, F.; Stunnenberg, H.G.; et al. Indole-derived psammaplin A analogues as epigenetic modulators with multiple inhibitory activities. *J. Med. Chem.* **2012**, *55*, 9467–9491. [CrossRef]
43. Hentschel, F.; Lindel, T. Synthesis of oximinotyrosine-derived marine natural products. *Synthesis* **2010**, *2*, 181–204.
44. Martins, A.; Vieira, H.; Gaspar, H.; Santos, S. Marketed marine natural products in the pharmaceutical and cosmeceutical industries: Tips for success. *Mar. Drugs* **2014**, *12*, 1066–1101. [CrossRef] [PubMed]
45. Malve, H. Exploring the ocean for new drug developments: Marine pharmacology. *J. Pharm. Bioallied. Sci.* **2016**, *8*, 83–91. [CrossRef]
46. Blunt, J.W.; Carroll, A.R.; Copp, B.R.; Davis, R.A.; Keyzers, R.A.; Prinsep, M.R. Marine natural products. *Nat. Prod. Rep.* **2018**, *35*, 8–53. [CrossRef]
47. Datta, D.; Talapatra, S.N.; Swarnakar, S. Bioactive compounds from marine invertebrates for potential medicines-an overview. *Int. Lett. Nat. Sci.* **2015**, *34*, 42–61. [CrossRef]
48. Lindequist, U. Marine-derived pharmaceuticals-challenges and opportunities. *Biomol. Ther.* **2016**, *24*, 561–571. [CrossRef]
49. Gerwick, W.H.; Moore, B.S. Lessons from the past and charting the future of marine natural products drug discovery and chemical biology. *Chem. Biol.* **2012**, *19*, 85–98. [CrossRef]
50. Kanase, H.R.; Singh, K.M. Marine pharmacology: Potential, challenges, and future in India. *J. Med. Sci.* **2018**, *38*, 49–53.
51. Shinde, P.; Banerjee, P.; Mandhare, A. Marine natural products as source of new drugs: A patent review (2015–2018). *Expert Opin. Ther. Pat.* **2019**, *29*, 283–309. [CrossRef] [PubMed]
52. Song, X.; Xiong, Y.; Qi, X.; Tang, W.; Dai, J.; Gu, Q.; Li, J. Molecular targets of active anticancer compounds derived from marine sources. *Mar. Drugs* **2018**, *16*, 175. [CrossRef] [PubMed]
53. Calcabrini, C.; Catanzaro, E.; Bishayee, A.; Turrini, E.; Fimognari, C. Marine sponge natural products with anticancer potential: An updated review. *Mar. Drugs* **2017**, *15*, 310. [CrossRef] [PubMed]
54. Li, T.; Ding, T.; Li, J. Medicinal purposes: Bioactive metabolites from marine-derived organisms. *Mini Rev. Med. Chem.* **2019**, *19*, 138–164. [CrossRef] [PubMed]
55. Singh, R.; Sharma, M.; Joshi, P.; Rawat, D.S. Clinical status of anti-cancer agents derived from marine sources. *Anticancer Agents Med. Chem.* **2008**, *8*, 603–617. [CrossRef]
56. Adrian, T.E. Novel marine-derived anti-cancer agents. *Curr. Pharm. Des.* **2007**, *13*, 3417–3426. [CrossRef]
57. Jaiganesh, R.; Sampath Kumar, N.S. Marine bacterial sources of bioactive compounds. *Adv. Food Nutr. Res.* **2012**, *65*, 389–408.
58. Peng, J.; Li, J.; Hamann, M.T. The marine bromotyrosine derivatives. *Alkaloids Chem. Biol.* **2005**, *61*, 59–262.
59. Godert, A.M.; Angelino, N.; Read, A.W.; Morey, S.R.; James, S.R.; Karpf, A.R.; Sufrin, J.R. An improved synthesis of psammaplin A. *Bioorg. Med. Chem. Lett.* **2006**, *16*, 3330–3333. [CrossRef]
60. García, J.; Franci, G.; Pereira, R.; Benedetti, R.; Nebbioso, A.; Rodríguez-Barrios, F.; Gronemeyer, H.; Altucci, L.; de Lera, A.R. Epigenetic profiling of the antitumor natural product psammaplin A and its analogues. *Bioorg. Med. Chem.* **2011**, *19*, 3637–3649. [CrossRef]
61. Nicolaou, K.C.; Hughes, R.; Pfefferkorn, J.A.; Barluenga, S.; Roecker, A.J. Combinatorial synthesis through disulfide exchange: Discovery of potent psammaplin A type antibacterial agents active against methicillin-resistant *Staphylococcus aureus* (MRSA). *Chem. Eur. J.* **2001**, *7*, 4280–4295. [CrossRef]
62. Hoshino, O.; Murakata, M.; Yamada, K. A convenient synthesis of a bromotyrosine derived metabolite, psammaplin A, from *Psammaplysilla* sp. *Bioorg. Med. Chem. Lett.* **1992**, *2*, 1561–1562. [CrossRef]
63. Hentschel, F.; Sasse, F.; Lindel, T. Fluorescent analogs of the marine natural product psammaplin A: Synthesis and biological activity. *Org. Biomol. Chem.* **2012**, *10*, 7120–7133. [CrossRef] [PubMed]
64. Kottakota, S.K.; Benton, M.; Evangelopoulos, D.; Guzman, J.D.; Bhakta, S.; McHugh, T.D.; Gray, M.; Groundwater, P.W.; Marrs, E.C.; Perry, J.D.; et al. Versatile routes to marine sponge metabolites through benzylidene rhodanines. *Org. Lett.* **2012**, *14*, 6310–6313. [CrossRef] [PubMed]
65. Hong, S.; Shin, Y.; Jung, M.; Ha, M.W.; Park, Y.; Lee, Y.J.; Shin, J.; Oh, K.B.; Lee, S.K.; Park, H.G. Efficient synthesis and biological activity of Psammaplin A and its analogues as antitumor agents. *Eur. J. Med. Chem.* **2015**, *96*, 218–230. [CrossRef] [PubMed]

66. Hong, S.; Lee, M.; Jung, M.; Park, Y.; Kim, M.Y.; Park, H.G. Efficient synthetic method of Psammaplin, A. *Tetrahedron Lett.* **2012**, *53*, 4209–4211. [CrossRef]
67. Oh, K.B.; Oh, M.N.; Kim, J.G.; Shin, D.S.; Shin, J. Inhibition of sortase-mediated *Staphylococcus aureus* adhesion to fibronectin via fibronectin-binding protein by sortase inhibitors. *Appl. Microbiol. Biotechnol.* **2006**, *70*, 102–106. [CrossRef] [PubMed]
68. Franci, G.; Folliero, V.; Cammarota, M.; Zannella, C.; Sarno, F.; Schiraldi, C.; Lera, A.R.; Altucci, L.; Galdiero, M. Epigenetic modulator UVI5008 inhibits MRSA by interfering with bacterial gyrase. *Sci. Rep.* **2018**, *8*, 13117. [CrossRef] [PubMed]
69. Lee, B.C.; Lee, A.; Jung, J.H.; Choi, S.H.; Kim, T.S. In vitro and in vivo anti-vibrio vulnificus activity of psammaplin a, a natural marine compound. *Mol. Med. Rep.* **2016**, *14*, 2691–2696. [CrossRef] [PubMed]
70. Salam, K.A.; Furuta, A.; Noda, N.; Tsuneda, S.; Sekiguchi, Y.; Yamashita, A.; Moriishi, K.; Nakakoshi, M.; Tsubuki, M.; Tani, H.; et al. Psammaplin A inhibits hepatitis C virus NS3 helicase. *J. Nat. Med.* **2013**, *67*, 765–772. [CrossRef] [PubMed]
71. Richard, K.; Williams, D.E.; de Silva, E.D.; Brockman, M.A.; Brumme, Z.L.; Andersen, R.J.; Tietjen, I. Identification of novel HIV-1 latency-reversing agents from a library of marine natural products. *Viruses* **2018**, *10*, 348. [CrossRef]
72. Mallol, A.; Santaló, J.; Ibáñez, E. Psammaplin A improves development and quality of somatic cell nuclear transfer mouse embryos. *Cell Reprogram.* **2014**, *16*, 392–406. [CrossRef] [PubMed]
73. Mallol, A.; Piqué, L.; Santaló, J.; Ibáñez, E. Morphokinetics of cloned mouse embryos treated with epigenetic drugs and blastocyst prediction. *Reproduction* **2016**, *151*, 203–214. [CrossRef] [PubMed]
74. Hiusen, T.J.; Kamble-Shripat, T. Delayed toxicity of two chitinolytic enzyme inhibitors (Psammaplin A and Pentoxifylline) against eastern subterranean termites (Isoptera: Rhinotermitidae). *J. Entomol. Sci.* **2013**, *106*, 1788–1793. [CrossRef]
75. Husen, T.J.; Kamble, S.T. An evaluation of chitinase inhibitors, psammaplin A and pentoxifylline, treated diets against the eastern subterranean teimite (Isoptera: Rhinotermitidae). *J. Entomol. Sci.* **2014**, *49*, 228–245. [CrossRef]
76. Saguez, J.; Hainez, R.; Cherqui, A.; Van Wuytswinkel, O.; Jeanpierre, H.; Lebon, G.; Noiraud, N.; Beaujean, A.; Jouanin, L.; Laberche, J.C.; et al. Unexpected effects of chitinases on the peach-potato aphid (*Myzus persicae* Sulzer) when delivered via transgenic potato plants (*Solanum tuberosum* Linné) and in vitro. *Transgenic. Res.* **2005**, *14*, 57–67. [CrossRef] [PubMed]
77. Francis, F.; Saguez, J.; Cherqui, A.; Vandermoten, S.; Vincent, C.; Versali, M.F.; Dommès, J.; De Pauw, E.; Giordanengo, P.; Haubruge, E. Purification and characterisation of a 31-kDa Chitinase from the myzus persicae aphid: A target for hemiptera biocontrol. *Appl. Biochem. Biotechnol.* **2012**, *166*, 1291–1300. [CrossRef] [PubMed]
78. Saguez, J.; Dubois, F.; Vincent, C.; Laberche, J.C.; Sangwan-Norreel, B.S.; Giordanengo, P. Differential aphicidal effects of chitinase inhibitors on the polyphagous homopteran *Myzus persicae* (Sulzer). *Pest. Manag. Sci.* **2006**, *62*, 1150–1154. [CrossRef]
79. Thoms, C.; Schupp, P.J. Activated chemical defense in marine sponges—A case study on aplysinella rhax. *J. Chem. Ecol.* **2008**, *34*, 1242–1252. [CrossRef]
80. Al Mamun Bhuyan, A.; Signoretto, E.; Lang, F. Triggering of suicidal erythrocyte death by psammaplin A. *Cell. Physiol. Biochem.* **2016**, *39*, 908–918. [CrossRef]
81. Kim, H.J.; Kim, J.H.; Chie, E.K.; Young, P.D.; Kim, I.A.; Kim, I.H. DNMT (DNA methyltransferase) inhibitors radiosensitize human cancer cells by suppressing DNA repair activity. *Radiat. Oncol.* **2012**, *7*, 39. [CrossRef] [PubMed]
82. Charkie, J. Psammaplin A: A putative adjuvant for DNA damaging therapies. *J. Cancer Sci. Ther.* **2014**, *6*, 505–509. [CrossRef]
83. Kim, H.J.; Kim, T.H.; Seo, W.S.; Yoo, S.D.; Kim, I.H.; Joo, S.H.; Shin, S.; Park, E.S.; Ma, E.S.; Shin, B.S. Pharmacokinetics and tissue distribution of psammaplin A, a novel anticancer agent, in mice. *Arch. Pharm. Res.* **2012**, *10*, 1849–1854. [CrossRef] [PubMed]
84. Nebbioso, A.; Pereira, R.; Khanwalkar, H.; Matarese, F.; García-Rodríguez, J.; Miceli, M.; Logie, C.; Kedinger, V.; Ferrara, F.; Stunnenberg, H.G.; et al. Death receptor pathway activation and increase of ROS production by the triple epigenetic inhibitor UVI5008. *Mol. Cancer Ther.* **2011**, *10*, 2394–2404. [CrossRef] [PubMed]

85. Mora, F.D.; Jones, D.K.; Desai, P.V.; Patny, A.; Avery, M.A.; Feller, D.R.; Smillie, T.; Zhou, Y.D.; Nagle, D.G. Bioassay for the identification of natural product-based activators of peroxisome proliferator-activated receptor-γ (PPARγ): The marine sponge metabolite psammaplin A activates PPARγ and induces apoptosis in human breast tumor cells. *J. Nat. Prod.* **2006**, *69*, 547–552. [CrossRef] [PubMed]
86. Baud, M.G.; Leiser, T.; Petrucci, V.; Gunaratnam, M.; Neidle, S.; Meyer-Almes, F.J.; Fuchter, M.J. Thioester derivatives of the natural product psammaplin A as potent histone deacetylase inhibitors. *Beilstein. J. Org. Chem.* **2013**, *9*, 81–88. [CrossRef] [PubMed]
87. Salaroglio, I.C.; Mujumdar, P.; Annovazzi, L.; Kopecka, J.; Mellai, M.; Schiffer, D.; Poulsen, S.A.; Riganti, C. Carbonic anhydrase XII inhibitors overcome P-glycoprotein-mediated resistance to temozolomide in glioblastoma. *Mol. Cancer Ther.* **2018**, *17*, 2598–2609. [CrossRef]
88. Hall, D.G.; Manku, S.; Wang, F. Solution- and solid-phase strategies for the design, synthesis, and screening of libraries based on natural product templates: A comprehensive survey. *J. Comb. Chem.* **2001**, *3*, 125–150. [CrossRef]
89. Nicolaou, K.C.; Hughes, R.; Pfefferkorn, J.A.; Barluenga, S. Optimization and mechanistic studies of psammaplin A type antibacterial agents active against methicillin-resistant *Staphylococcus aureus* (MRSA). *Chem. Eur. J.* **2001**, *7*, 4296–4310. [CrossRef]
90. Andjouh, S.; Blache, Y. Parallel synthesis of a bis-triazoles library as psammaplin A analogues: A new wave of antibiofilm compounds? *Bioorg. Med. Chem. Lett.* **2019**, *29*, 614–618. [CrossRef]
91. Baud, M.G.; Leiser, T.; Meyer-Almes, F.J.; Fuchter, M.J. New synthetic strategies towards psammaplin A, access to natural product analogues for biological evaluation. *Org. Biomol. Chem.* **2011**, *9*, 659–662. [CrossRef] [PubMed]
92. Baud, M.G.; Leiser, T.; Haus, P.; Samlal, S.; Wong, A.C.; Wood, R.J.; Petrucci, V.; Gunaratnam, M.; Hughes, S.M.; Buluwela, L.; et al. Defining the mechanism of action and enzymatic selectivity of psammaplin A against its epigenetic targets. *J. Med. Chem.* **2012**, *55*, 1731–1750. [CrossRef] [PubMed]
93. Khan, O.; La Thangue, N.B. HDAC inhibitors in cancer biology: Emerging mechanisms and clinical applications. *Immunol. Cell Biol.* **2012**, *90*, 85–94. [CrossRef] [PubMed]
94. Hentschel, F.; Raimer, B.; Kelter, G.; Fiebig, H.H.; Sasse, F.; Lindel, T. Synthesis and cytotoxicity of a diazirine-based photopsammaplin. *Eur. J. Org. Chem.* **2014**, *2014*, 2120–2127. [CrossRef]
95. El Bahhaj, F.; Désiré, J.; Blanquart, C.; Martinet, N.; Zwick, V.; Simoes-Pires, C.; Cuendet, M.; Gregoire, M.; Bertrand, P. Superacid and thiol-ene reactions for access to psammaplin analogues with HDAC inhibition activities. *Tetrahedron* **2014**, *70*, 9702–9708. [CrossRef]
96. Wen, J.; Bao, Y.; Niu, Q.; Liu, J.; Yang, J.; Wang, W.; Jiang, T.; Fan, Y.; Li, K.; Wang, J.; et al. Synthesis, biological evaluation and molecular modeling studies of psammaplin A and its analogs as potent histone deacetylases inhibitors and cytotoxic agents. *Bioorg. Med. Chem. Lett.* **2016**, *26*, 4372–4376. [CrossRef]

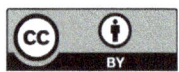 © 2019 by the authors. Licensee MDPI, Basel, Switzerland. This article is an open access article distributed under the terms and conditions of the Creative Commons Attribution (CC BY) license (http://creativecommons.org/licenses/by/4.0/).

MDPI
St. Alban-Anlage 66
4052 Basel
Switzerland
Tel. +41 61 683 77 34
Fax +41 61 302 89 18
www.mdpi.com

Marine Drugs Editorial Office
E-mail: marinedrugs@mdpi.com
www.mdpi.com/journal/marinedrugs

www.ingramcontent.com/pod-product-compliance
Lightning Source LLC
LaVergne TN
LVHW071951080526
838202LV00064B/6720